S0-BYJ-606

PREHOSPITAL EMERGENCY PHARMACOLOGY

Fourth Edition

BRYAN E. BLEDSOE, D.O., EMT-P
Medical Director, Emergency Services
Baylor Medical Center—Ellis County
Waxahachie, Texas
and
Clinical Assistant Professor of Emergency Medicine
University of North Texas Health Sciences Center
Fort Worth, Texas

DWAYNE E. CLAYDEN, EMT-P
Canadian Editor
Journal of Emergency Medical Services (JEMS)
and JEMS ON SCENE Canada
Calgary, Alberta, Canada
and
Paramedic, Highwood EMS
High River, Alberta, Canada

FRANK J. PAPA, D.O., Ph.D., F.A.C.E.P.
Professor of Emergency Medicine and Medical Education
Department of Medical Education
University of North Texas Health Sciences Center
Fort Worth, Texas

BRADY
Prentice Hall
Upper Saddle River, New Jersey 07458

Library of Congress Cataloging-in-Publication Data

Bledsoe, Bryan E., (date)
Prehospital emergency pharmacology / Bryan E. Bledsoe, Dwayne E. Clayden, Frank J. Papa. — 4th ed.
p. cm.
ISBN 0-8359-6065-X (alk. paper)
1. Medical emergencies. 2. Chemotherapy. 3. Drugs. I. Clayden, Dwayne E. II. Papa, Frank J., 1949– . III. Title.
[DNLM: 1. Emergencies. 2. Drug, Therapy. WB 105 B646P 1995]
RC86.7.B597 1995
616.02'5—dc20
DNLM/DLC
for Library of Congress 95-24665
CIP

Publisher: Susan Katz
Editorial Assistant: Carol Sobel
Director of Production and Manufacturing: Bruce Johnson
Manufacturing Buyer: Ilene Sanford
Managing Production Editor: Patrick Walsh
Production Editor/Compositor: BookMasters, Inc.
Printer/Binder: Courier, Westford, Mass.

Notice: The author and the publisher of this book have taken care to make certain that the equipment, doses of drugs and schedules of treatment are correct and compatible with the standards generally accepted at the time of publication. Nevertheless, as new information becomes available, changes in treatment and in the use of equipment and drugs become necessary. The reader is advised to carefully consult the instruction and information material included in the package insert of each drug or therapeutic agent, piece of equipment or device before administration. This advice is especially important when using new or infrequently used drugs. No endorsement by the American Heart Association or any of its committees is stated or implied, nor is there any suggested warranty of performance during the American Heart Association Advanced Cardiac Life Support Course. Prehospital Care Providers are warned that use of any drugs or techniques must be authorized by their medical advisor, in accord with local laws and regulations. The publisher disclaims any liability, loss, injury, or damage incurred as a consequence, directly or indirectly, of the use and application of any of the contents of this book.

Printed in the United States of America

10 9

ISBN 0-8359-6065-X

Prentice-Hall International (UK) Limited, *London*
Prentice-Hall of Australia Pty. Limited, *Sydney*
Prentice-Hall Canada Inc., *Toronto*
Prentice-Hall Hispanoamericana, S.A., *Mexico*
Prentice-Hall of India Private Limited, *New Delhi*
Prentice-Hall of Japan, Inc., *Tokyo*
Pearson Education Asia Pte. Ltd., *Singapore*
Editora Prentice-Hall do Brasil, Ltda., *Rio de Janeiro*

Contents

Preface to the Fourth Edition

Prehospital Emergency Pharmacology is a complete guide to the most common medications used in prehospital emergency care. The first edition was published in 1982 and quickly became a standard textbook in EMS libraries. The text is designed with two purposes in mind. First, it is a complete pharmacology teaching text. Second, it is a handy reference to the most common drugs and fluids used in prehospital care.

The fourth edition of *Prehospital Emergency Pharmacology* reflects the most extensive revision of the text to date. It has been extensively updated to reflect current trends in prehospital care as well as recent changes in Advanced Cardiac Life Support (ACLS) and Pediatric Advanced Life Support (PALS). Each chapter has been revised. A separate chapter on the autonomic nervous system has been added to help the student understand this important physiologic system. The biggest change in the fourth edition is the addition of Dwayne Clayden as a co-author. Dwayne is a paramedic and publisher from Calgary, and he brings a Canadian perspective to the text. His contribution is evident in the case studies and objectives.

We hope that *Prehospital Emergency Pharmacology* will prove a valuable aid to both the practicing paramedic and the paramedic student.

Dedication

First, to my wife Emma who has endured more than any person should be asked to. This whole "book business" takes a great deal of time. I thank her for her patience and her love. Also, to my children, Bryan and Andrea, who have also been patient through many books. They are finally old enough to understand what I do. They now tell me they are proud of what I do and have done.

Second, I appreciate the assistance and support of my coworkers who so often cover for me when I am out of town (often out of the hemisphere) and understand that I have to balance my life between my vocations and avocations.

Bryan E. Bledsoe, D.O.

To my wife Nancy whose confidence in me motivated me to reach higher. To our children Meagan, Lauren, and Matthew for their patience as I worked "in the office" on this book. And to my friends in EMS, especially Baxter and Bryan, thank you.

Dwayne Clayden

Authors' Note

As *Prehospital Emergency Pharmacology* enters its fourth edition, it is time again to acknowledge the many talented individuals who provided both support and assistance throughout all four editions of this text.

First, we would like to thank Susan Katz, publisher at Brady, for her assistance and support in this project. Sharon E. Anderson, Project Director with BookMasters, Inc. skillfully organized and supervised production of the fourth edition.

We would like to acknowledge the assistance provided by the reviewers of the fourth edition including Richard Cherry, M.Ed., EMT-P; Robert S. Porter, M.A., EMT-P; Paul Matera, M.D., EMT-P; and many others.

Photography for the fourth edition was provided by Ken Kerr, EMT-P with Urgent Image in Dandridge, Tennessee. His photographs are excellent and certainly enhance the fourth edition. DeKalb County Public Safety Department, EMS Division in Decatur, Georgia, provided equipment and models for the photography sessions. The models were Lt. Danny Harris, EMT-P and Robert Watts, Master Paramedic. Commander David Bean and Chief Jimmy Hagan served as the departmental facilitators. Jefferson County EMS in Dandridge, Tennessee, also provided assistance for the photography sessions. Seth McMillan, EMT-I, Joey Carlton, EMT-P, and Kara Kerr, R.N., EMT, served as models. Jack Cochoran, EMS Director, served as the departmental facilitator.

Finally, as with the three prior editions, we would like to thank Emma Bledsoe for her patience as well as her assistance in typing portions of the manuscript.

DISCLAIMER

The drugs presented in this text should only be administered under explicit medical control. EMS standards and levels of care vary significantly across this country and Canada. Paramedics should always refer to local standards and policies, as specified by the local medical director, regarding the administration of emergency medications and fluids. Some medications presented in this text may be appropriate for one system and inappropriate for another.

Every effort has been made to assure that information provided in this reference is accurate and complete at the time of publication. Dosages and routes are taken from the most recent American Heart Association *Advanced Cardiac Life Support (ACLS)* and *Pediatric Advanced Life Support (PALS)* standards, where applicable. Drugs not covered in ACLS and PALS standards are referenced to the *Physician's Desk Reference* or the American Medical Association's *Drug Evaluation.* Although the review process has been extensive, errors may be present. Also, the dosages, routes, and standards for emergency medications are revised periodically. THEREFORE, IT IS THE RESPONSIBILITY OF ALL INDIVIDUALS TO BE FAMILIAR WITH THE EMERGENCY MEDICATIONS AND FLUIDS USED IN THEIR SYSTEM AS SPECIFIED BY THE SYSTEM MEDICAL DIRECTOR. THIS IS TO INCLUDE THE INDICATIONS, CONTRAINDICATIONS, DOSAGES, AND ROUTES.

INFECTIOUS DISEASES

Infectious diseases such as Human Immunodeficiency Virus (HIV) infection, hepatitis B infection, and other illnesses pose an occupational risk for prehospital personnel. Because of this, all EMS personnel must adhere to the "Universal Precautions" for health care workers as published by the Centers for Disease Control. The use of Universal Precautions will serve to minimize the risk of infectious disease transmission. ALWAYS USE "UNIVERSAL PRECAUTIONS" IN ANY PATIENT CARE SITUATION.

chapter 1

General Information

OBJECTIVES

1. List four drug sources and give examples of each source.
2. Define the terms *pharmacology* and *pharmacologists.*
3. Identify drugs by their chemical name, generic name, trade name, and official name.
4. List four sources of drug information and demonstrate how to find a medication in one of these references.
5. List several examples of both liquid and solid drugs.

INTRODUCTION

Drugs are chemical agents used in the diagnosis, treatment, or prevention of disease. The study of drugs and their actions on the body is called *pharmacology.* Scientists who study the effects of drugs on the body are called *pharmacologists.* It is through experimental pharmacology that medicine has made many of its most profound advances.

HISTORICAL CONSIDERATIONS

The use of drugs in the treatment of various medical disorders is as old as the practice of medicine itself. Written records of drug use date back to early

Egyptian times. Hippocrates, generally considered the father of modern medicine, wrote extensively on the use of drugs, although he rarely used them in the care of his patients. Following the Renaissance, healers began to take a somewhat more scientific approach to disease, and found that certain drugs were useful in treating some disorders but not others. Drug therapy was largely *empiric*, and physicians were frequently unsure which body systems the drugs affected.

One common additive to early medications was the purple foxglove plant. A common flowering plant, the purple foxglove was first described in 1250 A.D. by Welsh physicians. It was long thought to be a diuretic because of its role in the treatment of dropsy, an old term used to describe the generalized body edema associated with congestive heart failure. In 1785 William Withering described the use of the purple foxglove plant in the treatment of dropsy and other disorders. Although he did not associate the improvement seen in the treatment of dropsy as being due to the foxglove's effect on the heart, he did note its effectiveness. He wrote, "It has a power over the motion of the heart to a degree yet unobserved in any other medicine." It was not until 1800 that the effect of foxglove specifically on the heart was actually described and its suspected action as a diuretic was finally discarded.

Digitalis is the active agent in foxglove. Digitalis tends to increase myocardial contractile force. It was this increase in cardiac performance, with subsequently improved renal perfusion and filtration, that caused a reduction in the body swelling, and not its diuretic effect as earlier thought. Even today digitalis remains one of the most commonly prescribed medications in the treatment of congestive heart failure and other cardiovascular disorders.

Medicine changed dramatically in the early part of the twentieth century with the discovery of antibiotics. Prior to the introduction of the sulfa class antibiotics in 1935, physicians had virtually no effective therapy for infections. Penicillin became widely available in the early 1940s, thus providing physicians a versatile yet inexpensive antibiotic. Additional antibiotics were subsequently developed. The introduction of antibiotic therapy resulted in a significant decrease in mortality and a resultant increase in life expectancy in the United States and other developed countries.

DRUG SOURCES

Drugs are derived from four primary sources—plant, animal, mineral, and synthetic. Emergency medications derived from *plant sources* include morphine sulfate and atropine sulfate among others. Morphine is used to treat moderate to severe pain. It is made from parts of the opium plant, which is native to Turkey and other parts of the Middle East. In addition to morphine, heroin, codeine, and many other analgesic preparations are derived from the opium plant. However, because of their psychotropic effects, these drugs are subject to abuse. They also can result in physical and psychological dependence.

Atropine sulfate, another drug derived from plant sources, is used in the treatment of slow heart rates and in certain types of toxicological emergencies. Atropine is derived from the deadly nightshade plant (*Atropa bel-*

ladonna). This plant is native to central and southern Europe but cultivated widely in North America.

Examples of drugs derived from *animal sources* include insulin and oxytocin. Both of these agents are endocrine hormones extracted from desiccated endocrine glands of mammals. Insulin is used in the treatment of diabetes mellitus, whereas oxytocin is used to induce labor and treat certain types of vaginal bleeding.

Two emergency medications come from *mineral (inorganic) sources*. They are sodium bicarbonate ($NaHCO_3$) and magnesium sulfate ($MgSO_4$). Sodium bicarbonate is occasionally used to treat severe metabolic acidosis as well as being an adjunct in certain toxicological emergencies. Magnesium sulfate is used in the treatment of eclampsia, a life-threatening seizure associated with pregnancy, as well as in certain cardiac emergencies.

Most drugs on the market today are synthetically derived. The term *synthetic* means that they are made by combining two or more simpler compounds. Common examples of emergency drugs that are synthetically manufactured include lidocaine (Xylocaine), bretylium tosylate (Bretylol), diazepam (Valium), and many others. Lidocaine and bretylium tosylate are used to treat cardiac dysrhythmias. Valium is used to treat seizures, anxiety, and other neuropsychiatric disorders.

A new technology, called *genetic engineering*, has allowed mass production of drugs that are identical to human hormones. This process, also called *recombinant DNA technology,* involves taking genetic material (DNA) from one organism and placing it into another. This technology is used to manufacture insulin, hepatitis B vaccine, and several other products. Insulin is manufactured by taking the genetic code for human insulin and placing it into the cells of selected bacteria. These bacteria can then be grown in large quantities, thus producing a large amount of insulin at relatively low cost (see Figure 1-1).

DRUG LEGISLATION

Before a drug can be marketed, it must undergo extensive testing. This testing generally involves two phases, animal studies and clinical patient studies. Only after these extensive tests, and with governmental approval, can drugs be placed on the market. Even after clinical usage, the effectiveness of the drugs must be closely monitored. The Food and Drug Administration (FDA) is the federal agency responsible for approval of drugs before they are made available to the general public.

The FDA enforces rigid standards imposed by various legislation. In 1906 Congress enacted the Pure Food and Drug Act. In addition to establishing the FDA, this act prohibited the sale of medicinal preparations that had little or no use and restricted the sale of drugs with a potential for abuse. The Pure Food and Drug Act named the *United States Pharmacopeia (USP)* and the *National Formulary (NF)* as official drug standards. Any drug bearing the official title USP or NF must conform to rigid standards regarding purity, preparation, and dosage.

The Pure Food and Drug Act was not as all encompassing as its planners had envisioned it to be. For several years stronger drug laws were

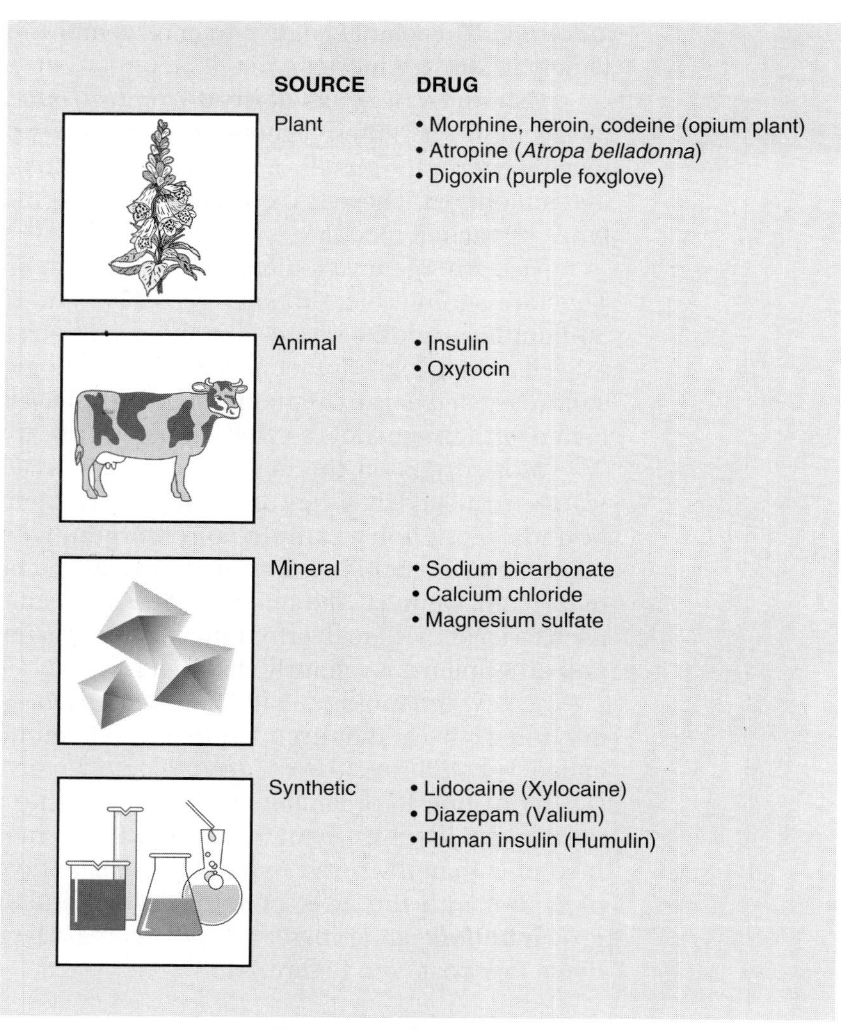

SOURCE
DRUG
Plant
• Morphine, heroin, codeine (opium plant)
• Atropine (*Atropa belladonna*)
• Digoxin (purple foxglove)
Animal
• Insulin
• Oxytocin
Mineral
• Sodium bicarbonate
• Calcium chloride
• Magnesium sulfate
Synthetic
• Lidocaine (Xylocaine)
• Diazepam (Valium)
• Human insulin (Humulin)

Figure 1-1 Drug sources.

debated both in Congress and state legislatures. Finally, in 1938, Congress enacted the Federal Food, Drug and Cosmetic Act. Among the more important features of this act was the truth-in-labeling clause. The act required that the label name all the ingredients and include directions for the drug's use. The label must also indicate whether the preparation contains habit-forming drugs and, if so, in what percentage.

NARCOTICS

A problem almost as old as medicine itself is abuse and addiction to certain drugs. Narcotics are among the drugs most frequently abused. Recognizing the need to control the sale of narcotics, the federal government enacted the Harrison Narcotic Act in 1914. This act served to control the importation, manufacture, and sale of the opium plant and its derivatives. It also controlled the derivatives of the coca plant. The primary drug derived from the coca plant is cocaine. As a result of this act, these drugs, as well as other drugs added to the list later, could be obtained only with special prescriptions. Only physicians who qualified and attained a special narcotic license could prescribe this class of drugs.

In 1970 major revisions were made in the use and control of narcotics and other drugs. This law, the Comprehensive Drug Abuse Prevention and Control Act of 1970 (commonly called the Controlled Substance Act of 1970), classifies the drugs used in medicine into five different schedules. A summary of the five schedules follows:

Schedule I. Drugs in this schedule have a high potential for abuse and no accepted medical use. Drugs in this class include some derivatives of the opium plant (heroin), marijuana, synthetic opiates, and hallucinogenic drugs (LSD). These drugs are generally used only in research.

Schedule II. Drugs in this schedule have a high potential for abuse, yet have accepted medical uses. Some opium preparations, some amphetamines, synthetic narcotics, and cocaine are included in this group. Emergency drugs used by paramedics classified in Schedule II include morphine sulfate and meperidine (Demerol).

Schedule III. Drugs having a lesser degree of abuse potential and accepted medical indications are classified as Schedule III. Drugs containing some narcotic ingredients are usually placed in this class. Codeine is a popular narcotic used to enhance the analgesic effects of other analgesic drugs. An example of this mixture is acetaminophen with codeine (Tylenol #3).

Schedule IV. Drugs having a low potential for abuse, but which may cause physical or psychological dependence, are placed in Schedule IV. Many of the depressants, stimulants, and sedatives are classified as Schedule IV. Valium is an example of a Schedule IV drug.

Schedule V. Schedule V drugs are drugs that have low potential for abuse. Cough medications containing codeine as well as certain antidiarrheal agents that contain opiates are classified as Schedule V drugs.

The Controlled Substances Act mandates that prescriptions for Schedule II drugs cannot be refilled. Moreover, it requires that prescriptions for Schedule II drugs be filled within 72 hours. Prescriptions for drugs in this class cannot be called into the pharmacy over the telephone (except in special situations). Prescriptions for drugs in Schedules III and IV may be refilled up to 5 times within 6 months. Prescriptions for Schedule V drugs may be refilled at the discretion of the physician.

Responsibility for enforcing the Controlled Substances Act rests with the Drug Enforcement Administration (DEA). Only physicians approved by the DEA may write prescriptions for scheduled drugs. The physician must indicate his or her DEA number on the prescription. Many states have enacted laws further regulating controlled substances.

MEDICAL CONTROL

Medication administration is one of the skills that separates advanced life support from basic life support providers. With this added skill come added responsibilities. The appropriate administration of a drug can often mean the difference between life and death in patients with serious emergencies. On the other hand, administration of the wrong drug, or the wrong dose, can cause adverse effects or even death. Thus, it is imperative that advanced life support personnel have a thorough understanding of the medications used in their EMS system.

Medical Director

The EMS system will retain a *medical director* who will be actively involved in, and ultimately responsible for, all clinical and patient care. All prehospital medical care provided by non-physicians is considered an extension of the medical director's license. Every prehospital ambulance or rescue service must have a medical director who is responsible for that service. Prehospital care providers are designated agents of the medical director, regardless of whose employees they may be. For this reason, the medical director determines which providers may care for patients within the system. The medical director is the ultimate authority in all direct- and indirect-medical control issues.

Direct Medical Control

Direct medical control, also known as on-line medical control, exists when prehospital providers communicate directly with a physician. The physician's direction is usually based on established protocols for managing specific problems. This physician assumes responsibility and gives treatment orders for patients. Direct medical control physicians should be experienced in emergency medicine. They should have completed a training program that emphasizes system particulars, treatment protocols, and communications policies and procedures. Once they have become proficient in these areas, they should go through a formal certification process. They should also be required to ride with crews to get a feel for the realities of prehospital field medicine.

Indirect Medical Control

Indirect medical control, also known as off-line medical control, includes training and education, protocol development, audit, chart review, and quality assurance. To be effective, medical control must have official and clearly defined authority with power to discipline, or limit, the activities of those who deviate from the established standard of care.

Treatment Protocols

Treatment protocols are designed by the off-line medical control system to provide a standardized approach to common patient problems and a consistent level of medical care. When treatment is based on such protocols, the on-line physician assists prehospital personnel in interpreting the patient's complaint, understanding the findings of their evaluation, and applying the appropriate treatment protocol.

The medications and intravenous fluids used in prehospital care can only be administered on the order of a licensed physician. Orders for prehospital treatment may be either verbal or written. Verbal orders may take place over EMS radios, cellular telephones, or in person. Written orders are usually presented as *prehospital standing orders* or *prehospital treatment protocols*. Standing orders are written directives that may be carried out without, or prior to, contacting medical control. Protocols are treatment guidelines. They may incorporate standing orders or they may require contact with medical control prior to initiating advanced life support therapy.

DRUG NAMES

Drugs are identified by four different names: chemical, generic, trade, and official. The most elemental name is the *chemical name*. Because drugs are usually chemically complex in nature, so too are the chemical names. The *generic name*, usually an abbreviated version of the chemical name, is frequently used. Manufacturers of pharmaceuticals rarely refer to drugs by their generic name. Instead, they devise a name for a drug that is based on its chemical name or on the type of problem it is used to treat. This is referred to as the *trade name*. Trade names are always capitalized whereas generic names are not. In recent years, controversy has developed regarding generic and nongeneric drugs. When writing a prescription, a physician can order the drug either by the trade name or the generic name. Until recently, the pharmacist had to fill the drug as written. Now, in many states, the pharmacist may substitute a less-expensive generic drug for the prescription. Generic drugs are, as a rule, not inferior in quality. They are usually cheaper because they are manufactured by lesser-known companies with minimal advertising and production costs. The fourth method of naming a drug is the *official name*. The official name is followed by the initials USP or NF, which are official publications that list drugs conforming to standards set forth by the publication. The official name is usually the same as the generic name. An example of the four names of a specific drug is as follows:

Chemical Name: *ethyl 1-methyl-4-phenylisonipecotate hydrochloride*
Generic Name: meperidine hydrochloride
Trade Name: Demerol Hydrochloride
Official Name: meperidine hydrochloride, USP

DRUG REFERENCES

Several publications provide valuable information concerning drugs. These include the following:

AMA Drug Evaluation. This manual, which is published by the American Medical Association, provides information on all drug groups and includes dosages, prescribing information, and usage.

Physicians' Desk Reference (PDR). The PDR is a valuable reference. It contains information concerning most of the drugs on the market today and a very useful product identification guide showing actual size and color pictures of commonly prescribed drugs. The PDR is published yearly by the Medical Economics Company. Drug information is provided to the Medical Economics Company by the various manufacturers. Thus, there are several drugs, particularly older drugs, which are not listed in the PDR.

Hospital Formulary. The Hospital Formulary is a loose-leaf book published by the American Society of Hospital Pharmacists. Its loose-leaf format allows it to be constantly updated, and it is available in all hospital pharmacies and in most emergency departments.

Drug Inserts. The pamphlets packaged with most drugs are good sources of information. They can be collected and put into a notebook for personal use.

DRUG FORMS

Drugs come in many forms. Each form has its advantages and disadvantages. For example, drugs taken by mouth tend to have a slow and unpredictable rate of absorption and thus a slower rate of onset. Drugs given intravenously, although rapidly acting, are much more difficult to administer. The following are some common drug preparations.

Liquid Drugs

Liquid drugs usually consist of a powder dissolved in a liquid. The drug is referred to as the *solute.* The liquid into which it is dissolved is called the *solvent.* In liquid drug preparations, the primary difference from one preparation to another is the solvent.

Solutions. Solutions are preparations that contain the drug dissolved in a solvent, usually water (for example, 5% dextrose in water).

Tinctures. Tinctures are drug preparations whereby the drug was extracted chemically with alcohol. They will usually contain some dilute alcohol (for example, tincture of iodine).

Suspensions. Suspensions are drugs that do not remain dissolved. After sitting for even short periods, these drugs will tend to separate. They must always be shaken well before use (for example, penicillin preparations).

Spirits. Spirit solutions contain volatile chemicals dissolved in alcohol (for example, spirit of ammonia).

Emulsions. Emulsions are preparations in which an oily substance is mixed with a solvent into which it does not dissolve. When mixed, it forms

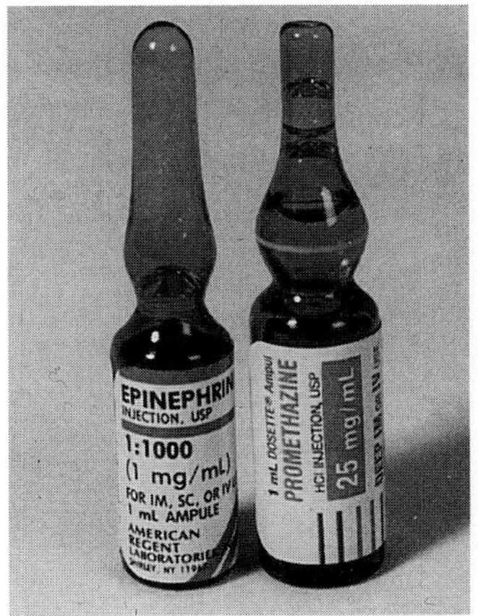

Figure 1-2 Ampules.

globules of fat floating in the solvent. This is similar to what occurs in oil and vinegar salad dressing.

Elixirs. Elixirs are preparations that contain the drug in an alcohol solvent. Flavoring, often cherry, is added to improve the taste (for example, Tylenol Elixer).

Syrups. Often drugs are suspended in sugar and water to improve the taste. These are referred to as syrups (for example, cough syrup).

Liquid drugs administered into the body through either intramuscular, subcutaneous, or intravenous routes are called *parenteral drugs*. Most drugs used in emergency medicine are parenteral. Because they are introduced into the body, they must be sterile. They are packaged in several types of containers. Sterile parenteral containers designed to carry a single patient dose are called *ampules* (see Figure 1-2). Generally, the tops of the ampules are broken, and the drug is drawn into a syringe for administration.

In emergency medicine most drugs given parenterally are in *prefilled syringes* (see Figure 1-3). These preparations save time by avoiding the problems inherent to ampules. Wyeth manufactures a type of syringe called *Tubex* (see Figure 1-4). This syringe is designed for a disposal cartridge containing the desired drug and is reusable. Several of the medications used in the emergency department and the field, including morphine and meperidine, are frequently carried in Tubex form.

Vials are another type of container for parenteral drugs (see Figures 1-5 and 1-6). Vials may contain a single dose or multiple dosages. Many drugs used in emergency medicine are supplied in vials.

Solid Drugs

Solid drugs are usually administered orally, although many can be administered rectally. They include the following:

Pills. Pills are drugs that are shaped into a form that makes them easy to swallow.

Powders. Powders are drugs in powdered form. They are not as popular as pills, yet some are still in use (for example, B.C. Powder).

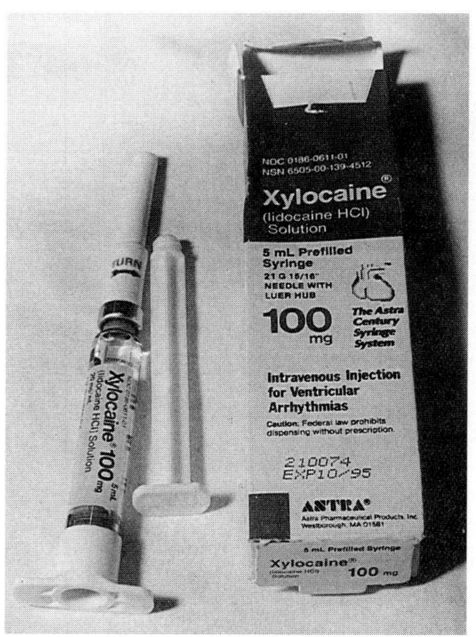

Figure 1-3 Prefilled syringes.

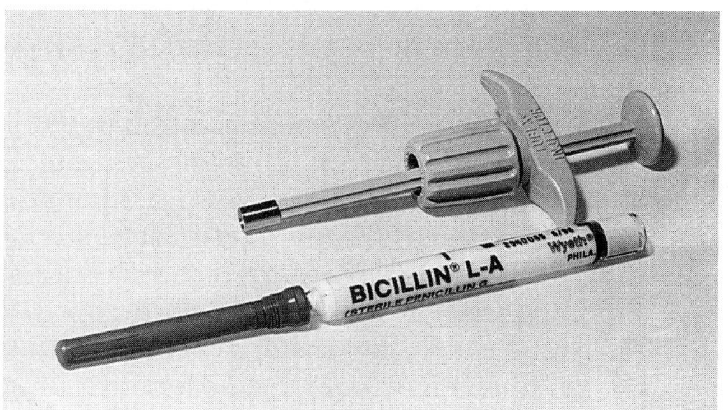

Figure 1-4 Tubex syringes.

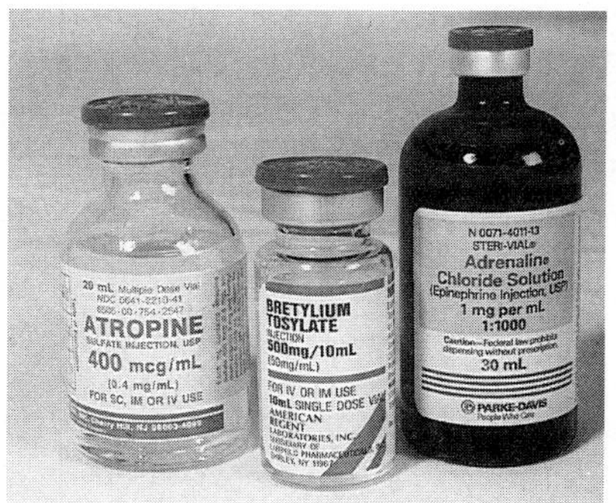

Figure 1-5 Multi-dose vials.

Capsules. Capsules consist of gelatin containers into which a powder is placed. The gelatin dissolves, liberating the powder (for example, Dalmane capsules) into the gastrointestinal tract.

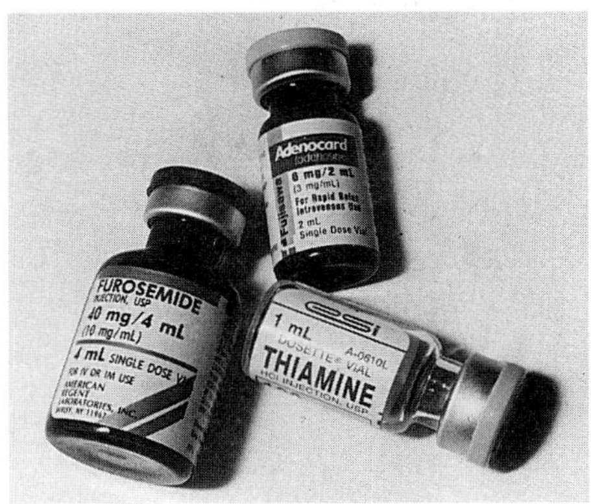

Figure 1-6 Single-dose vials.

Tablets. Tablets are similar to pills. They are composed of a powder that has been compressed into an easily swallowed form and are often covered with a sugar coating to improve taste.

Suppositories. Suppositories are mixed into a base that is solid at room temperature (approximately 70°F). When placed into the body, either rectally or vaginally, they dissolve and are then absorbed into the surrounding tissue.

COMMON PHARMACOLOGICAL TERMINOLOGY AND ABBREVIATIONS

It is common to use abbreviations in pharmacology. This serves to expedite paper work and promote efficiency. The abbreviations used in pharmacology are fairly standard. It is important to be familiar with these abbreviations and with some of the common terminology applicable to the field of emergency pharmacology (see Table 1-1).

Important Pharmacological Terminology

Antagonism. Antagonism signifies the opposition between two or more medications (for example, between Narcan and morphine).

Bolus. A bolus is a single, oftentimes large dose of medication (for example, lidocaine bolus, which is often followed by a lidocaine infusion).

Contraindications. Contraindications are the medical or physiological conditions present in a patient that would make it harmful to administer a medication of otherwise known therapeutic value.

Cumulative Action. A cumulative action occurs when a drug is administered in several doses, causing an increased effect. This is usually due to a quantitative buildup of the drug in the blood.

Depressant. A depressant is a medication that decreases or lessens a body function or activity.

Habituation. Habituation is the physical or psychological dependence on a drug.

Hypersensitivity. Hypersensitivity is a reaction to a substance that is normally more profound than seen in the normal population (for example, allergic reaction to penicillin).

Idiosyncrasy. An idiosyncrasy is an individual reaction to a drug that is unusually different from that seen in the rest of the population.

Indication. An indication refers to the medical condition(s) in which the drug has proven to be of therapeutic value.

Potentiation. Potentiation is the enhancement of one drug's effects by another (for example, barbiturates and alcohol).

Refractory. Patients who do not respond to a drug are said to be refractory to the drug (for example, a patient with premature ventricular contractions who does not respond to lidocaine).

Side Effects. Side effects are the unavoidable, undesired effects frequently seen even in therapeutic drug dosages.

Stimulant. A stimulant is a drug that enhances or increases a bodily function (for example, caffeine in coffee).

Synergism. Synergism is the combined action of two drugs. The action is much stronger than the effects of either drug administered separately.

Therapeutic Action. A therapeutic action is the desired, intended action of a drug given in the appropriate medical condition.

Tolerance. When patients are receiving drugs on a long-term basis, they may require larger and larger dosages of the drug to achieve a therapeutic effect. This increased requirement is termed tolerance.

Untoward Effect. An untoward effect is a side effect that proves harmful to the patient.

TABLE 1-1

Common Abbreviations

Abbreviation	*Meaning*
$\bar{a}$	*ante* (before)
a.c.	*ante cibos* (before meals)
ACh	acetylcholine
ACLS	advanced cardiac life support
admin.	administer
α	alpha
ALS	advanced life support
AMA	against medical advice
AMI	acute myocardial infarction
amp.	ampule
APAP	acetaminophen
ASA	aspirin
β	beta
bid	*bis in die* (twice a day)
$\bar{c}$	*cum* (with)
Ca^{++}	calcium ion
$CaCl_2$	calcium chloride
caps	capsules
cc	cubic centimeter
CC	chief complaint
CHF	congestive heart failure
Cl^-	chloride ion
cm	centimeter
cm^3	cubic centimeter
c/o	complains of

TABLE 1-1 (continued)

Common Abbreviations

Abbreviation	*Meaning*
CO	carbon monoxide
CO_2	carbon dioxide
COPD	chronic obstructive pulmonary disease
CSM	carotid sinus massage
CVA	cerebrovascular accident
°	degree
°C	degrees Celsius
D/C	discontinue
↓	decrease
D_5W	5% dextrose in water
$D_{10}W$	10% dextrose in water
$D_{50}W$	50% dextrose in water
dig	digitalis
Dx	diagnosis
ECG	electrocardiogram
EKG	electrocardiogram (from German)
elix	elixir
EOA	esophageal obturator airway
=	equal to
et	and
ET	endotracheal
ETC	endotracheal combitube
ETOH	alcohol (ethyl)
°F	degrees Fahrenheit
♀	female
g	gram
gr	grain
>	greater than
gtt	*gutta* (drop)
gtts	*guttae* (drops)
HHN	hand-held nebulizer
hs	*hora somni* (at bedtime)
↑	increase
IC	intracardiac
IM	intramuscular
IO	intraosseous
IV	intravenous
IVP	intravenous push
IVPB	intravenous piggyback
K^+	potassium
kg	kilogram
KO	keep open
KVO	keep vein open
l	liter
lb	pound
<	less than
LR	lactated Ringer's
$MgSO_4$	magnesium sulfate
♂	male
MAX	maximum
MDI	metered dose inhaler
µ	micro
µgtt	microdrop
µg	microgram
mcg	microgram
µm	micrometer
mEq	milliequivalent
mg	milligram

TABLE 1-1 (continued)

Common Abbreviations

Abbreviation	*Meaning*
min	minute
ml	milliliter
mm	millimeter
MS	morphine sulfate
MSO_4	morphine sulfate
N_2O	nitrous oxide
Na^+	sodium ion
$NaHCO_3$	sodium bicarbonate
nitro	nitroglycerin
NKA	no known allergies
NKDA	no known drug allergies
NTG	nitroglycerin
Ø	null or none
O_2	oxygen
OD	overdose
OPP	organophosphate poisoning
OD	*oculus dexter* (right eye)
OS	*oculus sinister* (left eye)
OU	*oculus utro* (both eyes)
oz	ounce
$\bar{p}$	*post* (after)
pc	*post cibos* (after eating)
PAC	premature atrial contraction
PAT	paroxysmal atrial tachycardia
PEA	pulseless electrical activity
pedi	pediatric
PJC	premature junctional contraction
po	*per os* (by mouth)
pr	*per rectus* (by rectum)
prn	*pro re nata* (when necessary)
PSVT	paroxysmal supraventricular tachycardia
$\bar{q}$	*quisque* (every)
qd	*quisque die* (every day)
qh	*quisque hora* (every hour)
qid	*quarter in die* (four times a day)
qod	every other day
qt	quart
®	registered trademark
RL	Ringer's lactate
Rx	treatment
$\bar{s}$	*sine* (without)
SC	subcutaneous
SK	streptokinase
sol	solution
SpO_2	oxygen saturation (oximetry)
SQ	subcutaneous
stat	*statim* (now or immediately)
SVN	small volume nebulizer
tid	*ter in die* (three times a day)
tPA	tissue plasminogen activator
TKO	to keep open
u	unit
ut dict	*ut dictum* (as directed)
y/o	year old

SUMMARY

Drugs are chemical agents used in the diagnosis, treatment, or prevention of disease. They are necessary for successful emergency care. It is important to be familiar with the commonly used emergency medications and with the terminology and abbreviations used in medicine so that communication with other medical personnel will be efficient and professional. Overall, it is essential to appreciate the inherent danger of any and all drugs, and to use them properly. The rule to remember is: *When in doubt, do no harm.*

KEY WORDS

drug. A chemical agent used in diagnosis, treatment, and prevention of disease.

Drug Enforcement Administration (DEA). Federal agency with responsibility for enforcing the Controlled Substances Act.

empiric. Skill or knowledge based entirely on experience.

enteral. Administration of a drug via the gastrointestinal tract.

Food and Drug Administration (FDA). The federal agency responsible for approval of drugs before they are made available to the general public.

genetic engineering. Genetic engineering, also called recombinant DNA technology, involves taking genetic material (DNA) from one organism and placing it into another.

medical director. A licensed physician who serves as the chief medical officer of an EMS service or system. Each paramedic functions under the license of the system medical director.

National Formulary. The Pure Food and Drug Act named the National Formulary (NF) and the United States Pharmacopeia (USP) as official drug standards. Any drug bearing the official title NF or USP must conform to a rigid set of standards regarding purity, preparation, and dosage.

off-line medical control. Off-line medical control, also known as *indirect medical control,* is the establishment of system policies and procedures, such as training, chart review, protocol development, audit, and quality improvement.

on-line medical control. On-line medical control, also known as *direct medical control,* is communication between field personnel and a medical control physician, with the medical control physician providing immediate direction for on-scene care.

parenteral. Routes of administering drugs into the body without going through the digestive tract.

pharmacologist. Scientist who studies the effects of drugs on the body.

pharmacology. The study of drugs and their actions on the body.

recombinant DNA. Recombinant DNA, also called genetic engineering, involves taking genetic material (DNA) from one organism and placing it into another.

solute. A powder (drug) that is dissolved in a liquid (solvent).

solvent. The liquid into which a drug (solute) is dissolved.

standing orders. Written directives that may be carried out without, or prior to, contacting medical control.

synthetic. Substance made by combining two or more simpler compounds.

treatment protocols. Treatment guidelines for prehospital care. They may incorporate standing orders or may require contact with medical control prior to initiating advanced life support therapy.

United States Pharmacopeia. The Pure Food and Drug Act named the United States Pharmacopeia (USP) and the National Formulary (NF) as official drug standards. Any drug bearing the official title USP or NF must conform to a rigid set of standards regarding purity, preparation, and dosage.

chapter 2

Pharmacokinetics and Pharmacodynamics

OBJECTIVES

1. Define pharmacokinetics and pharmacodynamics.
2. Define drug absorption.
3. Explain the factors involved in drug absorption.
4. Explain the factors that can affect drug distribution.
5. Explain biotransformation.
6. List and explain how a drug is eliminated from the body.

INTRODUCTION

To exert its desired biochemical and physiological effects on the body, a drug must reach its targeted tissues in a suitable form and in a sufficient concentration. The study of how drugs enter the body, reach their site of action, and are eventually eliminated is termed *pharmacokinetics*. Once drugs reach their targeted tissues, they begin a chain of biochemical events that ultimately lead to the physiological changes desired. These biochemical and physiological events are called the drug's *mechanism of action*.

The study of drug actions is termed *pharmacodynamics*. This chapter addresses the fundamentals of both pharmacokinetics and pharmacodynamics as they apply to prehospital emergency care.

PHARMACOKINETICS

To produce its desired effects, a drug must be present in the appropriate concentration at its various sites of action. Lidocaine, a drug commonly used in the treatment of life-threatening ventricular dysrhythmias, must reach its target—cardiac tissue—rapidly and in a sufficient concentration to suppress the dysrhythmia. Several factors influence the concentration of a drug at its site of action. These factors include *absorption* of the drug into the circulatory system; *distribution* of the drug throughout the body; *biotransformation* of the drug into its active form, if required; and finally, *elimination* of the drug from the body. It is important to point out that all of these factors do not play a role in every medication used in prehospital care. A fundamental understanding of each of these factors is essential.

Drug Absorption

Absorption is the process of movement of a drug from the site of application to the extracellular compartment of the body. The duration and intensity of a drug's action is directly related to the rate of absorption of the drug. Many factors affect drug absorption. These include:

- solubility of the drug,
- concentration of the drug,
- pH of the drug,
- site of absorption,
- absorbing surface area, and
- blood supply to the site of absorption.

The *solubility* is the tendency of a drug to dissolve. The human body is approximately 60% water. Thus, drugs given in water solutions are more rapidly absorbed than those given in oil-based solutions, suspensions, or solid forms.

The *concentration* of a drug also affects the rate of absorption. Drugs administered in high concentrations are absorbed much more rapidly than drugs administered in low concentrations.

Another factor that affects drug absorption is the *pH* of a drug. The pH refers to how acidic or how basic (alkaline) the drug is. Most drugs are either weak acids or weak bases. Acidic drugs tend to be more rapidly absorbed when placed into an acidic environment (such as the stomach). Alkaline drugs, on the other hand, are more rapidly absorbed when placed into an alkaline environment (such as the kidneys).

The *site of absorption* directly affects the rate of drug absorption. Once administered, drugs must pass through the various biological membranes until they reach the circulation. Drugs placed on the skin (transdermal route) must pass through several cell layers before reaching the circulatory system. On the other hand, drugs placed on mucous membranes (intranasal route) have much fewer cell layers through which to pass. Thus, drug absorption through mucous membranes is faster than drug absorption through the skin. It is sometimes useful to have slow absorption of a drug. A common

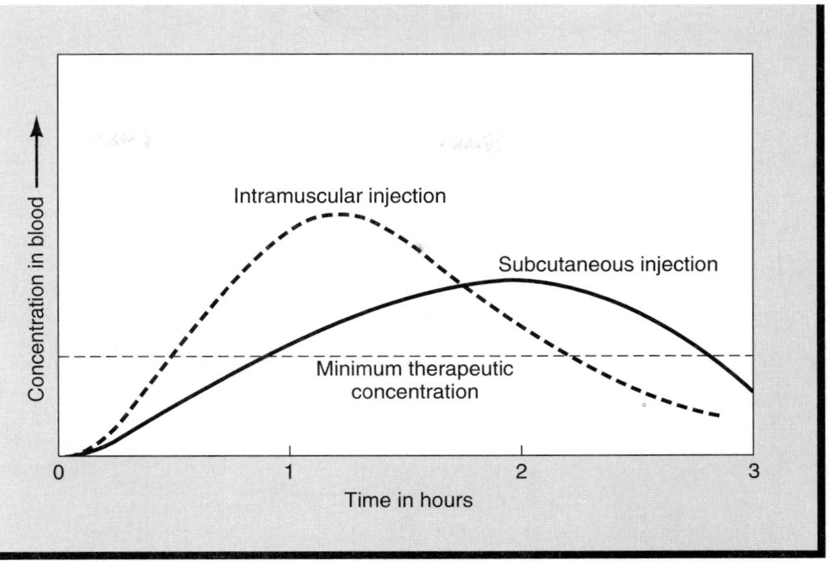

Figure 2-1 Comparison of drug levels following intramuscular and subcutaneous injections of the same drug.

emergency drug where prolonged absorption is desired is nitroglycerin. In these cases, nitroglycerin can be placed on the skin where it is slowly absorbed over a prolonged period of time.

The *surface area* of the absorbing surface is an important determinant of the rate of drug absorption. Drugs are absorbed quite rapidly from large surface areas. Inhaled medications are quickly distributed across the vast pulmonary epithelium. Drugs administered by this route are rapidly absorbed into the circulation. In fact, some studies have shown that the rate of drug absorption through the inhaled route is nearly as rapid as administration by the intravenous route.

Finally, drug absorption is related to *blood supply* to the site of absorption. Some areas of the body have very rich blood supplies while other areas do not. Medications placed in areas with rich blood supplies, such as the tissues under the tongue (sublingual), have rapid absorption. Medications placed in areas with poor blood supply, such as the fatty tissues (subcutaneous), have slower absorption. Muscle, as a rule, is more richly supplied with blood vessels than is subcutaneous tissue. Therefore, one would expect a drug to be absorbed more rapidly from muscle than from subcutaneous tissue (see Figure 2-1).

Knowledge of the various rates of drug absorption from each of the various routes is essential. Epinephrine 1:1,000, a drug commonly used in the management of acute allergic reactions, is generally given by the subcutaneous route. The reasons for choosing this site are many. First, epinephrine 1:1,000 is a potent and concentrated drug. Rapid absorption of a large quantity of this drug into the circulation would certainly accentuate epinephrine's side effects such as tachycardia, trembling, and elevated blood pressure. Second, the therapeutic effects of epinephrine are fairly brief. The slower absorption obtained with subcutaneous injection allows prolonged release of the drug into the circulation, thus maintaining the desired effects for a longer period (see Table 2-1).

TABLE 2-1

Comparison of Rates of Drug Absorption of Various Routes of Administration

Route	*Rate of Absorption*
Oral	Slow
Subcutaneous	Slow
Topical	Moderate
Intramuscular	Moderate
Intralingual	Rapid
Rectal	Rapid
Sublingual	Rapid
Endotracheal	Rapid
Inhalation	Rapid
Intraosseous	Immediate
Intravenous	Immediate
Intracardiac	Immediate

Systemic blood flow can also affect drug absorption. Factors that may *delay* absorption from parenteral sites include shock, acidosis, and peripheral vasoconstriction secondary to such things as hypothermia. Factors such as peripheral vasodilation, which can occur in hyperthermia and fever, may *increase* the rate of drug absorption.

Drug absorption may be minimized by injecting the medication directly into the circulatory system by the intravenous route. The desired effects are seen much sooner, and the eventual blood levels of the drug are much more predictable. Because of this, most critical-care medications are given intravenously (see Figure 2-2).

Distribution

Distribution is the process whereby a drug is transported from the site of absorption to the site of action. Once a drug is in the circulatory system, it is distributed throughout the various body tissues. Several factors can affect drug distribution. These include:

- cardiovascular function,
- regional blood flow,
- drug storage reservoirs, and
- physiological barriers.

As with drug absorption, drug distribution is dependent on *cardiovascular function*. Following administration and absorption, the drug is initially distributed to highly perfused body areas such as the brain, heart, kidneys, and liver. Delivery of the drug to the gastrointestinal system, skin, muscles, and fat is generally much slower. In certain conditions, such as shock and congestive heart failure, cardiac output will fall. When this occurs, drug distribution will become much slower and much more unpredictable. When cardiac output is markedly diminished, some body

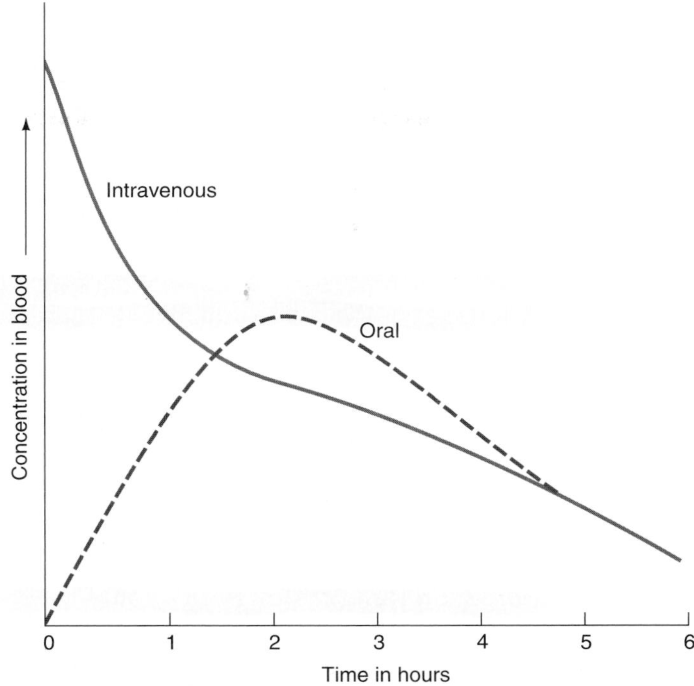

Figure 2-2 Comparison of drug levels following intravenous and oral administration of the same drug.

areas will be minimally perfused, and drug delivery to these areas will be negligible.

Variances in *regional blood flow* can also affect drug distribution. For example, in cardiogenic shock blood flow to the kidneys is often diminished. Medications that act specifically on the kidneys, such as diuretics, may not reach the kidneys in an adequate concentration to be effective.

Various compartments of the body can serve as potential *drug reservoirs*. These reservoirs store drugs by binding the drug to proteins present within the tissue in question. This action tends to delay the drug's onset of action and prolongs its duration of effect. There are two types of storage reservoirs: *plasma reservoirs* and *tissue reservoirs*.

Following absorption, many drugs will bind to proteins present in the blood plasma. The most common plasma protein involved in drug binding is *albumin*. However, other plasma proteins, such as hemoglobin and globulins, are utilized as well. This binding of drug to protein is usually reversible. The extent of binding depends upon the physical properties of the drug itself. Some drugs are highly bound while others have limited binding. The portion of the drug that is bound to plasma proteins is called the *bound drug* while the unbound portion is often referred to as the *free drug*. The degree to which a drug is bound is referred to as the *binding capacity*. Binding of a drug to plasma proteins tends to limit its concentration in the tissues.

Drugs can also accumulate in the various tissues of the body. Common tissue reservoirs include fat, bone, and muscle tissue. Once in these compartments, the drug will bind to proteins and similar substances. As with plasma protein binding, tissue binding is usually reversible. Some body compartments, such as the muscle tissue, can represent a sizable drug reservoir. Many drugs are lipid-soluble (fat-soluble). These drugs concentrate in the fatty tissues of the body resulting in a prolonged drug effect.

Drug distribution is also affected by *physiological barriers*. Physiological barriers inhibit the movement of certain substances while permitting the passage of others. One of the most important physiological barriers is the *blood-brain barrier*. The blood-brain barrier is an effective boundary between the central nervous system and the peripheral nervous system. Delivery of drugs and other substances to the brain is limited by the blood-brain barrier. It allows entry of certain drugs and is considered a protective mechanism of the brain. Drugs that are protein bound or in an ionized form are weak penetrators of the blood-brain barrier.

Biotransformation

Biotransformation, also called *metabolism*, is the process by which active drugs are converted to an inactive form. In certain situations, biotransformation may serve to convert an inactive drug into an active form. Most drugs used in medicine are active as administered. In order to be removed from the body, they must be converted to an inactive form. In addition, they must often be made water-soluble so that they can be excreted by the body. The process of biotransformation results in chemical variations of the drugs called *metabolites*. Biotransformation usually occurs in the liver although it can occur in other body tissues such as the kidneys, plasma, and nervous system.

Biotransformation begins immediately following introduction of the drug into the body. Certain drugs are rapidly biotransformed while others are not. For example, the emergency drug epinephrine is active as administered. However, it is very rapidly metabolized to inactive forms before elimination. Because of this rapid biotransformation, epinephrine must be readministered approximately every 3–5 minutes if still required.

Some drugs are inactive when administered. Once they have been absorbed, they must be converted to an active form, either in the blood or by the target tissue. The inactive precursor is referred to as a *prodrug*. Several drugs used in prehospital care must be converted into an active form before they can exert their desired effects. Diazepam (Valium), a drug used in the treatment of seizures, is relatively inactive as administered. Once in the body it is converted to its active metabolite, *desmethyldiazepam*, which then induces the desired effects (see Figure 2-3).

Elimination

Drugs are eventually eliminated from the body in either their original form or as metabolites. Drugs may be excreted by the kidneys into the urine, by the liver into the bile, by the intestines into the feces, or by the lungs with the expired air. The rate of elimination varies with the medication and the state of the body. During shock states, the kidneys are poorly perfused.

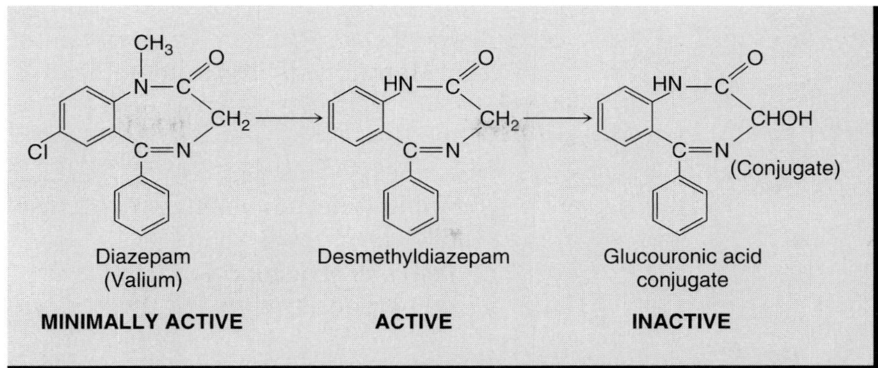

Figure 2-3 Metabolites of Diazepam.

Drugs that are primarily eliminated by the kidneys will then remain present in the body for longer periods. The slower the rate of elimination, the longer the drug stays in the body.

PHARMACODYNAMICS

Once a drug has arrived at the target tissue, it must induce the desired biochemical or physiological response. Most drugs must bind to *drug receptors* to cause their desired response. Drug receptors are generally proteins present on the surface of the cell membrane. When a drug combines with the drug receptor, a physiological response occurs. Drug receptors are often compared with "locks," whereas drugs are the "keys" that fit these locks. Once the drug is bound to the receptor (that is, the "key" is inserted in the "lock"), biochemical actions begin that ultimately lead to the desired response. Drugs that bind to a receptor and cause a response are referred to as *agonists*. Certain drugs, however, may bind to a receptor and not cause a response. Because of their presence on the receptor, they keep other drugs from binding. Drugs such as these are referred to as *antagonists*. The tendency of a drug to combine with a specific drug receptor is referred to as the drug's *affinity*. The power of a drug to produce a therapeutic effect is called the drug's *efficacy*. Drugs that are agonists have both affinity and efficacy. Drugs that are antagonists have affinity but not efficacy, as they do not produce a physiological response. Classic illustrations of this principle are the drugs epinephrine and propranolol (Inderal). Epinephrine, once administered, is transported to its various target tissues—namely, the heart, the lungs, and the peripheral blood vessels. Once at these target tissues it finds and binds to its receptors, which are called *beta receptors*. If the drug is able to bind to these beta receptors, then the desired physiological response will be seen. Several drugs themselves are inactive but can bind to beta receptors in much the same manner as epinephrine. These drugs are referred to as *beta blockers*, and the prototype drug of this group is propranolol. If a beta blocker has already bound to the receptor, then epinephrine cannot bind, and the desired effect is effectively blocked (see Figures 2-4 and 2-5). A more detailed discussion of beta receptors and beta blockers can be found in Chapter 5.

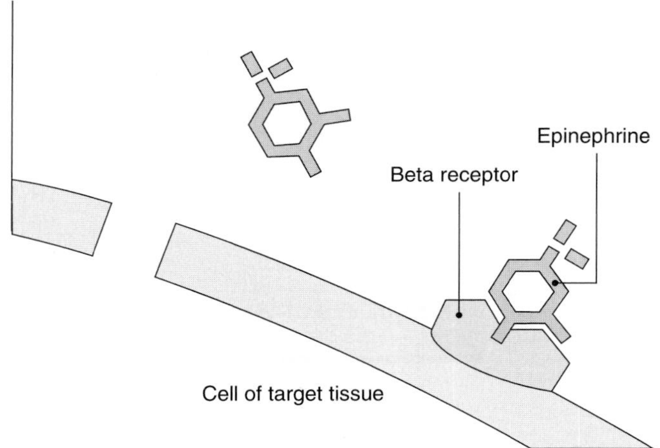

Figure 2-4 Epinephrine interacting with β receptor.

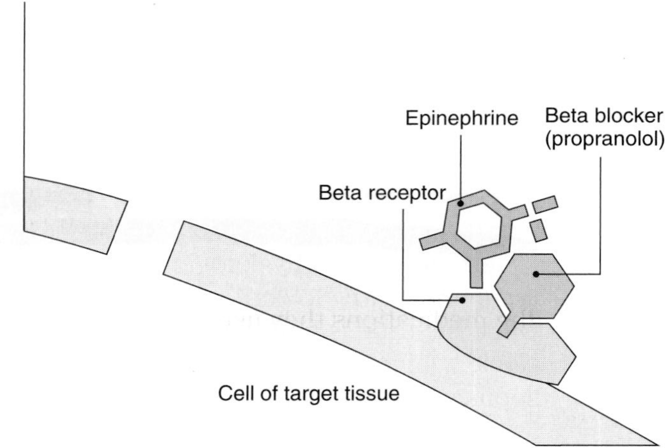

Figure 2-5 β Receptor blocked by propranolol.

Once again, for a medication to be effective it must reach a certain concentration at the target tissue. The minimal concentration of a drug necessary to cause the desired response is referred to as the *therapeutic threshold* or *minimum effective concentration*. A concentration below this therapeutic threshold will not induce a clinical response. There is also a point at which the drug concentration can get high enough to be toxic or even fatal. The general goal of drug therapy is to give the minimum concentration of a drug necessary to obtain the desired response (see Figure 2-6).

The difference between the minimum effective concentration and the toxic level varies significantly from drug to drug. The difference between these two concentrations is referred to as the *therapeutic index* and is usually obtained in the laboratory. Certain drugs, such as digitalis, have very little difference between the effective dose and the toxic dose. Such drugs

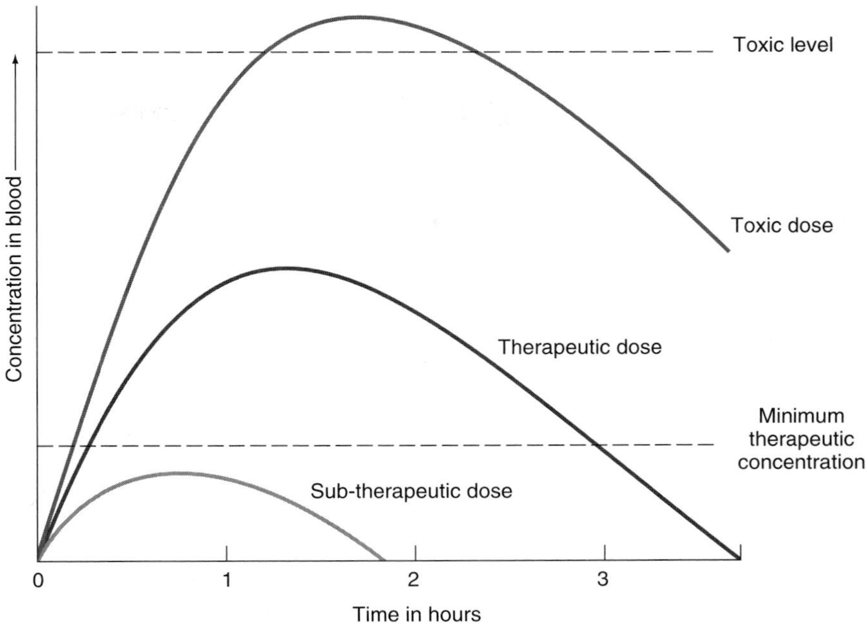

Figure 2-6 Comparison of blood levels following subtherapeutic, therapeutic, and toxic doses of the same drug.

are said to have a low therapeutic index. Drugs such as naloxone (Narcan), the narcotic antagonist, have a significant margin between the effective dose and the toxic dose and are said to have a high therapeutic index. Prehospital care providers should be familiar with the therapeutic indices of the medications they use.

SPECIAL CONSIDERATIONS IN DRUG THERAPY

Age, pregnancy, and lactation are important considerations in drug therapy. Both children and the elderly are particularly susceptible to the adverse effects of drugs. Because of this, drug dosages often must be modified for persons in these age groups. Likewise, special precautions must be taken when administering medications to a pregnant patient, as many medications will also affect the fetus. Certain drugs are excreted into the breast milk, which becomes a particular concern in mothers who are breast feeding their infants. The following sections discuss these special considerations in drug therapy.

Pediatric Patients

Children are typically smaller than adults, and drug dosages must be reduced accordingly. Pediatric drug dosages are typically based on the child's body weight or body surface area (BSA). Because of this, it is essential that prehospital personnel determine or approximate a child's weight before administering a medication. Often, the parents can provide an approximate weight from a recent doctor's visit. In emergencies the child's body weight can be estimated by determining the child's age and finding the average body weight for that age on a reference table.

Neonates (infants from birth to four weeks) are a special concern. Common sites of drug metabolism and elimination, such as the liver and kidneys, are not well developed in neonates. Because of this, both drug metabolism and excretion may be impaired. Drug dosages for neonates must often be modified to reflect these factors.

The American Heart Association (AHA) and the American Academy of Pediatrics (AAP) publish recommended drug dosages for most emergency medications. Often, the doses of common emergency drugs are listed on easy to use reference cards. To use these, simply look up the child's age or weight. Below the age or weight are the recommended dosages for common emergency drugs.

Another popular device for determining pediatric drug dosages is the Braslow Tape. To use the Braslow Tape, you simply unfold it and place it alongside the supine child. You then measure the child from the top of the head to the bottom of the feet. The tape is divided into various color coded drug dosage charts based on the child's length (which is directly related to the child's weight and body surface area). You simply use the dosage chart that corresponds to the child's length. In addition to drug dosages, the Braslow Tape contains recommended endotracheal tube sizes, defibrillator settings, and other important emergency information.

Geriatric Patients

The elderly are the fastest growing segment of our population and are frequent users of the EMS system. The aging process begins at the cellular level and affects virtually every body system. Common physiological effects of aging include:

- decreased cardiac output,
- decreased renal function,
- decreased brain mass,
- decreased total body water,
- decreased body fat,
- decreased serum albumin, and
- decreased respiratory capacity.

These changes can lead to altered pharmacodynamics and pharmacokinetics for many medications. With aging, the rate of metabolism and the excretion of medications can be significantly decreased. In addition, there is often decreased protein-binding due to decreased serum albumin. These factors combine to increase the relative potency of a drug. Because of this, the dosages of many medications must be reduced when administered to an elderly patient.

The elderly are more apt to suffer from more than one disease process at a time. In addition, they may be on chronic medications, which may affect

TABLE 2-2

Food and Drug Administration Pregnancy Safety Classification

Category A
Drugs for which controlled studies in humans have demonstrated no fetal risks. There are few category A drugs. Examples include multivitamins and prenatal vitamins.
Category B
Drugs for which animal or human studies have not demonstrated a significant risk. This category includes drugs for which animal studies indicate no fetal risks but for which there are no human studies, or drugs for which adverse effects have been demonstrated in animal studies but not in well-controlled human studies.
Category C
Drugs for which there are no adequate studies, either animal or human, or drugs for which there are adverse fetal effects in animal studies but no available human data.
Category D
Drugs for which there is evidence of fetal risk, but benefits are felt to outweigh these risks.
Category X
Drugs with proven fetal risks that clearly outweigh any benefits.

the emergency medications you need to administer in the prehospital setting. Multiple medical problems make drug dosing much more difficult. For example, treating a patient with congestive heart failure may be more difficult if the patient also has renal failure. In this case, the dosage of furosemide (Lasix) may need to be increased, while the dosage of morphine may need to be decreased. All factors must be considered before administering medications to the elderly.

Pregnancy and Lactation

Pregnancy presents two pharmacological problems. First, pregnancy causes a number of anatomical and physiological changes in the mother. These include:

- increased cardiac output,
- increased heart rate,
- increase in blood volume by up to 45%,
- decreased protein-binding,
- decreased hepatic metabolism, and
- decreased blood pressure.

These anatomical and physiological changes must be considered prior to administering medications or fluids to a pregnant patient.

The second consideration associated with pregnancy is that any medication administered to the mother has the potential to cross the placenta and affect the fetus. Some drugs cross the placenta rapidly while others do not. Thus, drugs should only be administered in pregnancy when the potential benefits outweigh the risks. The United States Food and Drug Administration (FDA) categorizes most drugs based upon their safety in pregnancy (see Table 2-2).

As with pregnancy, drug therapy can affect a breast feeding infant. Many medications are excreted readily into the breast milk. If the mother continues to breast feed while receiving these medications, the medications can be excreted into the breast milk and be ingested by the baby. If a breast feeding mother is to receive medications, she should be instructed to stop breast feeding and pump her breasts. She should dispose of the expressed milk until it is certain that the drug has been cleared from her system. During the time she is pumping her breasts, she should switch the infant to a commercial formula.

SUMMARY

A basic understanding of pharmacokinetics and pharmacodynamics is essential for prehospital personnel to anticipate the desired therapeutic effects as well as any possible side effects of the medications they administer. Such factors as rate of absorption, elimination, minimum therapeutic concentration, and toxic levels should be considered in all drugs.

KEY WORDS

absorption. The process whereby a drug is moved from the site of application into the body and into the extracellular fluid compartment.

affinity. The tendency of a drug to combine with a specific drug receptor.

agonist. A drug or other substance that binds with a specific drug receptor and causes a physiological response.

albumin. Protein found in almost all animal tissue. It constitutes one of the major proteins in human blood.

antagonist. A drug or other substance that blocks a physiological response or that blocks the action of another drug or substance.

binding capacity. The degree to which a drug is bound to tissue or plasma proteins.

biotransformation. Biotransformation, also called metabolism, is the process of changing a drug into a different form, either active or inactive, by the body.

blood-brain barrier. Protective mechanism that selectively allows the entry of selective compounds into the brain. It is an effective boundary between the central nervous system and the peripheral nervous system.

cumulative effect. A phenomenon that occurs when a drug is administered in several doses, causing an increased effect. It is usually due to a buildup of a drug in the blood.

distribution. The process whereby a drug is transported from the site of absorption to the site of action.

efficacy. The power of a drug to produce a therapeutic effect.

elimination. The process whereby a drug is removed from the body by excretion into the urine, feces, bile, saliva, sweat, breast milk, or expired air.

excretion. The elimination of waste products from the body. Excretion is often used interchangeably with the term elimination.

globulin. One of a broad category of simple proteins found in the body.

half life. The time required for a level of a drug in the blood to be reduced by 50 percent of its beginning level.

hemoglobin. An iron-containing compound found within the blood cell that is responsible for the transport and delivery of oxygen to the body cells.

loading dose. The initial dose of a drug given in a sufficient amount to achieve a therapeutic plasma level.

maintenance dose. The dose of a drug necessary to maintain a constant therapeutic plasma level.

metabolism. Metabolism is the sum total of all physical and chemical changes that occur within the body. In pharmacology it is often used interchangeably with the term biotransformation.

minimum effective concentration. The minimum amount of drug needed in the bloodstream to cause the desired therapeutic effect.

onset of action. The time interval between the administration of a drug and the first sign of its onset; onset of action is influenced by the physical and chemical properties of a drug as well as by its route of administration.

pH. A scientific method of expressing the acidity or alkalinity of a solution, which is the logarithm of the hydrogen ion concentration divided by 1. The higher the pH, the more alkaline the solution; the lower the pH, the more acidic the solution.

pharmacodynamics. The study of a drug's action upon the body.

pharmacokinetics. The study of how drugs enter the body, reach their site of action, and eventually are eliminated.

plasma (serum) level. The amount of the drug present in the plasma. The peak plasma level refers to the highest concentration produced by a specific dose.

solubility. The tendency of a drug to dissolve.

therapeutic index. The therapeutic index is an index of the drug's safety profile, which is determined by calculating the difference between the drug's therapeutic threshold and toxic level. It is typically determined in the laboratory.

therapeutic range. The difference between the minimal therapeutic and toxic concentrations of a drug. Drugs with a low therapeutic range present a higher risk of toxicity compared to drugs with a high therapeutic range. The therapeutic range is also referred to as the margin of safety.

therapeutic threshold. The minimum amount of drug needed in the bloodstream to cause a desired therapeutic effect.

toxic level. The plasma level at which severe adverse reactions are expected or likely.

toxicity. The degree to which a substance is poisonous. At high doses drugs can produce toxic effects that are not seen at low doses.

chapter 3

Administration of Drugs

OBJECTIVES

1. State the necessary components of a verbal or standing order.
2. Explain the five rights of drug administration.
3. Explain the advantages and disadvantages of alimentary versus parenteral administration.
4. List and explain three alimentary tract routes.
5. List and explain 9 parenteral routes.
6. Describe the landmarks for and demonstrate the technique for administering drugs via the subcutaneous route.
7. Describe the landmarks for and demonstrate the technique for administering drugs via the intramuscular route.
8. Describe the technique for administering IV medications by the IV bolus and IV piggyback administration routes.
9. Describe the technique for administering medications via the endotracheal tube route.
10. Describe the technique for administering medications via an intraosseous infusion.
11. Describe the different methods of administering medications through inhalation therapy.

INTRODUCTION

In the field of emergency medicine, medications must be administered promptly, in the correct dose, and by the correct route. Many drugs, although having therapeutic value when given by the appropriate route, can be fatal when given by another. Norepinephrine, for example, is a potent drug used to treat severe hypotension. It is designed to be given by slow, intravenous infusion. If given in an intravenous bolus, however, it may be fatal. This admonition applies to most medications used in emergency medicine.

The emergency scene is often hectic. Paramedics must often prepare and administer medications in the worst of environments. Because of this, it is essential that all prehospital personnel develop safe habits regarding drug preparation and drug administration. This serves to protect the patient as well as the paramedic.

This chapter will present the procedures for medication preparation and administration of medications used in emergency medical practice.

DRUG PREPARATION AND ADMINISTRATION

Prehospital personnel are responsible for preparing and administering many emergency drugs and fluids. The selection and administration of a particular medication is dependent upon an accurate and complete patient assessment. The results of this assessment must be relayed to medical control or applied to prehospital treatment protocols or standing orders. An inaccurate or incomplete patient assessment may lead to administration of the wrong drug.

The first step in medication administration is the medication order. The order may be in the form of a direct verbal order or through written standing treatment orders. The order will generally specify the following:

- medication desired,
- dose desired,
- administration route, and
- administration rate.

If possible, verbal medication orders should be written down as soon as they are received. After receiving the order, the paramedic should repeat the entire order back to the medical control physician. This assures that there is no misunderstanding related to the medication order. A typical medication order interchange is:

> ***Medical Control:*** "Start an IV of lactated Ringer's solution at 125 milliliters per hour and administer 5 milligrams of diazepam intravenously over one minute."
>
> ***Medic 1:*** "Confirming an IV of lactated Ringer's solution at 125 milliliters per hour and 5 milligrams of diazepam intravenously over one minute."
>
> ***Medical Control:*** "Affirmative Medic 1."

In systems that utilize standing orders, review the appropriate standing order. Confirm the ordered medication, dosage, route, and rate of medication administration. If possible, have another crew member review and double-check the standing order. Prepare and administer the medication as detailed in the standing order

It is essential to use good judgment regarding medication administration. Paramedics should always carefully evaluate the orders they receive. Occasionally, orders will be received that differ from accepted local prehospital protocols. In these cases, contact medical control and advise them of the discrepancy. If, after discussion of the discrepancy, the medical control physician does not change the order, paramedics should follow the order. The exception to this, of course, are orders that the paramedic feels will harm the patient. If you feel a particular medication or dose will harm the patient, notify the medical control physician that you are withholding the drug, and give the reason for doing so. Document well the circumstances surrounding the controversy and submit them to the system medical director for resolution. Although you are responsible to the medical control physician, you have a higher duty to protect the health and well-being of your patient.

Five Rights of Medication Administration

After you have received the medication or fluid order, you should then administer the drug in question. In performing drug administration, you should adhere to the ***five rights of medication administration:***

- right patient,
- right medication,
- right dose,
- right route, and
- right time.

Right Patient. Assuring that the right patient receives the right drug is usually not a problem in prehospital care as there is typically only one patient being treated. However, there may be circumstances where more than one patient is undergoing treatment. This is especially true in multiple casualty incidents (MCIs) where there may be many patients involved. In cases where there are multiple patients, it is prudent to use some label to distinguish patients. Some systems prefer to use the patient's last name. However, it is not uncommon for members of one family to be involved in an emergency. Each family member will usually have the same last name and some will have the same first names (i.e., William and William, Jr.). In these cases, it is best to assign numbers (i.e., Patient #1, Patient #2) or letters of the alphabet to each patient (i.e., Patient "A," Patient "B") to avoid confusion..

Confusion regarding multiple patients is more of a problem for medical control than for individual paramedics. A multiple casualty incident may utilize several ambulances, often with similar call signs. Each ambulance will contact medical control regarding the patient or patients they are

TABLE 3-1

Universal Precautions

Emergency response personnel should practice Body Substance Isolation (BSI), a strategy that considers ALL body substances potentially infectious. To achieve this, all emergency personnel should utilize personal protective equipment (PPE). Appropriate PPE should be available on every emergency vehicle. The minimum recommended PPE includes the following:

- *gloves.* Disposable gloves should be standard equipment for all emergency response personnel. They should be donned by all personnel BEFORE initiating any emergency care. When an emergency incident involves more than one patient, the paramedic should attempt to change gloves between patients, if possible. When gloves have been contaminated, they should be removed as soon as possible. To properly remove contaminated gloves, grasp one glove approximately one inch from the wrist. Without touching the inside of the glove, pull the glove half-way off and stop. With that half-gloved hand, pull the glove on the opposite hand completely off. Place the removed glove in the palm of the other glove, with the inside of the removed glove exposed. Pull the second glove completely off with the ungloved hand, only touching the inside of the glove. Always wash hands after gloves are removed, even when the gloves appear intact.
- *masks and protective eyewear.* Masks and protective equipment should be present on all emergency vehicles and used in accordance with the level of exposure encountered. Masks and protective eyewear should be worn together whenever blood spatter is likely to occur, such as arterial bleeding, childbirth, endotracheal intubation, invasive procedures, oral suctioning, and clean-up of equipment that requires heavy scrubbing or brushing. Masks should be worn by the paramedic and placed on the patient when the potential for airborne transmission of disease exists.
- *HEPA respirators.* Due to the resurgence of tuberculosis (TB), prehospital personnel should take measures to protect themselves from TB infection through use of a high-efficiency particulate air (HEPA) respirator. The HEPA respirator should be of a design approved by the National Institute of Occupational Safety and Health (NIOSH). It should fit snugly and be capable of filtering out the tuberculosis bacillus. The HEPA respirator should be worn when caring for patients with confirmed or suspected TB. This is especially true when performing "high hazard" procedures such as administration of nebulized medications, endotracheal intubation, or suctioning on a patient with suspected or confirmed TB.
- *gowns.* Gowns serve to protect clothing from splashes of blood. If large splashes of blood are expected, such as occur with childbirth, impervious gowns should be worn.
- *resuscitation equipment.* Disposable resuscitation equipment should be the primary means of artificial ventilation in emergency care. Such items should be used once, then disposed of.

Remember, the proper use of personal protective equipment ensures effective infection control and minimizes risk. Use ALL protective equipment recommended for any particular situation to ensure maximum protection. Consider ALL body substances potentially infectious and ALWAYS practice body substance isolation.

transporting. Care should be taken to distinguish the patients and units to avoid confusion and possible medication error. This can be minimized by using effective scene management techniques such as the Incident Command System. In these cases, each patient will be designated with a number or letter at the time of triage. Radio communications, both initial and subsequent, should refer to the patient by this designation. This will help avoid confusion both in the field and at medical control.

Right Medication. A common error in prehospital drug administration is selection of the wrong medication. Most emergency medications are supplied in ampules, vials, or prefilled syringes. Many of these look similar in their external appearance. To assure that the right drug is selected, paramedics should carefully read the label. If the drug is supplied in a box, check the label on the box and compare it with the label on the vial or ampule itself after removing it from the box. *Never assume that a medication is correct simply because it is in the correct place in the drug box!* Always read and double check the label!

Drug preparations and concentrations can vary. In addition to checking the drug name, always check to assure that the drug concentration is the one you desire. This is especially true for drugs that are carried in differing concentrations (i.e., epinephrine 1:1,000 and epinephrine 1:10,000 or lidocaine 100 mg for intravenous bolus and lidocaine 1 gram for intravenous infusion).

Always check the expiration date of a drug prior to administration. In addition, hold the medication up to the light and inspect for discoloration or particles in the solution. Expired and discolored medications should be discarded. Routine (preferably daily) drug box inspections should detect any expired medications. However, always doublecheck the medication prior to administration.

Right Dose. Administration of the correct drug dose is crucial. Errors in dosage occur either when calculating the correct dose or in preparing the correct dose. Most drug orders are fairly straightforward and most medications are supplied in unit-dose forms. In these cases, drug dosage calculation and drug preparation are easy. However, many medications, especially those administered by intravenous infusion, are much more difficult to dose. In these cases, paramedics should refer to standardized dosage charts to assist with preparation and administration of the desired dose

Right Route. Most medications used in prehospital care are designed to be given by the intravenous route. However, certain medications can be given by other routes depending on the physician's orders. It is the paramedic's responsibility to know the various administration routes by which a particular drug can be administered. For example, the drugs hydroxyzine (Vistaril) and promethazine (Phenergan) are frequently used in the treatment of nausea. Promethazine can be administered both intravenously and intramuscularly. Hydroxyzine, in comparison, can only be administered by the intramuscular route.

Right Time. Most medication orders for prehospital care call for immediate ("stat") administration of the drug. These orders are generally one time orders. However, certain drugs may be repeated. This is especially true in cardiac arrest situations where drugs are administered at specific time intervals.

An important consideration is the rate at which a drug should be administered. This is usually expressed as the period of time over which the drug in question should be administered. Many drugs can be administered rapidly as an IV bolus. Others must be administered at a specific rate. Diazepam, for example, should never be administered faster than 1 milliliter per minute (5 milligrams per minute). The rate of drug administration is particularly crucial for intravenous infusion medications (i.e., lidocaine, dopamine, norepinephrine, etc.).

> Prior to administration, a drug should be checked at least three times: first, when it is removed from the drug box; second, when the drug is prepared; and third, immediately prior to administration.

GENERAL ADMINISTRATION ROUTES

The two primary channels for getting medications into the body are through the alimentary canal (or digestive tract) and by parenteral routes. In acute care medicine, administration is almost always parenteral because the onset of action is much quicker and, usually, more predictable.

The following is a comparison of the relative advantages and disadvantages of alimentary versus parenteral administration.

Alimentary Tract

Advantages

1. Simple
2. Safe
3. Generally less expensive
4. Low potential for infection

Disadvantages

1. Slow rate of onset
2. Cannot be given to unconscious or nauseated patients
3. The absorbed dosage may vary significantly because of actions of digestive enzymes and the condition of the intestinal tract.

Parenteral Route

Advantages

1. Rapid onset
2. Can be given to unconscious and nauseated patients
3. Absorbed dosage and action are more predictable.

Disadvantages

1. Administration often difficult and painful
2. Usually more expensive
3. Side effects usually more severe
4. Potential for infection

Alimentary Tract Routes

The common routes of alimentary tract administration used in general medical practice are as follows:

Oral. The best, and most convenient, way of administering drugs is by mouth. Most medical drugs are available in oral preparations. The effects of oral administration are often not seen until 30 to 45 minutes after administration.

Sublingual. Some drugs can be administered sublingually (that is, under the tongue). When administered in this fashion, the drug is placed under the tongue where it quickly dissolves. The drug is then absorbed into the vast capillary network present in the mucous membranes. Nitroglycerin, a drug frequently used in the management of angina pectoris, is administered by this route.

Rectal. Rectal administration may have both local and systemic effects. It may be necessary to administer some medications rectally, especially if the patient is nauseated. The rectal route is frequently used in infants and children who may not be able to swallow oral medications. Absorption of rectally administered drugs is generally somewhat slower than by the oral route.

Parenteral Routes

Any method of administration that does not involve passage through the digestive tract is termed parenteral. Parenteral routes include the following:

Topical. Certain drugs can be placed on the skin where they are slowly absorbed into the capillary network underneath the skin. The rate of onset varies, but the duration of action is prolonged. This route is often used to administer nitroglycerin in the emergency setting.

Intradermal. Drugs can be injected into the dermal layer of the skin. The amount of medication that can be given via this route is limited, and systemic absorption (into the blood stream) is very slow. Generally, this route is reserved for diagnostic skin tests, like allergy testing.

Subcutaneous. With subcutaneous administration, medications are injected into fatty, subcutaneous tissue under the skin and overlying muscle. The rate of absorption is slower than that seen with intramuscular and intravenous administration. Epinephrine 1:1,000, which is used in the treatment of acute asthma and other respiratory emergencies, is almost always administered subcutaneously. A maximum of 2 milliliters of a drug can be given subcutaneously.

Intramuscular. The most commonly used route of parenteral medication administration is the intramuscular route. The drug is injected into muscle tissue from which it is absorbed into the bloodstream. This method of administration has a predictable rate of absorption but is considerably slower than intravenous administration.

Intravenous. Most medications used in emergency medicine are designed to be administered intravenously. These can be in the form of an intravenous (IV) bolus or as a slow IV infusion, sometimes referred to as a piggyback infusion. The rate of absorption is rapid and predictable. Of all the routes frequently employed, however, IV administration of drugs has the most potential for causing adverse reactions.

Endotracheal. When an IV line cannot be started, it is sometimes possible to administer emergency medications down an endotracheal tube, which permits absorption into the capillaries of the lungs. It has been shown that this route has a rate of absorption as fast as the IV route. Drugs that can be administered endotracheally include epinephrine, lidocaine, naloxone, and atropine.

Sublingual Injection. In the rare instance where neither an IV line can be started nor an endotracheal tube inserted, certain drugs can be injected into the vast capillary network immediately under the tongue. Lidocaine is the agent most frequently given by this route.

Intracardiac. Injection of a medication directly into the ventricle of the heart is referred to as intracardiac administration. Because of the many complications associated with this procedure, it is reserved exclusively for life-threatening situations, such as cardiac arrest, when an IV line cannot be established nor an endotracheal tube placed.

Intraosseous. When an IV line cannot be started in children under 6 years of age, many emergency medications can be administered intraosseously. A needle can be placed in the anterior aspect of the proximal tibia through which medications and fluids can be administered. The onset of action is similar to IV administration.

Inhalational. Medications can be administered directly into the respiratory tree in cases of respiratory distress resulting from reversible airway disease including asthma and certain types of chronic obstructive pulmonary disease. These medications are usually nebulized into a water vapor and breathed with normal respiration.

Vaginal. Medications can be placed into the vagina where they are absorbed into surrounding tissues. Most vaginal medications are supplied in creams or vaginal suppositories. The onset of action is slow and the effects are generally limited to the lower female genital tract.

MEDICATION ROUTES USED IN EMERGENCY MEDICINE

Emergency medications are often administered parenterally by either the subcutaneous, intramuscular, intravenous, endotracheal, intraosseous, or inhalational route. Always use universal precautions in patient care, particularly with drug administration. This section outlines the procedure for administration by each of these routes.

Subcutaneous Injection

Epinephrine 1:1,000 is the emergency drug most frequently given subcutaneously. The procedure is as follows:

1. Receive order.
2. Confirm the order and write it down.
3. Prepare the necessary equipment and don gloves:
   - 1-cc syringe
   - needle (preferably 5/8 inch in length, 25 gauge)
   - alcohol preparation or other antibacterial swab
   - 4 × 4 gauze pad
   - medication

4. Explain to the patient what you are going to do. Be sure to warn him or her of any complications that might result from the administration.
5. Reconfirm that the patient is not allergic to the medication you are going to administer.
6. Examine the ampule of medication, reconfirming that it is correct. Hold it up to the light and inspect for discoloration or particles in the solution. Do not administer if discolored or if particles are present.
7. "Shake down" the ampule. This will force the liquid to the lower portion of the ampule so that it can be broken without spillage of the drug.
8. Break the ampule using a 4 × 4 gauze pad to prevent injury.
9. Draw the medication into the syringe. Invert the syringe and expel any air present.
10. Choose a suitable site. The easiest and most accessible site is the subcutaneous tissue over the deltoid muscle in the arm (see Figure 3-1).
11. Pinch up the skin and insert the needle into the tissue at a 45 degree angle (see Figure 3-2).
12. Aspirate the syringe to assure that you are not in a blood vessel. If you get any blood return, you should withdraw the needle and reattempt administration at another site.

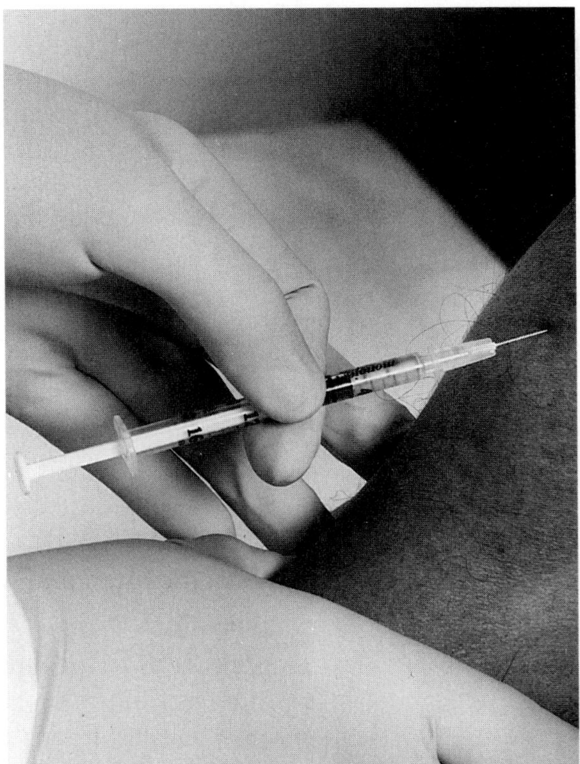

Figure 3-1 Subcutaneous injection.

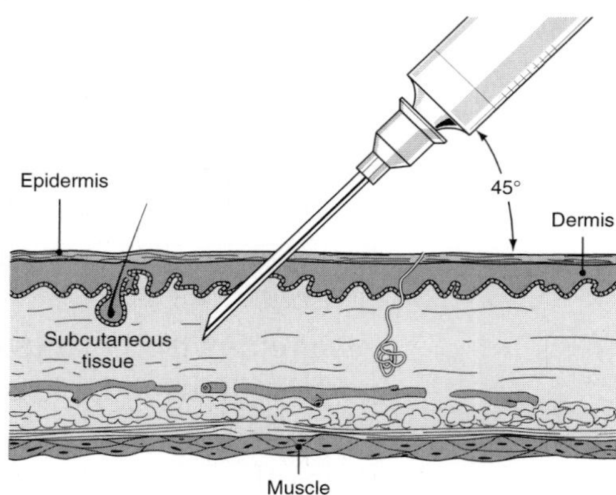

Figure 3-2 Needle properly inserted in subcutaneous tissue.

13. Inject the medication slowly.
14. Remove the syringe. Do not recap the needle.
15. Apply pressure to the site.
16. Cover with an adhesive strip.
17. Confirm administration of the medication.
18. Closely monitor the patient for the desired therapeutic effect and possible side effects.

Intramuscular Injection

Intramuscular injection is useful when rapid drug action is not required. The most common muscles into which drugs are administered are the deltoid and the gluteal. A maximum of 1 milliliter of medication can be given into the deltoid, whereas 10 milliliters can be given into the gluteal.

Medications can be given intramuscularly using the standard syringe, the Tubex system, or prefilled syringes. The procedure for intramuscular medication administration is as follows:

1. Receive order.
2. Confirm the order and write it down.
3. Prepare the necessary equipment and don gloves:
   - syringe of sufficient size to contain the medication
   - needle (preferably 3/4 to 1 inch in length, 21 to 25 gauge)
   - alcohol preparation or other antibacterial swab
   - 4 × 4 gauze pad
   - medication
4. Explain to the patient what you are going to do. Be sure to warn him or her of any complications that might result from the administration.
5. Reconfirm that the patient is not allergic to the medication you are going to administer.

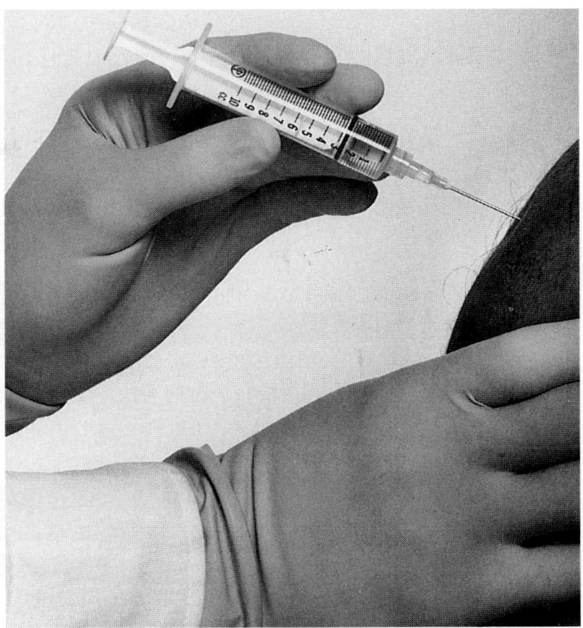

Figure 3-3 Intramuscular injection.

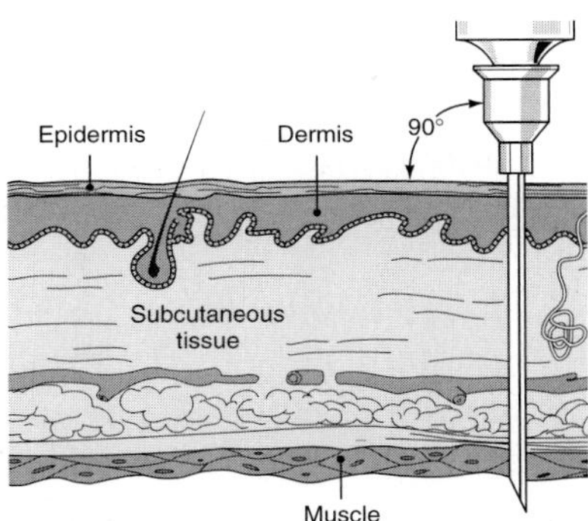

Figure 3-4 Needle properly inserted in muscle tissue.

6. Examine the ampule of medication, reconfirming that it is correct. Hold it up to the light and inspect for discoloration or particles in the solution. If the medication is discolored or contains particles, do not administer it.
7. "Shake down" the ampule. This will force the liquid to the lower portion of the ampule so that it can be broken without spillage of the drug.
8. Break the ampule using a 4 × 4 gauze pad to prevent injury.
9. Draw the medication into the syringe. Invert the syringe and expel any air present.
10. Choose a suitable site. The easiest and most accessible site is the deltoid muscle in the arm (see Figure 3-3).
11. Insert the needle into the tissue at a 90 degree angle (see Figure 3-4).
12. Aspirate the syringe to assure that you are not in a blood vessel. If you get any blood return, you should withdraw the needle and reattempt administration at another site.

13. Inject the medication slowly.
14. Remove the syringe. Do not recap the needle.
15. Apply pressure to the site.
16. Cover with an adhesive strip.
17. Confirm administration of the medication.
18. Closely monitor the patient for the desired therapeutic effect and possible undesired side effects.

It is important to note that, as a rule, patients presenting with a chief complaint of chest pain should not receive medications by the intramuscular route. Intramuscular injection of medication may cause an elevation of certain muscle enzymes that routinely circulate in the blood. In the emergency department these enzymes are frequently measured to determine whether the chest pain is of myocardial origin. An intramuscular injection in the prehospital phase of emergency medical care can cause a false elevation of these enzymes, which can subsequently confuse the emergency department physician as he or she attempts to determine the etiology of the chest pain. There may be occasions, however, when the medical control physician may permit intramuscular injections when no other immediate route is available and administration of the medication is essential.

Intravenous Administration

As mentioned previously, there are two distinct methods of IV medication administration: (1) the IV bolus and (2) slow IV infusion (sometimes called "piggyback").

Emergency medications administered by the IV bolus technique are usually administered with prefilled syringes. Many medications, however, are still available only in ampule or vial form.

In all but a few cases, it is essential that an IV be established before administering medications intravenously. This makes the repeated administration of intravenous medications less traumatic.

IV Bolus

1. Receive the order.
2. Confirm the order and write it down.
3. Prepare the necessary equipment and don gloves:
   - syringe of sufficient size to contain the medication
   - needle (preferably 1 inch long, 18 gauge)
   - alcohol preparation or other antibacterial swab
   - adhesive bandage strip
   - medication
4. Explain to the patient what you are going to do. Be sure to warn him or her of any complications that might arise as a result of the administration.
5. Reconfirm that the patient is not allergic to the medication that you are going to administer.
6. Examine the ampule of medication, reconfirming that it is correct. Hold it up to light and inspect for discoloration or particles in the

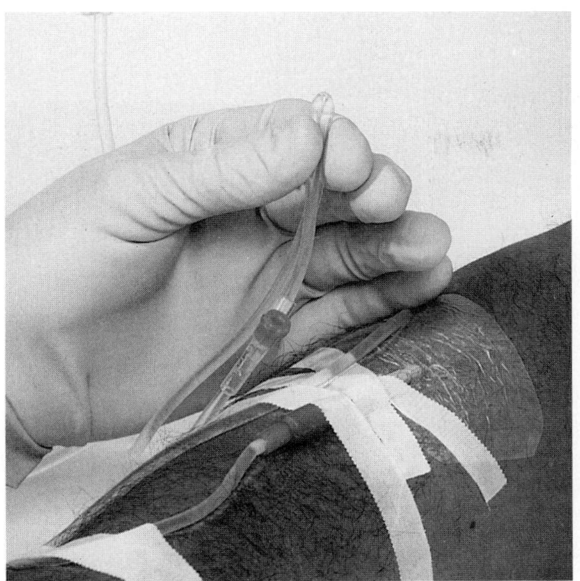

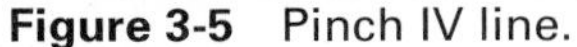

Figure 3-5 Pinch IV line.

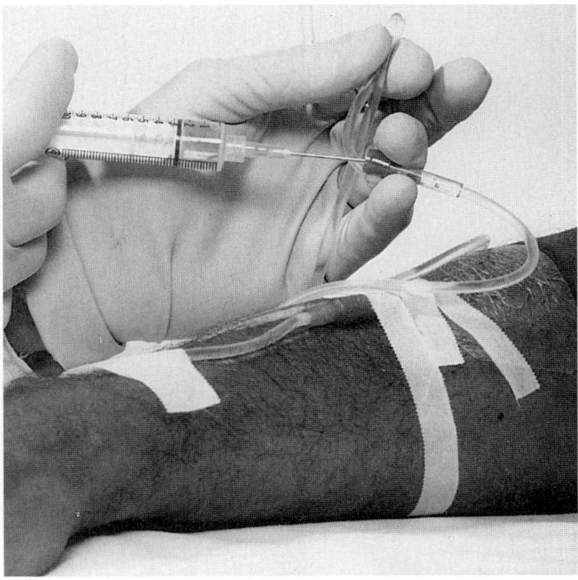

Figure 3-6 IV injection.

solution. Do not administer the medication if discolored or if particles are present.

7. "Shake down" the ampule. This will force the liquid to the lower portion of the ampule so that it can be broken without spillage of the drug.
8. Break the ampule using a 4 × 4 gauze pad to prevent injury.
9. Draw the medication into the syringe. Invert the syringe and expel any air.
10. Locate the medication port on the IV administration set, and cleanse it with antibacterial solution.
11. Insert the needle into the medication port.
12. Pinch the IV line off above the medication port (see Figure 3-5)
13. Administer the medication in a slow, deliberate fashion (see Figure 3-6).
14. Remove the needle and wipe the medication port with antibacterial solution.
15. Release the pinched line.
16. Confirm administration of the medication.
17. Closely monitor the patient for the desired therapeutic effects as well as any undesired side effects.

IV Piggyback

1. Receive the order.
2. Confirm the order and write it down.
3. Prepare the necessary equipment and don gloves:
   - medication
   - syringe to transfer the medication from the ampule to the diluent

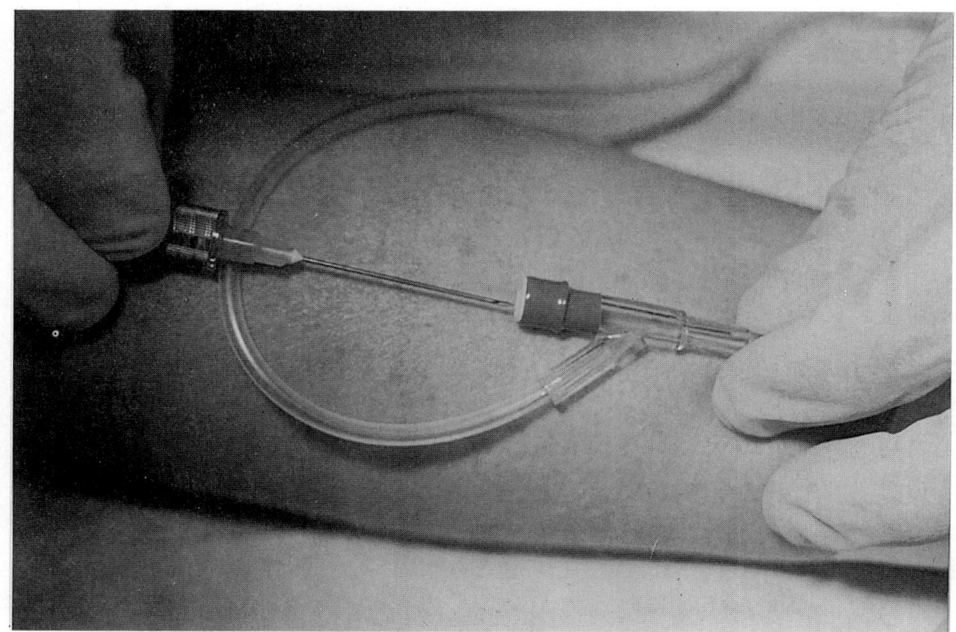

Figure 3-7 Insert the needle into the administration port of an established IV line.

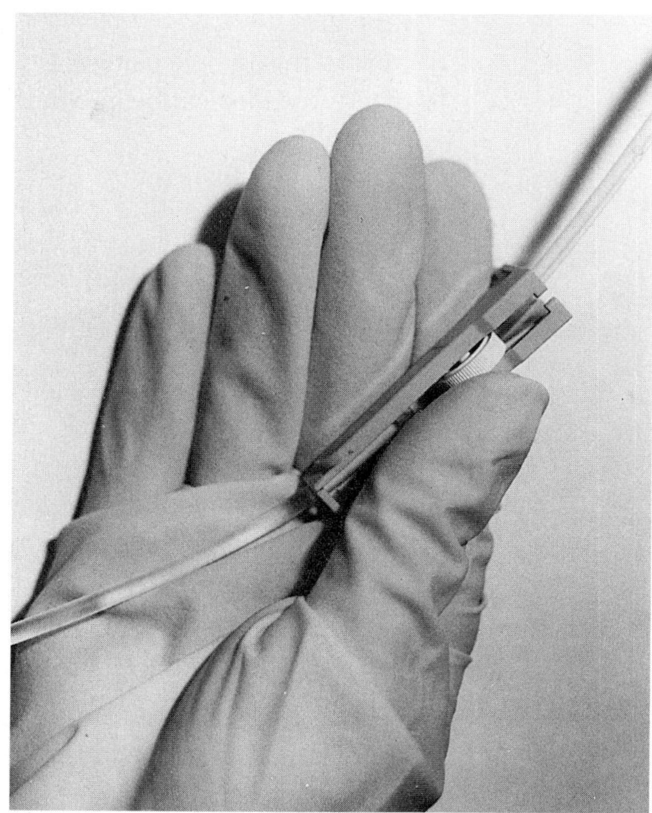

Figure 3-8 Following IV injection, adjust the flow rate.

- alcohol prep or other antibacterial scrub
- two 18-gauge, 1-inch needles
- label for the bag

4. Explain to the patient what you are going to do. Be sure to warn him or her of any complications that might arise as a result of the administration.
5. Reconfirm that the patient is not allergic to the medication that you are going to administer.
6. Examine the ampule of medication, reconfirming that it is correct. Hold it up to light and inspect for discoloration or particles in the solution. Do not administer if discolored or if particles are present.
7. "Shake down" the ampule. This will force the liquid to the lower portion of the ampule so that it can be broken without spillage of the medication.
8. Break the ampule using a 4×4 gauze pad to prevent injury.
9. Draw the medication into the syringe using aseptic technique. Invert and expel any air.
10. Cleanse the medication port on the IV bag into which the medication will be added.
11. Invert the bag and add the medication through the medication addition port.
12. Remove the needle and cleanse the medication addition port.
13. Invert the bag several times and place an administration set into it.
14. Bleed the air out of the administration set and attach a 1-inch, 18-gauge needle.
15. Cleanse the medication port on the administration set of the already established IV line and insert the needle (see Figure 3-7).
16. Tape the needle securely.
17. Adjust the flow rate of the piggyback infusion to the desired dose (see Figure 3-8).
18. Label the bag for emergency department personnel.
19. Confirm establishment of the infusion.
20. Closely monitor the patient for the desired therapeutic effects as well as any undesired side effects.

Endotracheal Administration

The endotracheal route is very effective and often forgotten in the emergency setting. When an IV cannot be established, and the patient is in dire need of lidocaine, naloxone, atropine, or epinephrine, which may be the case in cardiac arrest, these drugs may be instilled via the endotracheal tube. The rate of absorption is as fast as IV administration. When administering a medication via the endotracheal tube, the dose should be increased to 2 to 2.5 times the intravenous dose.

A common situation follows:

A patient is encountered in ventricular fibrillation and is immediately countershocked. The patient converts to an improved rhythm with a fair pulse. An IV line cannot be immediately established, however. The patient begins to have frequent multifocal premature ventricular contractions. Lidocaine can now be administered down the endotracheal tube to stabilize the rhythm until a peripheral line can be established.

The procedure is as follows:

1. Receive the order.
2. Confirm the order and write it down.
3. Prepare the prefilled medication syringe and don gloves.
4. Examine the ampule of medication, reconfirming that it is correct. Quickly hold it up to light and inspect for discoloration or particles in the solution. Do not administer if foreign bodies are present or if discolored.
5. Hyperventilate the patient in anticipation of administration.
6. Remove the bag-valve-mask unit and inject the medication down the tube (see Figure 3-9).
7. Replace the bag-valve-mask unit and resume ventilation.

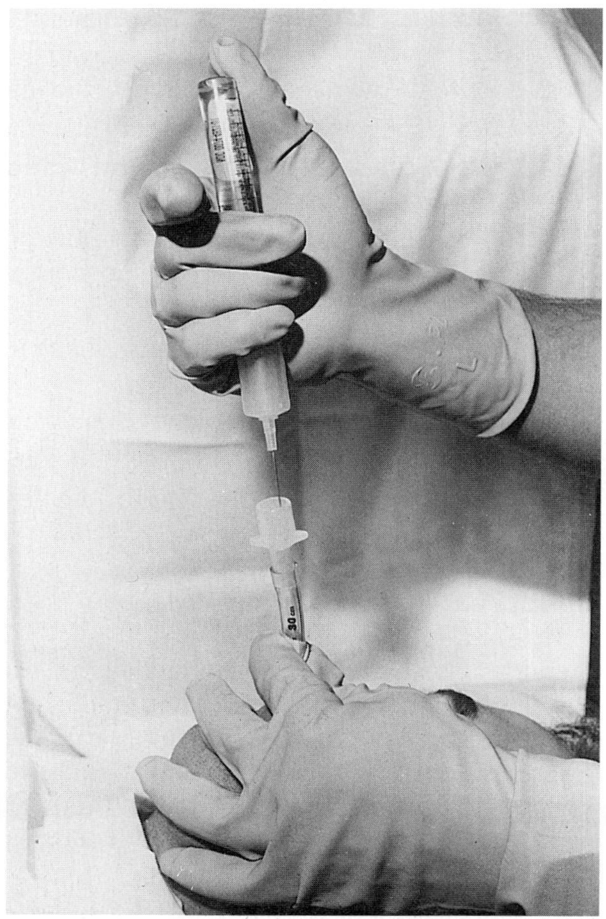

Figure 3-9 Endotracheal drug administration.

8. Monitor the patient for the desired therapeutic effect and any possible undesired side effects.

Use caution when administering endotracheal medications while using an end-tidal carbon dioxide detector. Some medications, when administered via the endotracheal route, may cause false end-tidal CO_2 readings.

Intraosseous Injection

It is often difficult to establish an IV line in children younger than 6 years of age. In instances in which an IV cannot be established, and the child needs emergency medications or fluids, an intraosseous line can be established. A needle is placed into the proximal tibia, approximately 1 to 3 centimeters below the tibial tuberosity, on the anterior surface. The needle is advanced through the cortex of the bone into the bone marrow cavity. Entry into the marrow cavity is evidenced by a lack of resistance after penetrating the bony cortex, the needle standing upright without support, the ability to aspirate bone marrow into a syringe connected to the needle, or the free flow of the infusion without significant subcutaneous infiltration. Fluids and drugs administered into the marrow cavity quickly enter the circulatory system. The onset of action of drugs administered by this route is similar to IV injection. Drugs that can be administered by this route include the catecholamines, lidocaine, atropine, and sodium bicarbonate, as well as fluids. *Intraosseous infusion is only indicated in children younger than 6 years of age and only when an IV line cannot be established.*

The procedure is as follows:

1. Receive the order.
2. Confirm the order and write it down.
3. Prepare the necessary equipment and don gloves:
   - medication
   - intravenous fluid
   - syringe
   - intraosseous needle or 16- to 18-gauge spinal needle (see Figure 3-10)
   - povidone iodine preparation
4. Examine the ampule, vial, or syringe of medication or fluid, and make sure it is correct. Also make sure it is not discolored and does not contain any particles. Do not administer if particles are present or if discolored.
5. Locate the anterior tibial tuberosity. Choose a spot approximately 1 to 3 centimeters below.
6. Prepare the area extensively with three povidone iodine preparations in a circular fashion.
7. Replace your gloves with sterile gloves.
8. Take the sterile needle and insert it into the bone at a perpendicular angle or angled slightly inferior. Stop insertion when a lack of resistance is felt (see Figures 3-11 and 3-12).

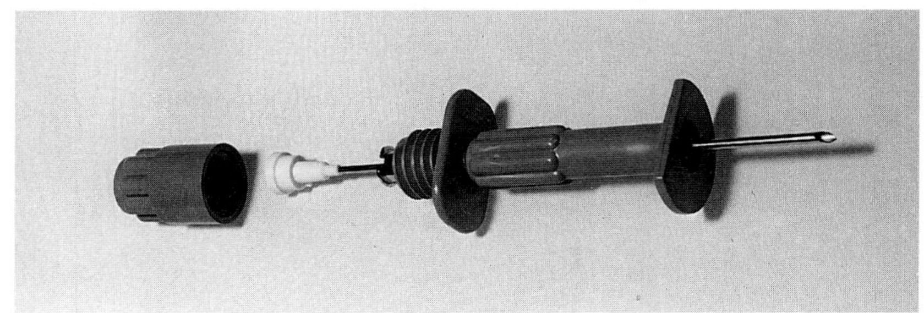
Figure 3-10 Intraosseous needle.

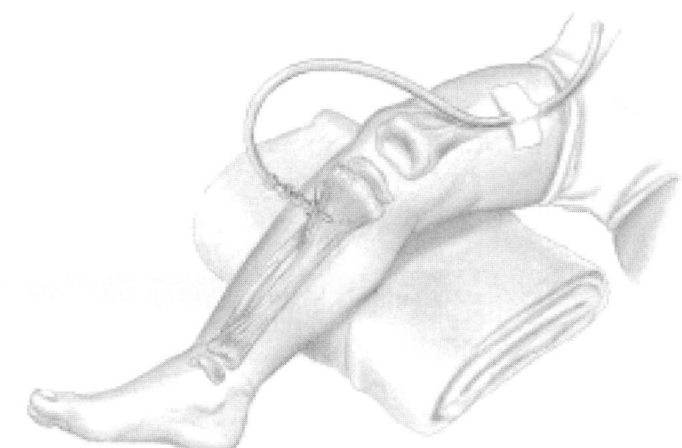
Figure 3-11 Insertion of intraosseous needle.

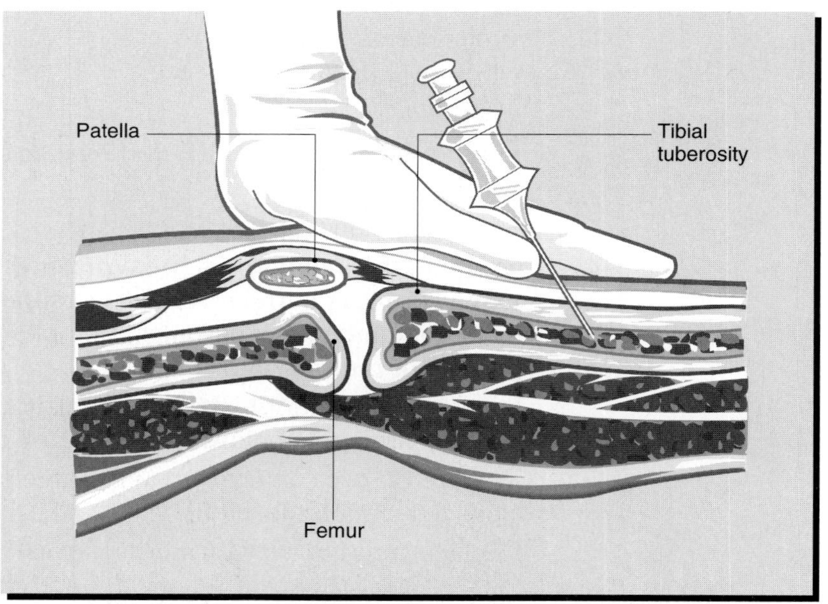

Figure 3-12 Intraosseous needle properly in place.

9. Place a syringe on the needle, and attempt to aspirate a small amount of marrow.
10. If the needle is properly placed (that is, it stands upright without support or you are able to aspirate marrow), attach it to an IV line and the desired fluid. Do not administer IV fluid unless ordered, and then only in doses of 20 milliliters per kilogram.
11. Administer the medication.
12. Remove the syringe. Do not recap the needle. Dispose of the needle and syringe properly.
13. Closely monitor the child for the desired effects as well as any side effects.
14. Secure the intraosseous needle before movement of the child.

Inhalational Administration

Many medications used in the treatment of respiratory emergencies are administered by inhalation. The most common example of this is oxygen. In addition, there are medications that are designed to be administered into the respiratory tree. The most common of these are the bronchodilators. These include metaproterenol (Alupent), racemic epinephrine, isotharine (Bronkosol), ipatropium (Atrovent), and albuterol (Ventolin). By administering these drugs directly into the respiratory tree, they can quickly reach their site of action with minimal absorption delays.

The following are three common methods for administering these medications:

Metered Dose Inhalers. Metered dose inhalers are aerosolized forms of the medication in a small canister. Most bronchodilators are supplied in this form. Many patients have these at home and use them routinely. The canister is attached to a mouthpiece. The patient places his or her lips around the mouthpiece, begins to inhale, and presses the canister. When the canister is pressed, a metered amount of the drug is delivered in aerosol form. The amount of drug delivered is accurate and limited. Metered dose inhalers are designed for single-patient use (see Figure 3-13).

Spinhaler, Rotohaler. These commercial devices are designed for patients who have difficulty operating the metered dose inhalers. Special capsules are placed in the device. When inhaled, the capsules release medication that is delivered to the respiratory tree (see Figure 3-14).

Small-volume Nebulizer. Small-volume nebulizers, also called updraft or hand-held nebulizers, are the most commonly used method of administering inhaled medications in the emergency setting. The nebulizer has a chamber into which a solution of the medication, usually diluted with 2 to 3 milliliters of sterile saline, is placed. Oxygen or compressed air is blown past the chamber causing the medication to be aerosolized. The patient inhales the aerosolized medication with each breath. This method of bronchodilator administration is advantageous because it delivers supplemental oxygen, delivers the medication over a 5- to 10-minute interval, and is supplied in single-dose ampules (see Figures 3-15 and 3-16).

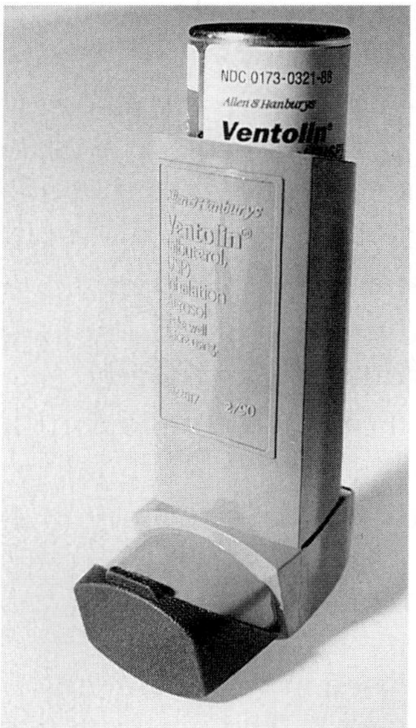

Figure 3-13 Metered dose inhaler.

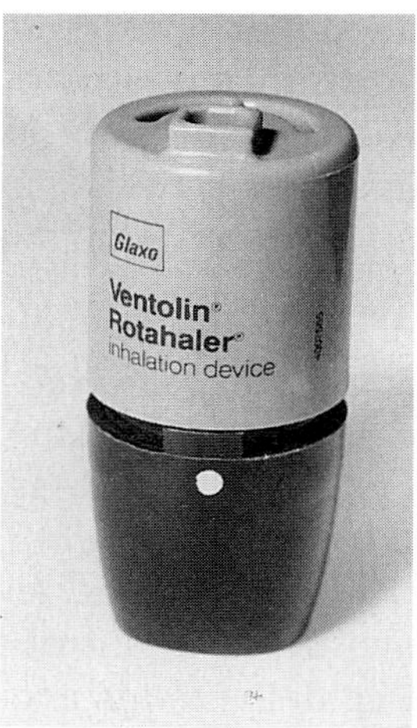

Figure 3-14 Spinhaler (Ventolin Rotahaler).

SUMMARY

It is essential that acute care personnel be competent with all of the medication routes used in emergency medicine. These skills can be developed only after repeated practice in the classroom and the clinical setting. It is important to be familiar with all of the medications used in routine prehospital care in your system and the routes by which they are administered. If there is any doubt concerning an order or an administration route, consult the medical control physician or a drug reference source. Each time you administer a medication you should assure you have met each of the five "rights" of medication administration: Right patient, right medication, right dose, right route, and right time.

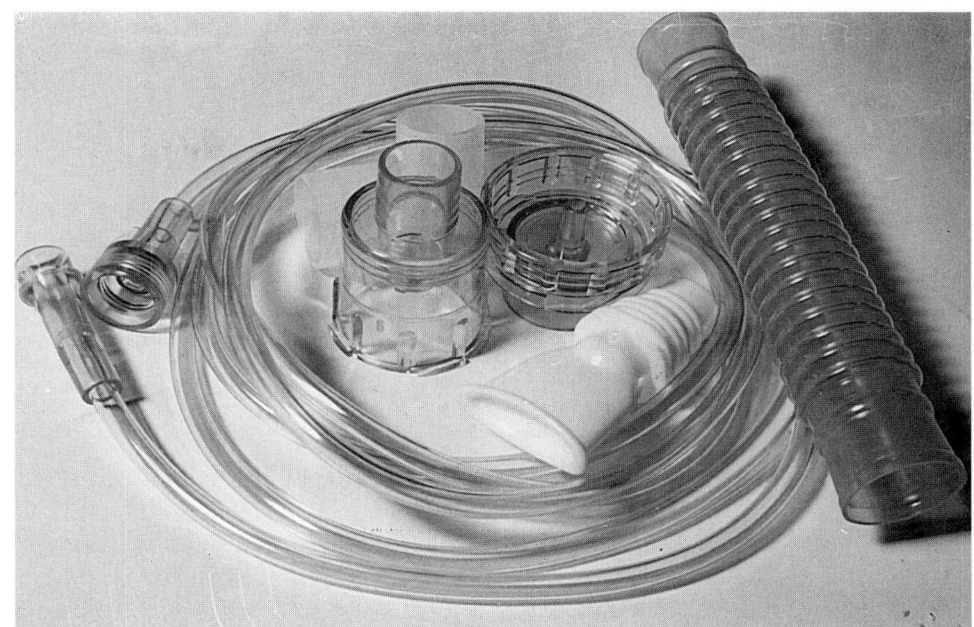

Figure 3-15 Small volume nebulizer.

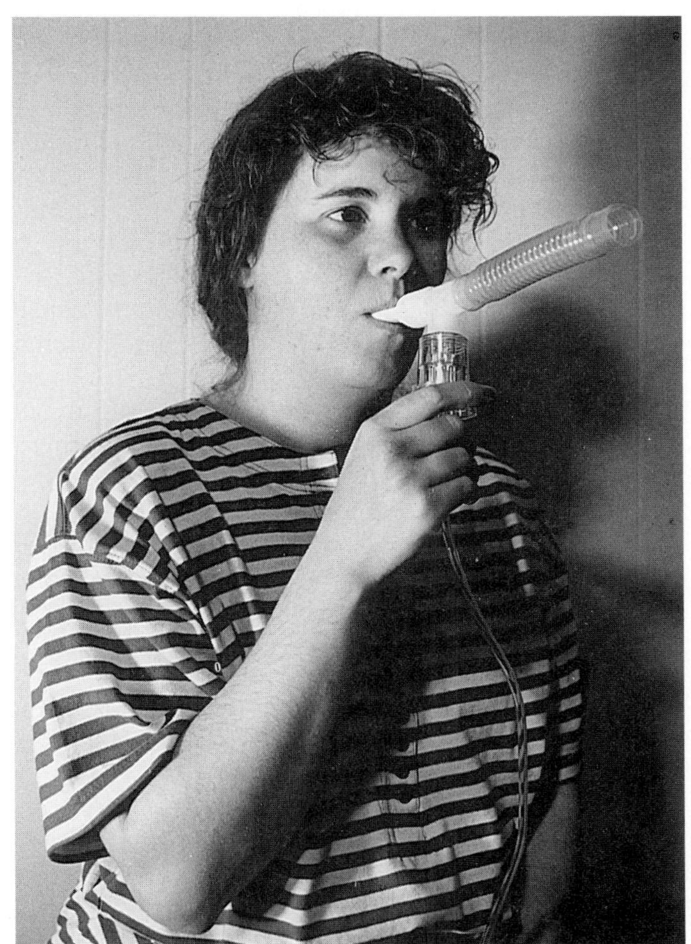

Figure 3-16 Medication administration via a small volume nebulizer.

This book is not a substitute for a rigorous classroom instruction session on medication administration. It is purely designed as a teaching aid for the student and as a reference source for others.

KEY WORDS

alimentary canal. The digestive tract.

bolus. A method of intravenous medication administration by which a drug is rapidly administered rather than infused over a period of time.

endotracheal. A route of medication administration by which drugs are administered down an endotracheal tube.

inhalation. Entrance of a substance into the body through the respiratory tract.

intracardiac. Administration of medications directly into the heart. This route is not recommended for prehospital care.

intradermal. A parenteral route of medication administration by which a drug is injected into the dermal layer of the skin.

intramuscular injection. A common parenteral route of medication administration by which a drug is injected into the skeletal muscle.

intraosseous. A route of fluid and drug administration where select medications or fluids are injected into the bone marrow. This route is considered an alternative to venous access in children under the age of 6.

intravenous. A commonly used parenteral route of medication administration by which a drug is injected directly into venous circulation.

intravenous infusion. A method of medication administration by which a drug or fluid is given over time.

metered dose inhaler. A device for administering medication by inhalation; it consists of a canister containing a liquid that, when activated, delivers the medication via a fine mist.

piggyback. A method of administering a medication by slow IV infusion.

rectal. An enteral route of medication administration by which a drug is instilled in the rectum.

stat. Latin abbreviation meaning "immediately."

subcutaneous. A common parenteral route of medication administration by which a drug is injected into the loose connective tissue between the dermis and the muscle.

sublingual. A route of medication administration by which a drug is absorbed across the rich blood supply of the tongue.

chapter 4

Drug Dosage Calculations

OBJECTIVES

1. Define "metric system."
2. Define the common metric prefixes.
3. Demonstrate the ability to do routine calculations and conversions using the metric system.
4. Calculate any given drug dose for medications used in your EMS system using the basic formula.
5. Calculate drug doses using variations of the basic formula.
6. Complete the practice problems using the basic formula and variations.

INTRODUCTION

Administration of the correct drug dosage is essential to proper medical care. Medications used in emergency medicine are available from many different manufacturers, many in different strengths, volumes, and containers. It is important to be familiar with the common emergency drug preparations. In addition, all personnel should be able to prepare the correct medication dose quickly from available ampules or vials regardless of drug concentration or volume.

Familiarity with the systems of measurement frequently used in medicine, especially the metric system, is essential. Conversion from one system to another is often required.

In this chapter common mathematical operations required to complete dosage calculations, as well as several formulas, are presented.

SYSTEM OF WEIGHTS AND MEASURES

The metric system is the principal system of weights and measures used in pharmacology. Tradition has caused some apothecaries' weights and measures to endure, however. The metric system is used worldwide as the standard system of weights and measures in both science and medicine. In recent years the U.S. government has begun the arduous transition from the English system to the metric system.

The metric system is a system of weights and measures devised by the French. The metric system is based on the unit 10. All units were either 10 times larger or 1/10 as large as the next unit. Because the metric system is based on 10, the conversion from one unit to another is fairly simple. The change from one set of units to another requires moving only a decimal point.

In making physical descriptions, three things need to be measured: mass, length, and volume. *Mass* is the quantity of matter present in a given substance. *Length* is the distance between two points. *Volume* is the space occupied by a given substance. The metric system has three fundamental units for the measurement of mass, length, and volume. The fundamental unit used for measuring mass is the *gram*; the fundamental unit used for measuring length is the *meter*; the fundamental unit used for measuring volume is the *liter*. All other metric units used to describe length, mass, and volume are derivatives of these three fundamental, or base, units. Instead of using a large number of zeros, a person making metric conversions can simply change the prefix. Common metric system prefixes include the following:

kilo- = 1000 (k)

hecto- = 100 (h)

deka- = 10 (D)

Fundamental unit = 1 (gram, liter, or meter)

deci- = 1/10 (d)

centi- = 1/100 (c)

milli- = 1/1000 (m)

micro- = 1/1,100,000 (μ)

The following prefixes are most frequently encountered: kilo-, centi-, milli-, and micro-.

Metric Conversions

To change a prefix, simply move the decimal point. Common examples of metric conversions follow:

1,000 liters = 1 kiloliter

1,000 grams = 1 kilogram

1/1000 gram = 1 milligram (0.001 gram = 1.0 milligram)

1/100 meter = 1 centimeter (0.01 meter = 1.0 centimeter)

Most of us learned only the English system of measurement while in school. To bring the metric system into perspective, the following are some common conversions with which we need to be familiar:

1 centimeter = 0.39 inches

1 meter = 39.37 inches

1 liter = 1.05 quarts

1 kilogram = 2.2 pounds

2.54 centimeter = 1.0 inch

Occasionally, orders will be received for certain drugs in the old apothecaries' system. The most common apothecary measure likely to be seen is the *grain*. Many physicians still routinely prescribe some medications, especially analgesics, in grains. Because most emergency drugs are supplied in metric measures, a conversion is required. The conversion is as follows:

1 grain = 60 milligrams

thus

1/4 grain = 15 milligrams

Another conversion often used in medicine is between cubic centimeters and milliliters. One milliliter of water occupies 1 cubic centimeter of space. Thus:

1 cubic centimeter (cm^3) = 1 milliliter (ml)

The term "cubic centimeter" is falling into disuse, with milliliter being the preferred term. Occasionally both may be seen.

Familiarity with the metric system, and its conversions, is essential. The following practice problems should be mastered before moving to the next section.

In addition to the trend in medicine toward the metric system, we are also seeing the switch from the use of the Fahrenheit system of temperature measurement to the Celsius system. The Celsius system is based on the physical properties of water. The freezing point was designated 0°C, which is 32°F. The boiling point of water was designated 100°C, which is 212°F. Thus, normal body temperature is either 98.6°F or 37°C. The conversion is as follows:

From Fahrenheit to Celsius:

$$(\text{Degrees Fahrenheit} - 32) \times 0.556 = \text{Degrees Celsius}$$

From Celsius to Fahrenheit:

$$(\text{Degrees Celsius} \times 1.8) + 32 = \text{Degrees Fahrenheit}$$

Example:

$$(98.6°\text{F} - 32) \times 0.556 = 37°\text{C}$$

$$37 \times 1.8 = 66.6 + 32 = 98.6°\text{F}$$

PRACTICE PROBLEMS

Convert the following:

1. 2 kilograms = ______ grams
2. 300 milligrams = ______ grams
3. 1.5 grams = ______ milligrams
4. 500 milliliters = ______ liters
5. 1 liter = ______ milliliters
6. 1/2 grain = ______ milligrams
7. 90 milligrams = ______ grains
8. 175°F = ______°C
9. 10°C = ______°F
10. 15 centimeters = ______ inches
11. 2 inches = ______ centimeters
12. 187 pounds = ______ kilograms
13. 95 kilograms = ______ pounds
14. 231 pounds = ______ kilograms
15. 35 kilograms = ______ pounds

(Answers can be found on page 62.)

DRUG CALCULATIONS

Each textbook has its own method of presenting the process of drug calculations. This text is no different. Most drug calculations required in prehospital care are generally quite similar. They range from simple parenteral calculations to more elaborate infusion calculations integrating time intervals into the process. When making a calculation, the following information will normally be available:

Desired Dose. The desired dose is the quantity of medication or fluid that the physician wants the patient to receive. This is usually expressed in milligrams, grams, or grains.

Concentration of Drug on Hand. The concentration of the drug on hand is the amount of the drug present in the ampule or vial. This is usually expressed in milligrams, grams, or grains.

Volume of Drug on Hand. The volume of the drug on hand is the amount of fluid within the ampule or vial into which the drug is dissolved. This is usually represented in milliliters.

Based on the information presented earlier, the calculation of the volume of the drug to be administered to the patient can be made. The following formula represents this relationship:

$$\text{VOLUME TO BE ADMINISTERED (X)} = \frac{\text{(VOLUME ON HAND) (DESIRED DOSE)}}{\text{(CONCENTRATION ON HAND)}}$$

EXAMPLE 1

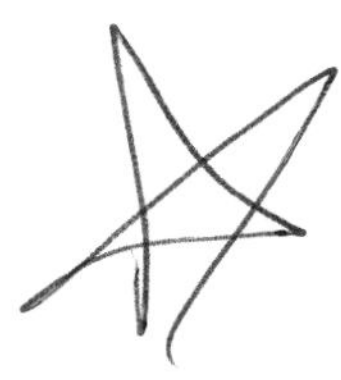

A physician wants 5 milligrams of parenteral Valium administered to a patient. The Valium ampule contains 10 milligrams of Valium in 2 milliliters of solvent. The following calculation must then be made (see Figure 4-1):

$$\text{VOLUME ADMIN (X)} = \frac{\text{(VOLUME ON HAND) (2 ml) (DESIRED DOSE) (5 mg)}}{\text{(CONCENTRATION ON HAND) (10 mg)}}$$

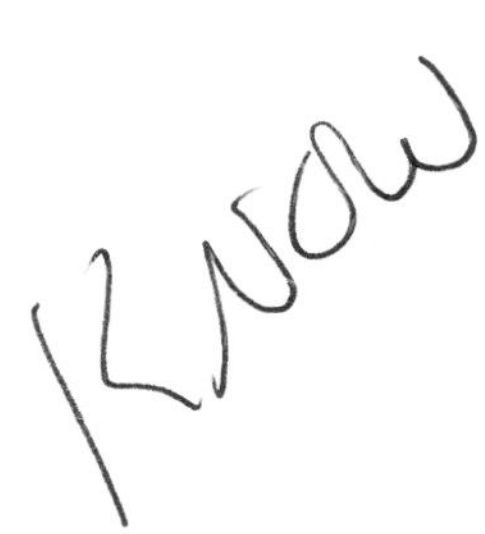

To solve, multiply:

$$X = \frac{(2\text{ ml})(5\text{ mg})}{(10\text{ mg})}$$

Thus:

$$X = \frac{10}{10}$$

Then:

$$X = 1\text{ ml}$$

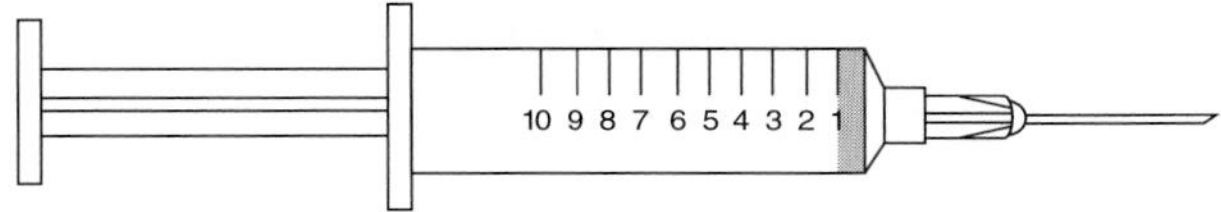

Figure 4-1 Correct dosage is 1 milliliter.

EXAMPLE 2

A physician wants 75 milligrams of lidocaine administered to a patient in an IV bolus. The drug is supplied in a prefilled syringe containing 100 milligrams of lidocaine in 5 milliliters of solvent. Calculate the number of milliliters to be administered. The calculation is as follows (see Figure 4-2):

$$X = \frac{(5 \text{ ml})(75 \text{ mg})}{(100 \text{ mg})}$$

Thus:

$$X = \frac{375}{100}$$

Then:

$$X = 3.75 \text{ ml}$$

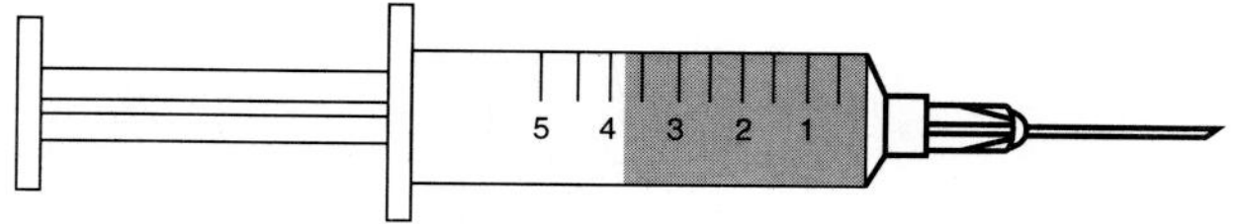

Figure 4-2 Correct dosage is 3.75 milliliters.

This formula holds true for all of the drug calculations routinely used in emergency medicine, but it works only if all of the measurements are in the same units.

Variations on a Theme

The formula presented earlier is useful for calculating the infusion rate of IV drips. All that is required is to multiply "X" times the drops per milliliter delivered by your set. The end result will be the number of drops per minute that needs to be delivered.

EXAMPLE 3

A physician wants 2 milligrams per minute of lidocaine administered to a patient. She orders 2 grams of lidocaine to be placed into 500 milliliters of 5% dextrose in water. A minidrip infusion set that delivers 60 drops per milliliter is being used. The problem can be solved as follows (see Figure 4-3):

$$\frac{(500 \text{ ml})(2 \text{ mg/min})}{(2000 \text{ mg})} \times 60 \text{ drops/ml} = X \text{ drops per minute}$$

Then:

$$\frac{(1000)}{(2000)} = 0.5 \times 60 \text{ drops/ml} = 30 \text{ drops/minute}$$

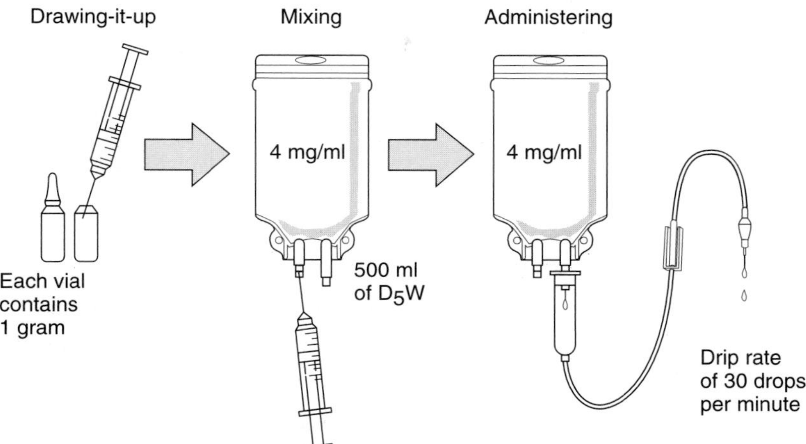

Figure 4-3 Correct dosage is 30 drops/minute.

Other Calculations

Sometimes an order will be received to administer a drug to a patient based on the patient's weight. The drug dosage must then be calculated based on the patient's weight. This can then be plugged into the formula.

EXAMPLE 4

A physician wants a patient to receive 5 milligrams per kilogram body weight of Bretylol. The patient weighs 220 pounds. The Bretylol is supplied in ampules containing 500 milligrams in 10 milliliters. How many milliliters of the drug should be administered?

To solve this problem, two preliminary calculations are required. First, the patient's weight must be converted to kilograms. Then, the patient's weight, in kilograms, must be multiplied by the number of milligrams per kilogram that is to be delivered. The calculation goes as follows (see Figure 4-4):

1. Convert pounds to kilograms:

$$\frac{220 \text{ lb}}{2.2 \text{ lb/kg}} = 100 \text{ kg}$$

2. Calculate the desired dose:

$$100 \text{ kilograms} \times 5 \text{ milligrams/kilogram} = 500 \text{ milligrams}$$

3. Calculate the volume to be administered using the formula:

$$X = \frac{(10\text{ ml})(500\text{ mg})}{(500\text{ mg})}$$

Then:

$$X = \frac{(5000)}{(500)} = 10\text{ ml}$$

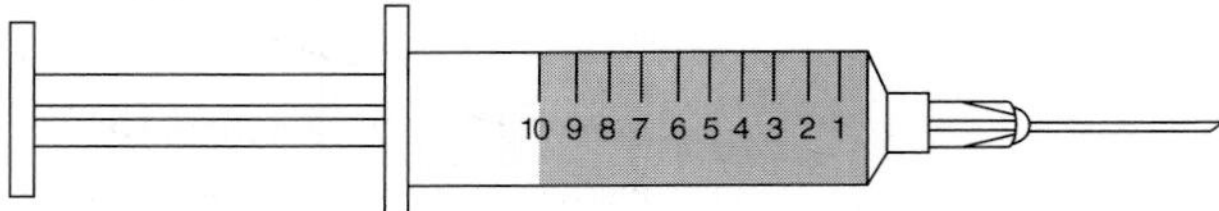

Figure 4-4 Correct dosage is 10 milliliters.

One additional calculation that is often made is to calculate the rate of infusion of an IV fluid not containing any medication.

EXAMPLE 5

The emergency physician wants a 1-liter bag of lactated Ringer's to be infused into a patient over 2 hours. The IV administration set delivers 10 drops per milliliter. How many drops per minute should be infused?

To solve this problem, the formula presented earlier is not used. Instead, the volume of fluid should be divided by the number of minutes over which the fluid is to be administered. Then, that value is multiplied by the rate of the set.

1. Convert hours to minutes:

$$2\text{ hours} \times 60\text{ minutes/hour} = 120\text{ minutes}$$

2. Divide the volume of fluid by the number of minutes:

$$\frac{1000\text{ ml}}{120\text{ minutes}} = 8.3\text{ milliliters/minute}$$

3. To determine the number of drops per minute:

$$8.3\text{ milliliters/minute} \times 10\text{ drops/milliliter} = 83\text{ drops/minute}$$

PRACTICE PROBLEMS

1. A physician wants you to administer 50 milligrams of lidocaine. Lidocaine is supplied in 5-milliliter ampules containing 100 milligrams of the drug. How many milliliters should you administer?
2. You are ordered to give a patient 1 mEq of sodium bicarbonate per kilogram of body weight. The patient weighs 77 pounds. If sodium bicarbonate is supplied in 50-milliliter syringes containing 50 mEq of the drug, how many milliliters should you administer?
3. You are to give a patient 0.8 milligrams of Narcan. Narcan is supplied in 1-milliliter ampules containing 0.4 milligram of the drug. How many milliliters should you administer?
4. You are to administer 3 milligrams per minute of lidocaine in an infusion. The physician asks you to place 1 gram of lidocaine in 1 liter of 5% dextrose in water. If you use a minidrip set that delivers 60 drops per milliliter, how many drops per minute would you deliver?
5. You are to administer 0.4 milligrams of 1:1,000 epinephrine. Epinephrine 1:1,000 contains 1 milligram of the drug in 1 milliliter of solvent. How many milliliters should you deliver?
6. You are to administer 1 liter of 0.9% sodium chloride over a 4-hour period. If you use an infusion set that delivers 10 drops per milliliter, how many drops per minute would you infuse?
7. You are to administer 5 milligrams per kilogram of Bretylol. Bretylol is supplied in ampules containing 500 milligrams of the drug in 10 milliliters of solvent. If the patient weighs 165 pounds, how many milliliters would you give?
8. A physician orders you to administer 1/2 of a gram of calcium chloride to a patient who overdosed on verapamil. If calcium chloride comes in a 10-milliliter syringe containing 1000 milligrams, how many milliliters would you administer?
9. You are ordered to administer 2 liters of lactated Ringer's over 6 hours. If the administration set you are going to use delivers 10 drops per milliliter, how many drops per minute should you infuse?
10. You are to deliver 15 micrograms per kilogram per minute of Intropin to a patient. The patient weighs 110 pounds. You are ordered to place 4 ampules of Intropin into 500 milliliters of 5% dextrose. Each ampule contains 200 milligrams. Using a minidrip set that delivers 60 drops per milliliter, how many drops per minute should you infuse?

(Answers can be found on page 62.)

SUMMARY

Drug calculations and the metric system will become easier with experience. It is a process that is used throughout clinical training as well as every day on the job. The fundamental skills presented in this chapter must be mastered before confidence in the system can be developed. Practice problems are always helpful.

PRACTICE PROBLEM ANSWERS

Page 56

1. 2000 grams
2. 0.3 gram
3. 1500 milligrams
4. 0.5 liter
5. 1,000 milliliters
6. 30 milligrams
7. 1.5 grains
8. 79.5°C
9. 50°F
10. 5.9 inches
11. 5 centimeters
12. 85 kilograms
13. 209 pounds
14. 105 kilograms
15. 77 pounds

Pages 60–61

1. 2.5 milliliters
2. 35 milliliters
3. 2 milliliters
4. 180 drops per minute
5. 0.4 milliliter
6. 41.6 drops per minute
7. 7.5 milliliters
8. 5 milliliters
9. 55.6 drops per minute
10. 28.1 drops per minute

Additional practice problems can be found in Appendix F.

chapter 5

Fluids, Electrolytes, and IV Therapy

OBJECTIVES

1. Identify the body's major fluid compartments and the proportion of total body water they contain.
2. List the major electrolytes and discuss the role they play in maintaining a fluid balance within the human body.
3. Define the following terms and explain the role each process plays in human fluid dynamics:
   - diffusion
   - osmosis
   - active transport
   - facilitated diffusion
4. Identify the major elements of the blood and describe their purpose.
5. List the various fluid replacement products and describe the advantages and disadvantages of field use.
6. Define hypotonic, hypertonic, and isotonic solutions.
7. State the size of catheter to be used.
8. State the type of IV catheter to be used.
9. Explain the different types of IV fluids that can be used.
10. State which IV administration sets should be used and in what circumstances.

11. List the possible sites an IV can be inserted and the rationale for each.
12. Demonstrate the procedure for inserting an IV.
13. Describe the procedure for collecting blood samples from an IV.

INTRODUCTION

One of the most important aspects of prehospital care is the administration of IV fluids and electrolytes. There are two major reasons for administering intravenous fluids during the prehospital phase of emergency medical care. The first is to immediately replace intravascular blood volume. The second is to provide an easily accessible route for the administration of lifesaving emergency drugs.

FLUIDS

Water is the most abundant substance in the human body. Approximately 60% of the total body weight is water, which is located within two fluid *compartments* (or spaces). The largest of these fluid compartments is the *intracellular fluid compartment (ICF)*. The intracellular compartment includes all fluids found within the cells. Three fourths of all body water is within the intracellular compartment. The remaining water can be found outside of the cell membrane in the *extracellular fluid compartment (ECF)*. There are two major components of the extracellular fluid compartment. The first is *intravascular fluid*. Intravascular fluid is found within the blood vessels and outside of the cell membranes. The other component of the extracellular fluid compartment is the *interstitial fluid*. The interstitial fluid is that fluid found outside the cell membrane, yet not within any defined blood vessels. The relationship of the various fluid compartments is illustrated as follows:

EXTRACELLULAR FLUID	15% of Total Body Weight
(Interstitial Fluid = 10.5% of Total Body Weight)	
(Intravascular Fluid = 4.5% of Total Body Weight)	
INTRACELLULAR FLUID	45% of Total Body Weight
TOTAL BODY WATER	60% of Total Body Weight

INTERNAL ENVIRONMENT

The internal environment is the extracellular fluid discussed earlier. The extracellular fluid bathes each body cell. There is an important balance that must be maintained regarding the internal environment. Whenever one aspect of the internal environment deviates from normal, as frequently occurs in injury and illness, the body will immediately respond and return to normal. The body's tendency to maintain all of its physiological activities in proper balance, including the internal environment, is called *homeostasis*.

ELECTROLYTES

In addition to the body fluids, there are also important chemicals that are required for life. These chemicals are divided into two main classes: *electrolytes* and *nonelectrolytes*. Chemicals that take on an electrical charge when placed into water are called electrolytes. Chemicals that do not take on an electrical charge are called nonelectrolytes. All electrolytes are measured in quantities called *milliequivalents (mEq)*. Sodium bicarbonate, a common emergency drug, is an electrolyte. When placed into water, it quickly divides into charged particles or ions. All dosages of sodium bicarbonate are calculated in milliequivalents. Certain electrolytes, when dissolved in water, take on a positive charge. These are called *cations*. Examples of common cations include sodium (Na^{+}), potassium (K^{+}), magnesium (Mg^{++}), and calcium (Ca^{++}). Electrolytes that take on a negative charge are called *anions*. Examples of anions found within the body include chlorine (Cl^{-}), bicarbonate (HCO_3^{-}), phosphate (HPO_4^{-}), and most of the organic (carbon based) molecules. In addition to the fluid balance mentioned earlier, electrical neutrality must be carefully maintained between cations and anions.

CELL PHYSIOLOGY

To maintain physiological homeostasis, there must be an exchange of electrolytes and water materials across the membrane of the cell. The cell membrane is very complex. It is said to be *semipermeable*, meaning that it allows certain compounds to pass readily across it while restricting the passage of others. Many materials must pass across the cell membrane including oxygen, carbon dioxide, nutrients, fluids, and electrolytes. There are three major ways to move substances across the cell membrane: *diffusion*, *facilitated diffusion*, and *active transport*. Diffusion is a passive process, whereas facilitated diffusion and active transport require energy expenditure by the cell (see Figure 5-1).

Diffusion

Diffusion occurs when concentrations of various substances become higher on one side of the semipermeable cell membrane. When this difference occurs, an *osmotic gradient* is created. The side of the cell membrane with the higher concentration is said to be *hypertonic* with respect to the other side. Conversely, the side of the membrane with the lower concentration is said to be *hypotonic* in relation to the other (see Figure 5-2).

When both sides of the cell membrane have an equal concentration of the substance in question, the system is said to be *isotonic*. These concepts underpin the rationale for IV therapy. IV fluids with a solute concentration less than that of blood are said to be hypotonic solutions. An example of a hypotonic solution is 0.45% sodium chloride (1/2 normal saline).

Substances that have a solute concentration equal to that of blood are said to be *isotonic*. Lactated Ringer's and 0.9% sodium chloride are examples of isotonic fluids. An example of a hypertonic solution is 50% dextrose in water. Although not a classical "IV fluid," it plays a major role in prehospital

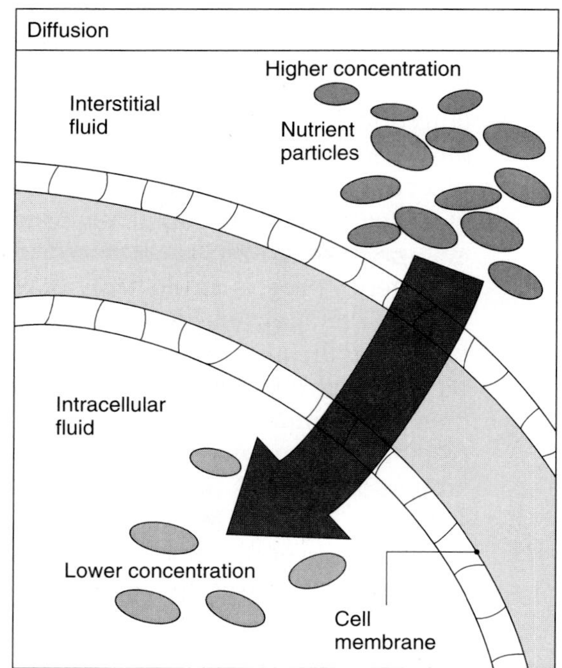

Figure 5-1 Diffusion. The solute moves from the area of higher concentration to the area of lower concentration.

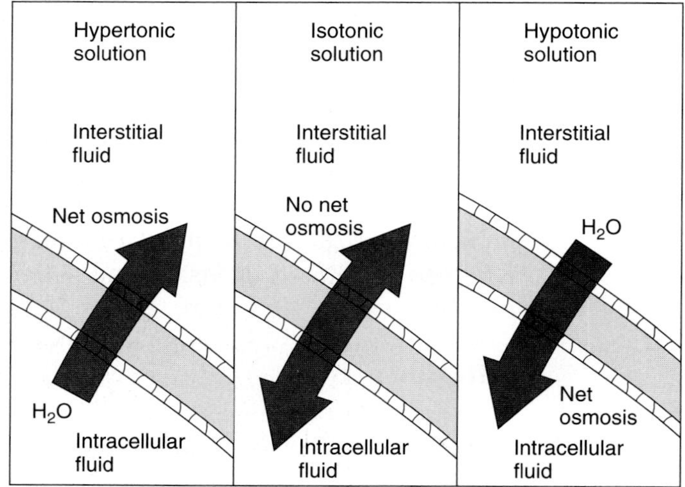

Figure 5-2 Relationship and effects of hypotonic, isotonic, and hypertonic solutions.

care. One of the most important substances that passes across the cell membrane is water. Water will diffuse readily across the cell membrane from an area of higher water concentration to an area of lesser water concentration. The diffusion of water in this manner is called *osmosis* (see Figure 5-3).

Facilitated Diffusion

Certain molecules can move across the cell membrane by a process known as *facilitated diffusion*. Glucose is an example of such a molecule. Facilitated diffusion requires the assistance of "helper proteins" on the surface

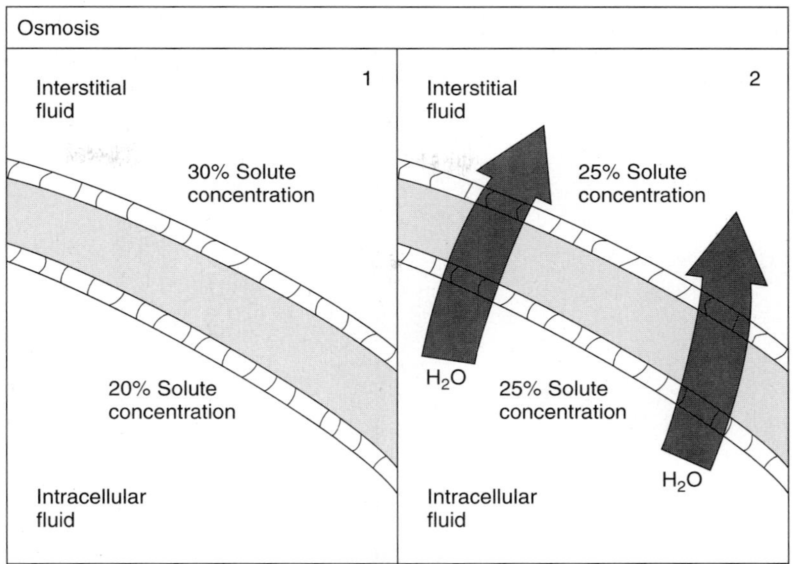

Figure 5-3 Osmosis. Water moves across the cell membrane to equalize concentrations.

of the cell membrane. These proteins, once activated, bind to the glucose molecule. After binding, the protein changes its configuration and transports the glucose molecule into the cell where it is released. The transport protein is then ready for another glucose molecule. Depending on the substance being transported, facilitated diffusion may or may not require energy.

Active Transport

Sometimes it is desirable for the body to maintain a gradient along a cell membrane. This is especially true regarding the ions sodium (Na^+) and potassium (K^+). To sustain life, the concentration of sodium outside the cell membrane must be significantly higher than that inside the cell. Also, the concentration of potassium must be maintained at a much higher level within the cell. To maintain the gradient, the sodium must be pumped out of the cell and potassium must be pumped into the cell. Both of these processes require energy. This is an example of active transport.

BLOOD

One of the most important aspects of the extracellular fluid, and thus the internal environment, is blood. Blood is responsible for transport of oxygen (O_2) to cells and carbon dioxide (CO_2) from cells.

There are two major aspects of blood: fluid and cells. The fluid in which all of the blood cells are suspended is called *plasma* (see Figure 5-4).

There are three major classes of blood cells. The first are the red blood cells or *erythrocytes* (see Figure 5-5). Erythrocytes contain an important iron-containing protein called *hemoglobin*. Hemoglobin is responsible for the transport of oxygen and carbon dioxide.

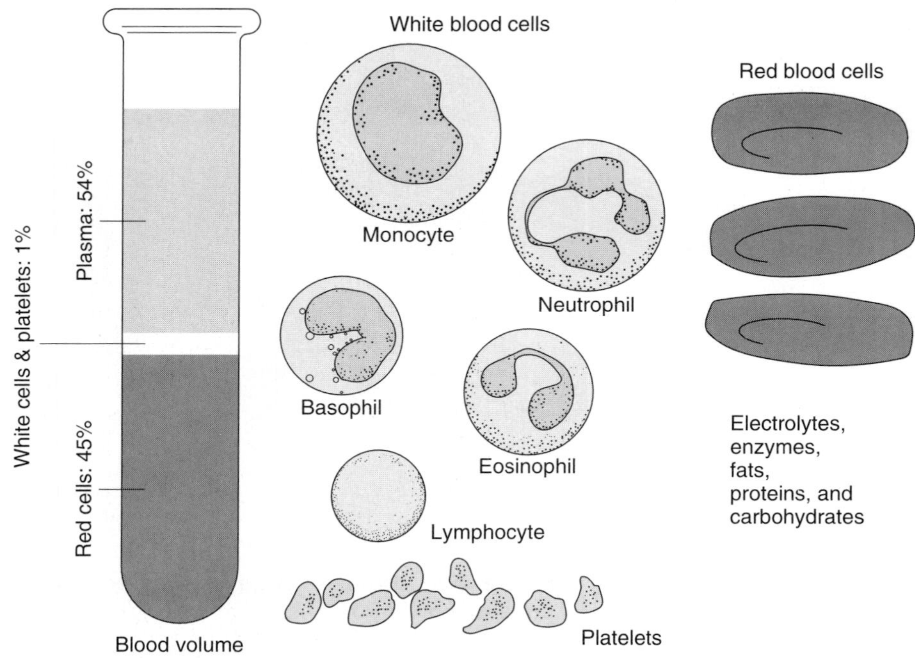

Figure 5-4 Various components of blood.

A significant percentage of blood, approximately 45 percent, is red blood cells. The percentage of red blood cells present is referred to as the *hematocrit*. White blood cells, or *leukocytes*, are the second type of cells found in the blood. The leukocytes are responsible for combating infection. The last type of blood cells present are the platelets, or *thrombocytes*, responsible for blood clotting.

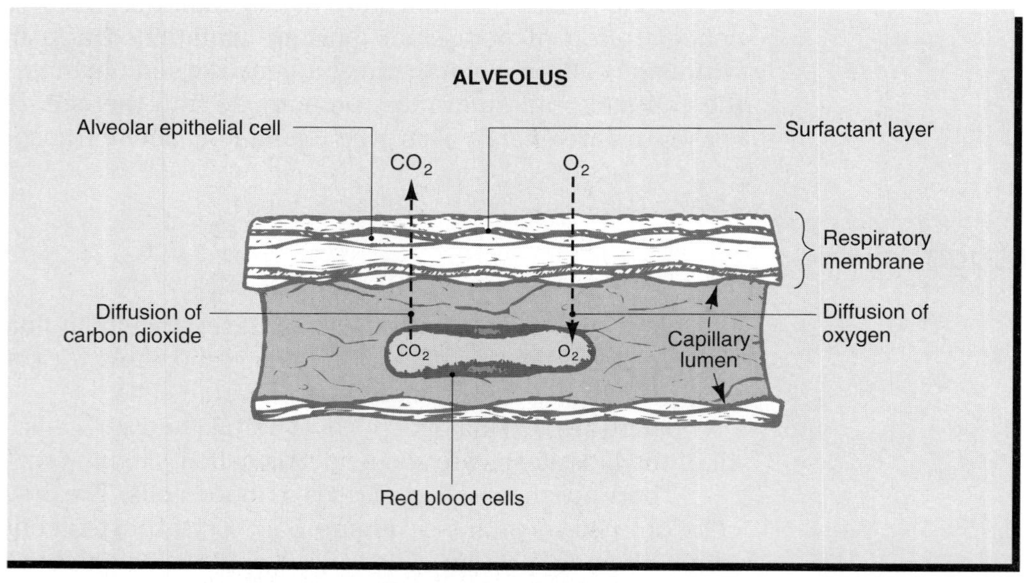

Figure 5-5 The red blood cell.

IV THERAPY

As mentioned earlier, there are two major indications for IV therapy. The first is to replace fluid losses, which may occur as a result of hemorrhage caused by trauma or from severe diarrhea, vomiting, heat exhaustion, and burns. It is best to replace the fluid losses with intravenous fluids of similar isotonicity.

There are two major classes of IV fluids: colloids and crystalloids. *Colloids* contain compounds of high molecular weight, usually proteins, which do not readily diffuse across the cell membrane. In addition, they exert *colloid osmotic pressure*, which means they tend to attract water into the intravascular space. Thus, a small amount of a colloid can be administered to a patient with a greater than expected increase in intravascular volume. This is because the colloid will draw water from the interstitial space and the intracellular compartment in order to increase the intravascular volume. Common examples of colloids include:

- *plasma protein fraction (Plasmanate)*. Plasmanate is a protein-containing colloid. The principle protein present is albumin, which is suspended, along with other proteins, in a saline solvent.
- *salt-poor albumin*. Salt-poor albumin contains only human albumin. Each gram of albumin holds approximately 18 milliliters of water in the blood stream.
- *Dextran*. Dextran is not a protein but a large sugar molecule with osmotic properties similar to albumin. It comes in two molecular weights (40,000 and 70,000 Daltons). Dextran 40 has two to two and one-half times the colloid osmotic pressure of albumin.
- *hetastarch (Hespan)*. Hetastarch, like Dextran, is a sugar molecule with osmotic properties similar to protein. It does not appear to share many of Dextran's side effects.

Colloid replacement therapy, at present, does not have a role in prehospital care except under rare circumstances. Colloid products are expensive and have a short shelf life.

Crystalloids contain only water and electrolytes. These substances will all readily diffuse across the cell membrane. Crystalloids are the primary solutions used in prehospital intravenous fluid therapy. There are multiple fluid preparations. It is often helpful to classify them according to the *tonicity* related to plasma:

- *isotonic solutions*. Isotonic solutions have electrolyte composition similar to blood plasma. When placed into a normally hydrated patient, they will not cause a significant fluid or electrolyte shift.
- *hypertonic solutions*. Hypertonic solutions have a higher solute concentration than plasma. These fluids will tend to cause a fluid shift out of the intracellular compartment into the extracellular compartment when administered to a normally hydrated patient. Later, there will be a diffusion of solute in the opposite direction.

- *hypotonic solutions*. Hypotonic solutions have less of a solute concentration when compared to plasma. When administered to a normally hydrated patient, they will cause a movement of fluid from the extracellular compartment into the intracellular compartment. Later, solutes will move in an opposite direction.

You will choose replacement fluids based on patient needs and the patient's underlying problem. As a rule, hemorrhage occurs so fast that there is not time for a significant fluid shift between the extracellular and intracellular space. Because of this, replacement fluids are most commonly isotonic. It is for this reason that you will use lactated Ringer's and normal saline most often. If the patient is dehydrated due to fluid loss from diarrhea or fever, then there is a greater deficit of water than sodium. In this case, you may be asked to use hypotonic fluids such as half-normal saline.

Some replacement fluids contain a single element, such as sodium chloride or dextrose, while others contain multiple elements. Solutions, such as lactated Ringer's, are designed so that the concentration of electrolytes is very similar to that of the plasma. It is because of this that these are referred to as *balanced salt solutions*.

Three of the most commonly used solutions in prehospital care include lactated Ringer's solution, 0.9 sodium chloride (normal saline), and 5% dextrose in water (D_5W).

- *lactated Ringer's*. Lactated Ringer's solution is an isotonic, electrolyte solution. It contains sodium chloride, potassium chloride, calcium chloride, and sodium lactate in water.
- *normal saline*. Normal saline is an electrolyte solution containing sodium chloride in water that is isotonic with extracellular fluid.
- *5% dextrose in water*. D_5W is a hypotonic, glucose solution used to keep a vein open and to supply calories necessary for cell metabolism. While it has an initial effect of increasing the circulatory volume, glucose molecules rapidly move across the vascular membrane. The resultant free water will follow almost immediately, leaving little effect on circulating blood volume.

Both lactated Ringer's solution and normal saline are used to replace fluid volume because their administration causes an immediate expansion of the circulatory volume. However, as was noted earlier, due to the movement of the electrolytes and water, two thirds of either of these solutions is lost to the interstitial space within one hour. Lactated Ringer's solution is the better IV fluid for the patient who is losing blood. However, it is not compatible with whole blood, which will most likely be given when the patient arrives at the emergency department. In aggressive fluid resuscitation, it is recommended that you initiate two IV lines, one with lactated Ringer's solution and one with normal saline.

The second reason for initiating an IV infusion in the field is to provide a route for the administration of drugs. Although most IV fluids will work, 5% dextrose in water is usually chosen.

The following IV fluids are most frequently used in prehospital emergency care (see Table 5-1).

TABLE 5-1

Approximate Ionic Concentrations (mEq/l) and Calories per Liter

	Ionic Concentrations (mEq/l)							
	Sodium	*Potassium*	*Calcium*	*Chloride*	*Lactate*	*Calories per liter*	*Osmolarity*[a] *(mOsm/l)*	*pH Range*[b]
5% Dextrose Injection, USP	0	0	0	0	0	170	252	3.5–6.5
10% Dextrose Injection, USP	0	0	0	0	0	340	505	3.5–6.5
0.9% Sodium Chloride Injection, USP	154	0	0	154	0	0	308	4.5–7.0
Sodium Lactate Injection, USP (M/6 Sodium Lactate)	167	0	0	0	167	54	334	6.0–7.3
2.5% Dextrose & 0.45% Sodium Chloride Injection, USP	77	0	0	77	0	85	280	3.5–6.0
5% Dextrose & 0.2% Sodium Chloride Injection, USP	34	0	0	34	0	170	321	3.5–6.0
5% Dextrose & 0.33% Sodium Chloride Injection, USP	56	0	0	56	0	170	365	3.5–6.0
5% Dextrose & 0.45% Sodium Chloride Injection, USP	77	0	0	77	0	170	406	3.5–6.0
5% Dextrose & 0.9% Sodium Chloride Injection, USP	154	0	0	154	0	170	560	3.5–6.0
10% Dextrose & 0.9% Sodium Chloride Injection, USP	154	0	0	154	0	340	813	3.5–6.0
Ringer's Injection, USP	147.5	4	4.5	156	0	0	309	5.0–7.5
Lactated Ringer's Injection	130	4	3	109	28	9	273	6.0–7.5
5% Dextrose in Ringer's Injection	147.5	4	4.5	156	0	170	561	3.5–6.5
Lactated Ringer's with 5% Dextrose	130	4	3	109	28	180	525	4.0–6.5

[a]Normal physiolical isotonicity range is approximately 280–310 mOsm/l. Administration of substantially hypotonic solutions may cause hemolysis and administration of substantially hypertonic solutions may cause vein damage.

[b]pH ranges are USP for applicable solution, corporate specification for non-USP solutions.

(Adapted with permission from Travenol Laboratories, Inc., Deerfield, Illinois)

Plasma Protein Fraction (Plasmanate)

Class: Natural colloid

Description

Plasma protein fraction is a protein-containing colloid that is suspended in a saline solvent. The principal protein in plasma protein fraction is serum human albumin. Other proteins present include globulin and gamma globulin. Plasma protein fraction is prepared from large pools of human plasma. It is quite expensive and has a very short shelf life. Although rarely used in the prehospital phase of emergency medical care, plasma protein fraction is preferred by some emergency specialists in the management of hypovolemic states, especially burn shock. After a patient sustains a severe burn, fluid is lost from the blood into the surrounding tissue. Plasma protein fraction, because it remains in the circulating blood volume, is effective in maintaining adequate blood volume and blood pressure. It is usually used in combination with lactated Ringer's or normal saline.

Mechanism of Action

Plasmanate is a protein-containing colloid that remains in the intravascular compartment. It increases intravascular volume by attracting water from other fluid compartments by virtue of its colloid osmotic pressure.

Indications

- Hypovolemic shock, especially burn shock
- Hypoproteinemia (low protein states)

Contraindications

There are no major contraindications to plasma protein fraction when used in the treatment of life-threatening hypovolemic states.

Precautions

It is important to monitor constantly the response of the patient and adjust the rate of infusion accordingly. Monitor patient for elevated blood pressure and pulmonary edema during and following Plasmanate administration.

Side Effects

Chills, fever, urticaria (hives), nausea, and vomiting have all been reported with plasma protein fraction use.

Dosage

The plasma protein fraction infusion rate should be titrated according to the patient's hemodynamic response. In the management of shock secondary to burns, the physician's orders regarding the rate of administration must be closely followed. Standard formulas for IV fluid administration have been developed. The medical control physician will use these in judging the correct rate of intravenous administration.

Interactions

Solutions should not be mixed with or administered through the same administration sets as other intravenous fluids.

Route

Intravenous infusion

How Supplied

Plasma protein fraction is supplied in 250- and 500-milliliter bottles of a 5% solution. An administration set is usually attached.

Dextran

Class: Artificial colloid

Description

Dextran is a colloid differing significantly from plasma protein fraction. Instead of proteins, Dextran contains chains of sugars that are approximately the same molecular weight as serum albumin. Thus, because of their large molecular size, they remain within the circulating blood volume for an extended period. Although not as effective as plasma protein fraction, Dextran has proved effective as an adjunctive aid in the management of hypovolemic shock. Dextran is supplied in two molecular weights. Dextran 40 has an average molecular weight of approximately 40,000 Daltons. Dextran 40 is secreted by the kidneys much more readily than the higher molecular weight form, Dextran 70 (molecular weight of 70,000 Daltons). The higher molecular weight form tends to be broken down into glucose instead of being secreted in the Dextran form, as occurs with Dextran 40. The decision on which type of Dextran to use in prehospital care rests with the system medical director. Because Dextran is excreted through the urine, urine output is usually maintained with the administration of Dextran.

Mechanism of Action

Dextran is a sugar-containing colloid used as an intravascular volume expander. It remains in the intravascular compartment for approximately 12 hours. It increases intravascular volume by attracting water from other fluid compartments by virtue of its colloid osmotic pressure.

Indication

- Hypovolemic shock

Contraindications

Dextran should not be administered to patients who have a known hypersensitivity to the drug. It should not be administered to patients suffering congestive heart failure, renal failure, or known bleeding disorders.

Precautions

A major drawback to the use of Dextran is that it coats the red blood cells, thus preventing accurate blood typing and possibly hindering administration of whole blood if required. A tube of blood should be drawn before administering Dextran for blood typing at the hospital.

Allergic reactions, ranging from mild to severe anaphylaxis, have been known to occur following the administration of Dextran. If these occur, therapy should be immediately discontinued. In the case of mild reactions, the patient should be closely monitored, and emergency resuscitative drugs should be readily available. Severe allergic reactions may require the administration of epinephrine, diphenhydramine (Benadryl), and possibly corticosteroids.

It is usually preferable to use crystalloid solutions, such as lactated Ringer's, rather than Dextran, in the management of profound hypovolemic shock.

Side Effects

Rash, itching, dyspnea, chest tightness, and mild hypotension have all been reported with Dextran use. The incidence of these side effects is, however, very low and reactions are generally mild.

Increased bleeding time has also been reported with Dextran usage due to its interference with platelet function.

Interactions

Dextran should not be administered to patients who are receiving anticoagulants as it significantly retards blood clotting.

Dosage

The dosage of Dextran is titrated according to the patient's physiological response. In the management of burn shock, it is especially important to follow standard fluid resuscitation regimens to prevent possible circulatory overload.

Route

Intravenous infusion

How Supplied

Dextran 40 and Dextran 70 are supplied in 250- and 500-milliliter bottles.

Hetastarch (Hespan)

Class: Artificial colloid

Description

Hetastarch is an artificial colloid differing from both plasma protein fraction and Dextran. Hetastarch is derived from amylopectin and chemically resembles glycogen. The average molecular weight is approximately 450,000

Daltons, which gives it colloidal properties similar to that of human albumin. Intravenous infusion of hetastarch results in plasma volume expansion slightly greater than the amount infused.

Because the colloidal properties of hetastarch are quite similar to those of human albumin, it has proved effective in the management of hypovolemic shock, especially burn shock. It does not appear to share the blood typing problems seen with Dextran.

Mechanism of Action

Hetastarch is a starch-containing colloid used as an intravascular volume expander. Following administration, the plasma volume is expanded slightly in excess of the volume of hetastarch administered. This effect has been observed for up to 24 to 36 hours. Hetastarch increases intravascular volume by virtue of its colloid osmotic pressure.

Indications

- Hypovolemic shock, especially burn shock
- Septic shock

Contraindications

There are no major contraindications to hetastarch when used in the management of life-threatening hypovolemic states.

Precautions

It is important to constantly monitor the response of the patient and adjust the rate of infusion accordingly. Monitor the patient for signs of pulmonary edema and elevated blood pressure during and following hetastarch administration.

Large volumes of hetastarch may alter the body's coagulation mechanism. Hetastarch should be used with caution in patients receiving anticoagulants.

Side Effects

Nausea, vomiting, mild febrile reactions, chills, itching, and urticaria (hives) have been reported with hetastarch administration. Severe anaphylactic reactions have been rarely reported.

Interactions

Hetastarch should not be administered to patients who are receiving anticoagulants.

Dosage

The hetastarch infusion rate should be titrated according to the patient's hemodynamic response. In the management of burn shock, the physician's orders regarding the rate of administration must be closely followed. Standard formulas for colloid administration to burn patients have been developed. It is important to remember that a fall in blood pressure in burn shock occurs much later than with hemorrhagic causes.

Route

Intravenous infusion

How Supplied

Sterile 6% hetastarch in 0.9% sodium chloride is supplied in 500-milliliter bottles.

Lactated Ringer's (Hartman's Solution)

Class: Isotonic crystalloid solution

Description

Lactated Ringer's solution is one of the most frequently used IV fluids in the management of hypovolemic shock. It is an isotonic crystalloid solution containing electrolytes in the following concentrations:

Sodium (Na^+) 130 mEq/liter
Potassium (K^+) 4 mEq/liter
Calcium (Ca^{++}) 3 mEq/liter
Chloride (Cl^-) 109 mEq/liter

In addition to the electrolytes mentioned earlier, lactated Ringer's contains 28 mEq of lactate (lactic acid), which acts as a buffer.

Mechanism of Action

Lactated Ringer's replaces water and electrolytes.

Indications

- Hypovolemic shock
- Keep open IV

Contraindications

Lactated Ringer's should not be used in patients with congestive heart failure or renal failure.

Precautions

Patients receiving lactated Ringer's should be monitored to prevent circulatory overload.

Side Effects

Rare in therapeutic dosages

Interactions

Few in the emergency setting

Dosage

Crystalloids, such as lactated Ringer's, diffuse out of the intravascular space and into the surrounding tissues in less than an hour. Thus, it is often necessary to replace a liter of lost blood with 3 to 4 liters of lactated Ringer's.

In severe hypovolemic shock, lactated Ringer's should be infused through large-bore (14- or 16-gauge) IV cannulas. These infusions should be administered "wide open" until a systolic blood pressure of approximately 100 millimeters of mercury is achieved. When this blood pressure is attained, the infusion should be reduced to about 100 milliliters per hour. If the blood pressure falls again, then the infusion rate should be increased and adjusted accordingly. Adjunctive devices, such as the PASG and extremity elevation, may be used in the management of severe hypovolemic shock.

Route

Intravenous infusion

How Supplied

Lactated Ringer's is supplied in 250-, 500-, and 1000-milliliter bags and bottles.

5% Dextrose in Water (D_5W)

Class: Hypotonic dextrose-containing solution

Description

When vigorous fluid replacement is not indicated, 5% dextrose in water (D_5W) is frequently used. D_5W is ideal for providing a lifeline for the administration of intravenous drugs. D_5W is hypotonic, which prevents circulatory overload in patients with congestive heart failure.

Mechanism of Action

D_5W provides nutrients in the form of dextrose as well as free water.

Indications

- IV access for emergency drugs
- For dilution of concentrated drugs for intravenous infusion

Contraindications

D_5W should not be used as a fluid replacement for hypovolemic states.

Precautions

Dextrose-containing solutions are acidic and may produce local venous irritation. Subcutaneous administration from extravasation may result in tissue necrosis.

As with any IV fluid, it is important to watch for signs of circulatory overload when administering D_5W.

When treating hypoglycemia, it is imperative that a tube of blood be drawn before administering D_5W or 50% dextrose ($D_{50}W$).

Side Effects

Rare in therapeutic dosages

Interactions

D_5W should not be used with phenytoin (Dilantin) or amrinone (Inocor).

Dosage

D_5W is usually administered through a minidrip (60 drops/milliliter) set at a rate of "to keep open" (TKO).

Route

Intravenous infusion

How Supplied

D_5W is supplied in bags and bottles of 50, 100, 150, 250, 500, and 1000 milliliters.

10% Dextrose in Water ($D_{10}W$)

Class: Hypertonic dextrose-containing solution

Description

Ten percent dextrose in water ($D_{10}W$) is a hypertonic solution. Like D_5W, $D_{10}W$ is used only when vigorous fluid replacement is not indicated. $D_{10}W$ has twice as much carbohydrate as does D_5W, which makes it of use in the management of hypoglycemia.

Mechanism of Action

$D_{10}W$ provides nutrients in the form of dextrose as well as free water.

Indications

- Neonatal resuscitation
- Hypoglycemia

Contraindications

$D_{10}W$ should not be used as a fluid replacement for hypovolemic states.

Precautions

Dextrose-containing solutions are acidic and may produce local venous irritation. Subcutaneous administration from extravasation may result in tissue necrosis.

As with any IV fluid, it is important to be alert for signs of circulatory overload.

When treating hypoglycemia, it is imperative that a tube of blood be drawn before administering $D_{10}W$ or 50% dextrose ($D_{50}W$).

Side Effects

Rare in therapeutic dosages

Interactions

$D_{10}W$ should not be used with phenytoin (Dilantin) or amrinone (Inocor).

Dosage

The administration rate of $D_{10}W$ will usually be dependent on the patient's condition.

Route

Intravenous infusion

How Supplied

$D_{10}W$ is supplied in bottles and bags of 50, 100, 150, 250, 500, and 1000 milliliters.

0.9% Sodium Chloride (Normal Saline)

Class: Isotonic crystalloid solution

Description

The use of 0.9% sodium chloride, or normal saline as it is often called, has several applications in emergency medicine. Normal saline contains 154 milliequivalents per liter of sodium ions (Na^+) and approximately 154 milliequivalents per liter of chloride (Cl^-) ions. Because the concentration of sodium is near that of blood, the solution is considered isotonic.

Normal saline is especially useful in heat stroke, heat exhaustion, and diabetic ketoacidosis.

Mechanism of Action

Normal saline replaces water and electrolytes.

Indications

- Heat-related problems (heat exhaustion, heat stroke)
- Freshwater drowning
- Hypovolemia
- Diabetic ketoacidosis
- Keep open IV

Contraindications

The use of 0.9% sodium chloride should not be considered in patients with congestive heart failure as circulatory overload can be easily induced.

Precautions

Normal saline contains only sodium and chloride. When large amounts of normal saline are administered, it is quite possible for other important physiological electrolytes to become depleted. In cases in which large amounts of fluids may have to be administered, it might be prudent to use lactated Ringer's.

Side Effects

Rare in therapeutic dosages

Interactions

Few in the emergency setting

Dosage

The specific situation being treated will dictate the rate in which normal saline will be administered. In severe heat stroke, diabetic ketoacidosis, and freshwater drowning, it is quite likely that you will be called on to administer the fluid quite rapidly. In other cases, it is advisable to administer the fluid at a moderate rate (for example, 100 milliliters per hour).

Route

Intravenous infusion

How Supplied

Normal saline is supplied in 250-, 500-, and 1000-milliliter bags and bottles. Sterile normal saline for irrigation should not be confused with that designed for intravenous administration.

0.45% Sodium Chloride (1/2 Normal Saline)

Class: Hypotonic crystalloid solution

Description

One-half normal saline (0.45% sodium chloride) solution is a hypotonic crystalloid solution containing approximately one-half the concentration of sodium and chloride as does blood plasma.

Mechanism of Action

One-half normal saline replaces free water and electrolytes.

Indication

- Patients with diminished renal or cardiovascular function for which rapid rehydration is not indicated

Contraindications

Cases in which rapid rehydration is indicated

Precautions

One-half normal saline contains only sodium and chloride. When large amounts of one-half normal saline are administered, it is possible for other important physiological electrolytes to become depleted. In cases in which large amounts of fluids must be administered, it might be prudent to use lactated Ringer's.

Side Effects

Rare in therapeutic dosages

Interactions

Few in the emergency setting

Dosage

The specific situation and patient condition will dictate the rate at which one-half normal saline will be administered.

Route

Intravenous infusion

How Supplied

One-half normal saline is supplied in 250-, 500-, and 1000-milliliter bags and bottles.

5% Dextrose in 0.45% Sodium Chloride ($D_5$1/2NS)

Class: Hypertonic dextrose-containing crystalloid solution

Description

Five percent dextrose in 0.45% sodium chloride ($D_5$1/2NS) is a versatile fluid. It contains the same amount of sodium and chloride as does one-half normal saline. Dextrose has been added for its nutrient properties, providing 80 calories per liter.

Mechanism of Action

$D_5$1/2 NS replaces free water and electrolytes and provides nutrients in the form of dextrose.

Indications

- Heat exhaustion
- Diabetic disorders
- For use as a TKO solution in patients with impaired renal or cardiovascular function

Contraindication

$D_5$1/2NS should not be used when rapid fluid resuscitation is indicated.

Precautions

Dextrose-containing solutions are acidic and may produce local venous irritation. Subcutaneous administration from extravasation may result in tissue necrosis.

As with any IV fluid, it is important to watch for signs of circulatory overload when administering $D_5$1/2NS.

When treating hypoglycemia, it is imperative that a tube of blood be drawn before administering $D_5$1/2NS or 50% dextrose ($D_{50}W$).

Side Effects

Rare in therapeutic dosages

Interactions

$D_5$1/2NS should not be used with phenytoin (Dilantin) or amrinone (Inocor).

Dosage

The specific situation and patient condition will dictate the rate at which $D_5$1/2NS should be administered.

Route

Intravenous infusion

How Supplied

$D_5$1/2NS is supplied in bottles and bags containing 250, 500, and 1000 milliliters of the fluid.

5% Dextrose in 0.9% Sodium Chloride (D_5NS)

Class: Hypertonic dextrose-containing crystalloid solution

Description

Five percent dextrose in 0.9% normal saline is a hypertonic crystalloid to which 5 grams of dextrose per 100 milliliters of fluid has been added for its nutrient properties.

Mechanism of Action

D_5 NS replaces free water and electrolytes and provides nutrients in the form of dextrose.

Indications

- Heat-related disorders
- Freshwater drowning

- Hypovolemia
- Peritonitis

Contraindications

D_5NS should not be administered to patients with impaired cardiac or renal function.

Precautions

Dextrose-containing solutions are acidic and may produce local venous irritation. Subcutaneous administration from extravasation may result in tissue necrosis.

D_5NS contains only the electrolytes sodium and chloride. When large amounts of fluids must be administered, it might be prudent to use lactated Ringer's solution so as to prevent depletion of the other physiological electrolytes.

When treating hypoglycemia, it is imperative that a tube of blood be drawn before administering D_5NS or 50% dextrose ($D_{50}W$).

Side Effects

Rare in therapeutic dosages

Interactions

D_5NS should not be used with phenytoin (Dilantin) or amrinone (Inocor).

Dosage

The specific situation and patient condition will dictate the rate at which D_5NS is given.

Route

Intravenous infusion

How Supplied

D_5NS is supplied in bags and bottles containing 250, 500, and 1000 milliliters of the solution.

5% Dextrose in Lactated Ringer's (D_5LR)

Class: Hypertonic dextrose-containing crystalloid solution

Description

Five percent dextrose in lactated Ringer's (D_5LR) contains the same concentration of electrolytes as does lactated Ringer's. In addition to the electrolytes, however, 5 grams of dextrose per 100 milliliters of fluid has been added for nutrient properties. This added dextrose causes the solution to be hypertonic.

Mechanism of Action

D_5 LR replaces water and electrolytes and provides nutrients in the form of dextrose.

Indications

- Hypovolemic shock
- Hemmorhagic shock
- Certain cases of acidosis

Contraindications

D_5LR should not be administered to patients with decreased renal or cardiovascular function.

Precautions

Patients receiving D_5LR should be constantly monitored for signs of circulatory overload. It is essential that a blood sample be drawn before administering D_5LR to patients with hypoglycemia.

Dextrose-containing solutions are acidic and may produce local venous irritation. Subcutaneous administration from extravasation may result in tissue necrosis.

Side Effects

Rare in therapeutic dosages

Interactions

D_5LR should not be used with phenytoin (Dilantin) or amrinone (Inocor).

Dosage

In severe hypovolemic shock D_5LR should be infused through a large-bore catheter (14 or 16 gauge). This infusion should be administered "wide open" until a blood pressure of 100 millimeters of mercury is achieved. When the blood pressure is attained, the infusions should be reduced to 100 milliliters per hour. In other cases, the specific situation and patient condition will dictate the rate of administration.

Route

Intravenous infusion

How Supplied

D_5LR is supplied in bags and bottles containing 250, 500, and 1000 milliliters of the fluid.

INSERTION OF INDWELLING IV CATHETER

One of the earliest stages in the management of an acutely ill or injured patient is the placement of an IV catheter. In trauma cases an IV catheter will provide access for fluid resuscitation, whereas in medical disorders it will provide a route for drugs that must be given intravenously.

Before inserting an IV catheter, several decisions must be made to ensure the best possible care for the patient. They are the following:

1. What size catheter should be inserted?

When managing patients with trauma who require rapid fluid administration, it is imperative that a large catheter, either 14 or 16 gauge, be inserted. It is important to remember that patients who are likely to need whole blood on arrival at the hospital require a large-bore catheter.

2. What type of IV catheter should be inserted?

As a rule, an "over the needle" catheter is all that should be used in the prehospital setting. Butterfly catheters are usually too small to administer large amounts of fluids rapidly. Butterfly catheters should be carried for use in children, however. Occasionally, an adult with exceptionally small veins may be encountered and, in this case, a butterfly may be inserted if one of the other types of catheters cannot be placed.

3. What type of IV fluid should be used?

Usually, this decision will be left up to the base station physician. However, it is important to be familiar with the types of fluids that have been discussed in this chapter and anticipate the physician's order.

4. What type of administration set should be used?

There are two general types of IV administration sets. The macrodrip or standard set delivers in the neighborhood of 10 to 20 drops per milliliter depending on the manufacturer. Minidrip or microdrip sets deliver anywhere from 50 to 60 drops per milliliter depending on the manufacturer. If you are going to administer a large quantity of fluids, then you should use a macrodrip set. Any time you are going to administer a drug, you should use a minidrip set. This is especially true for piggyback drug infusions. Many systems also use Buretrol or Volutrol sets for administering aminophylline and similar drugs. If your system uses these sets, you should remember them when preparing to administer drugs like aminophylline.

5. Where should the IV be inserted?

Routinely, IV infusions should be started in the larger veins of the forearm. These are usually the most accessible and the least painful for the patient. When these veins are not available, as often occurs in shock and trauma, then any of the other peripheral sites should be attempted. The veins of the leg and the external jugular in the neck are considered peripheral veins. When treating medical or traumatic emergencies, the rule of thumb for starting an intravenous infusion is "any port in a storm."

Once these five decisions have been made, then the actual procedure of inserting the IV can begin. The procedure is as follows:

1. Receive the order.
2. Confirm the order and write it down.
3. Prepare the equipment and don gloves and protective eyewear:
   - Appropriate IV fluid
   - Appropriate administration set
   - Appropriate indwelling catheter
   - Extension IV tubing
   - Tourniquet
   - Antibiotic swab
   - 2 × 2 gauze pad
   - 1-inch tape
   - Antibiotic ointment
   - Short arm board

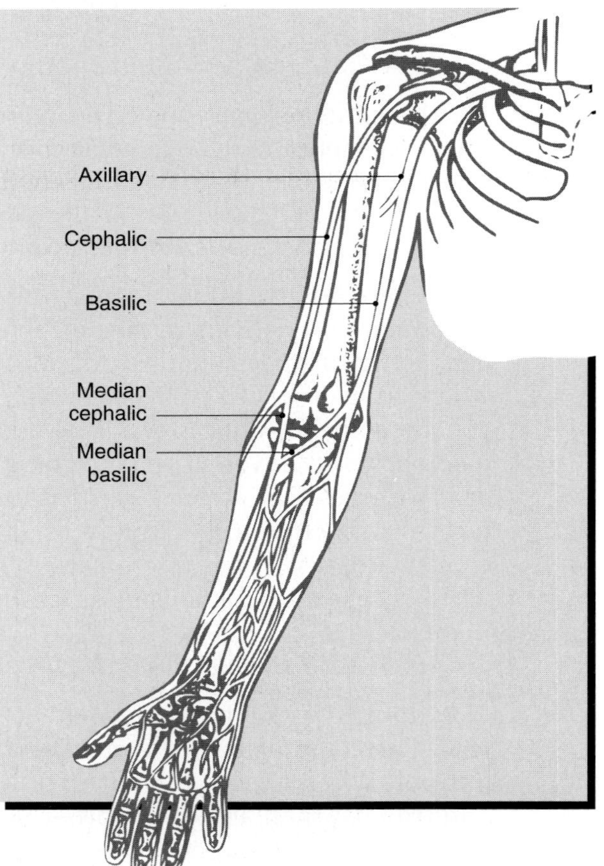

Figure 5-6 Veins of the arm.

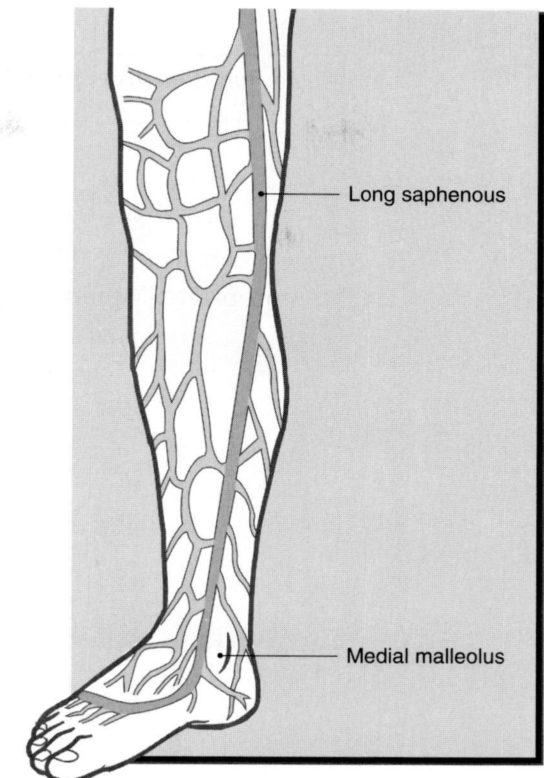

Figure 5-7 Veins of the leg.

4. Remove the envelope from the IV fluid.
5. Inspect the fluid, making sure that it is not discolored or containing any particulate matter; check that it contains the amount of fluid it should have. Do not administer if discolored, if particles are present, or if less than the indicated quantity of fluid is present.
6. Open and inspect the IV tubing.
7. Attach the extension tubing.
8. Close the clamp on the tubing.
9. Remove the sterile cover from the IV fluid and the administration set.
10. Insert the administration set into the IV fluid.
11. Squeeze the drip chamber to fill it with fluid.
12. Bleed all of the air out of the IV tubing.
13. Hang the bag on an IV pole (or have a bystander hold it) at the appropriate height.
14. Place the tourniquet on the patient to occlude venous flow only.
15. Select a suitable vein and palpate it (see Figures 5-6 and 5-7).
16. Prepare the site by cleansing it with an antibiotic swab.
17. Make the puncture using appropriate sterile technique, enter the vein, and advance the catheter (see Figures 5-8 through 5-10).
18. Take a blood sample.

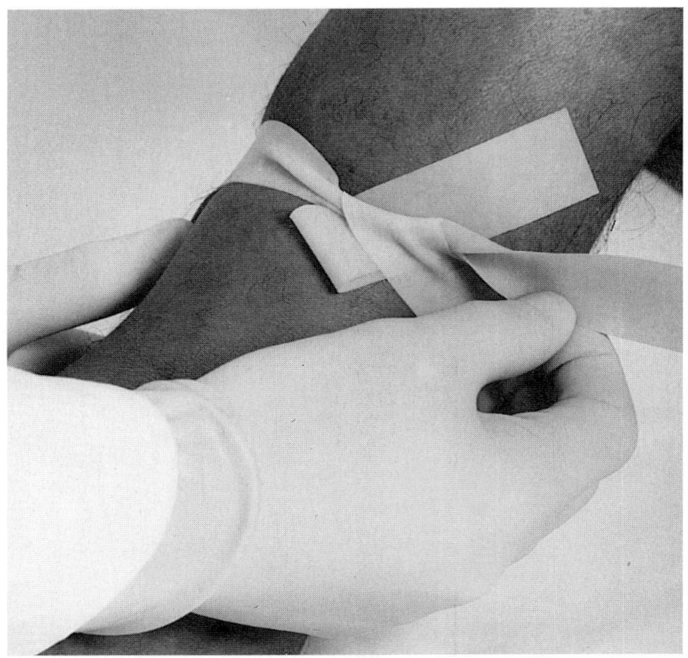

Figure 5-8 Apply the tourniquet to distend the vein.

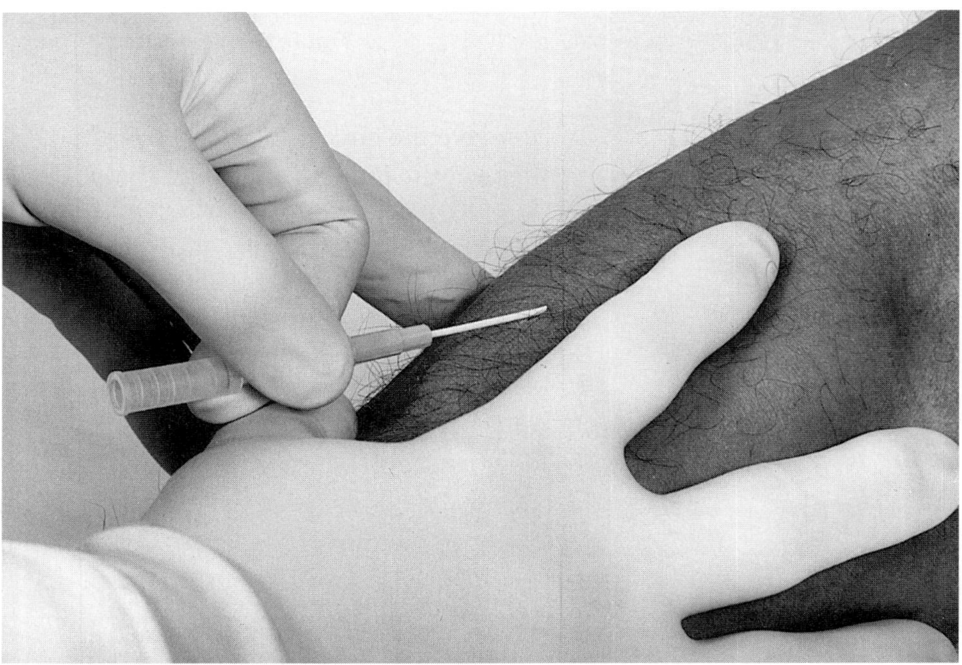

Figure 5-9 Puncture the skin and advance the catheter into the vein.

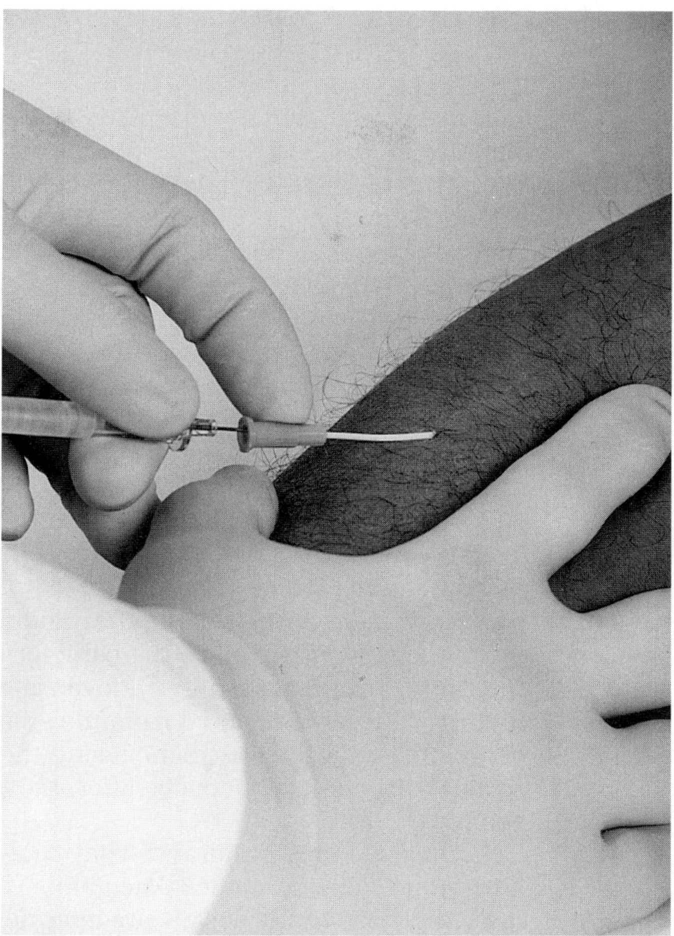

Figure 5-10 Gently advance the catheter into the vein.

19. Connect the IV tubing and slowly open the valve.
20. Remove the tourniquet.
21. Confirm that the fluid is flowing appropriately without any evidence of infiltration.
22. Apply an antibiotic ointment over the puncture and cover with a sterile 2 × 2 gauze pad or adhesive bandage.
23. Securely tape the IV catheter and tubing down.
24. Adjust the flow rate.
25. Apply a short arm board.
26. Place the blood sample in the appropriate tubes.
27. Label the IV bag with the patient's name, date, time the IV was initiated, gauge of the catheter, and your initials.
28. Confirm with medical control the successful completion of the IV.
29. Monitor the patient for the desired effects and any undesired ones as well.

COLLECTION OF BLOOD SAMPLES FOR LABORATORY ANALYSIS

It is becoming commonplace for prehospital personnel to obtain blood samples in the field for later laboratory analysis. There are several advantages to this. It will provide the emergency department physician with information about the patient before medical intervention. This is especially true in cases of suspected hypoglycemia when 50% dextrose is administered. In situations in which a patient may be trapped, or transport to the hospital is otherwise delayed, blood samples can be taken to the hospital before the patient so that blood can be typed and crossmatched, and ready when the patient eventually arrives in the emergency department. Any time a prehospital intervention might affect the subsequent care of the patient (for example, administering Dextran that may inhibit blood typing), always draw a blood sample according to local protocol.

Most commonly, blood samples are taken when an IV is started. Always follow universal precautions when caring for a patient, and especially when handling a blood sample. Gloves and goggles should be worn. After placing the IV catheter, and before connecting the IV line, a 10-milliliter syringe can be attached to the catheter and blood gently withdrawn from the vein. The syringe can be removed and the IV line connected. It is important to withdraw the blood from the syringe slowly. Withdrawing it rapidly can damage the blood cells causing them to rupture and leak their contents. This can erroneously alter the blood chemistries rendering the sample useless.

Once blood is withdrawn from a patient, it is usually placed into evacuated blood collection tubes (Vacutainer). These tubes have a vacuum that allows the tube to fill with a predetermined amount of blood. Most tubes contain a chemical to keep the blood from clotting. Each tube has a different color rubber top depending on its use and contents. The type of tube you may be asked to draw may vary from region to region. After you have withdrawn the blood as described earlier, place an 18-gauge needle on the syringe. Insert the needle into the rubber top and allow the tube to fill with blood. Do not attempt to overfill the tube or press on the plunger of the syringe. Allow the vacuum to fill the vial.

After you have filled the vials, invert them several times to mix the blood and the anticoagulant. Immediately write the patient's name, date, time drawn, your name, and incident number (if any) on the vial. Give the tubes to the appropriate emergency department personnel on arrival. Document on the patient report form the time the blood was drawn and to whom you gave it.

SUMMARY

As with the skills of medication administration, the insertion of an IV requires vigorous mannikin, classroom, and clinical training. This can only be accomplished under the supervision of a qualified instructor.

KEY WORDS

colloid. A substance of high molecular weight, such as plasma proteins. Colloids tend to remain in the intravascular space as opposed to crystalloids, which tend to diffuse out.

crystalloid. A solution containing crystalline substances, such as normal saline.

diffusion. The movement of solute (substances dissolved in a solution) from an area of greater concentration to an area of lesser concentration.

electrolytes. A chemical substance that dissociates into charged particles when placed in water.

erythrocytes. Red blood cells. The erythrocytes are responsible for transport of oxygen.

extracellular. The space outside the cell membrane.

hematocrit. A measure of the number of red blood cells found in the blood, stated as a percentage of the total blood volume.

homeostasis. The body's natural tendency to keep the natural environment constant.

hypertonic. A state in which a solution has a higher solute concentration on one side of a semipermeable membrane compared with the other side.

hypotonic. A state in which a solution has a lower solute concentration on one side of a semipermeable membrane compared to the other side.

intracellular. The space and materials within the cell membrane.

intravascular. The space within the blood vessels.

isotonic. A state in which solution on opposite sides of a semipermeable membrane are equal in concentration.

leukocytes. White blood cells. The leukocytes are responsible for fighting infection.

osmosis. The movement of a solvent (water) across a semipermeable membrane from an area of lesser (solute) concentration to an area of greater (solute) concentration; osmosis is a form of diffusion.

semipermeable membrane. A specialized biological membrane, such as that which encloses the body's cells, that allows passage of certain substances and restricts the passage of others.

chapter 6

The Autonomic Nervous System

OBJECTIVES

1. Describe the anatomy and physiology of the autonomic nervous system.
2. Compare sympathetic and parasympathetic actions.
3. Explain the function of the sympathetic nervous system.
4. List the four adrenergic receptors and explain the effect of each one on body organs.
5. Explain the function of the parasympathetic nervous system.

INTRODUCTION

The autonomic nervous system is a part of the peripheral nervous system and is responsible for control of involuntary or visceral bodily functions. It controls crucial cardiovascular, respiratory, digestive, urinary, and reproductive functions. It also plays a key role in the body's response to stress.

Many of the medications used in emergency care act directly or indirectly on the autonomic nervous system. Thus, it is essential that prehospital personnel have a good understanding of the structure and function of the autonomic nervous system. This chapter will discuss the anatomy and physiology of the autonomic nervous system as it applies to emergency pharmacological therapy.

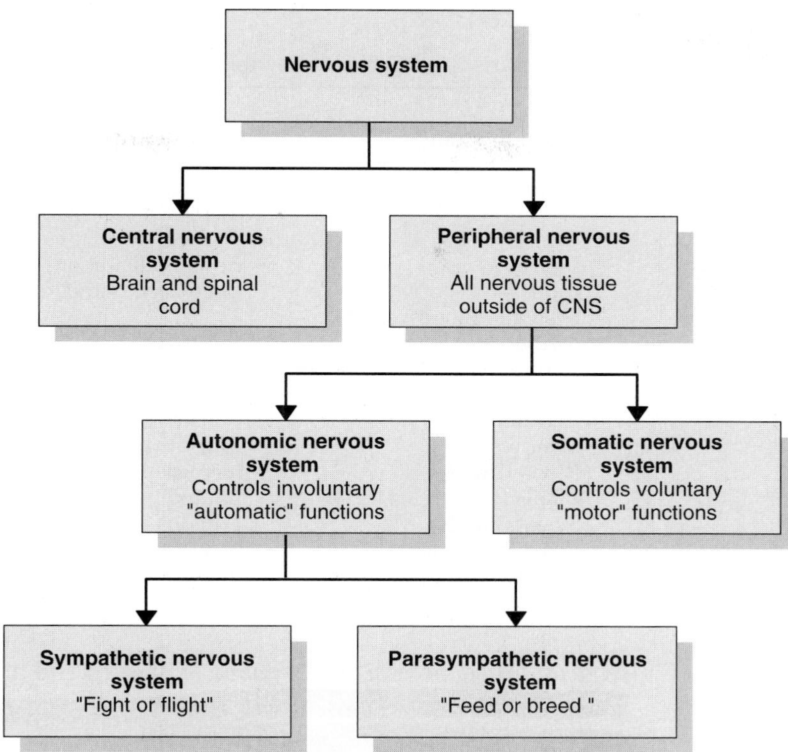

Figure 6-1 Functional organization of the nervous system.

THE AUTONOMIC NERVOUS SYSTEM

The *nervous system* is the body's principle control system. It regulates virtually all bodily functions via electrical impulses transmitted through nerves. Closely related to the nervous system is the *endocrine system*. Like the nervous system, the endocrine system is an important control system. However, unlike the nervous system, it exerts its effect on the body through the release of specialized chemical substances called *hormones*.

The nervous system is customarily divided into the central nervous system and the peripheral nervous system. The *central nervous system (CNS)* consists of the brain and spinal cord. In contrast, the *peripheral nervous system (PNS)* is composed of the cranial nerves and the peripheral nerves. The peripheral nervous system can be further divided into the somatic nervous system and the autonomic nervous system. The *somatic nervous system (SNS)* controls voluntary "motor" functions such as movement. The *autonomic nervous system (ANS)* controls involuntary "automatic" functions (see Figure 6-1).

The two functional divisions of the autonomic nervous system are the sympathetic nervous system and the parasympathetic nervous system. The *sympathetic nervous system* allows the body to function under stress. It is often referred to as the *fight or flight* aspect of the nervous system. The *parasympathetic nervous system*, on the other hand, primarily controls vegetative functions such as digestion of food. It is often referred to as the

TABLE 6-1

Comparison of Sympathetic and Parasympathetic Actions

Organ	*Sympathetic Stimulation*	*Parasympathetic Stimulation*
Heart	Increased rate	Decreased rate
	Increased contractile force	Decreased contractile force
Lungs	Bronchodilatation	Bronchoconstriction
Kidneys	Decreased output	No change
Systemic Blood Vessels		
Abdominal	Constricted	None
Muscle	Constricted (α)	None
	Dilated (β)	None
Skin	Constricted	None
Liver	Glucose release	Slight glycogen synthesis
Blood Glucose	Increased	None
Pupils	Dilated	Constricted
Sweat Glands	Copious sweating	None
Basal Metabolism	Increased up to 100%	None
Skeletal Muscle	Increased strength	None

feed or breed or *rest and repose* aspect of the autonomic nervous system. The parasympathetic nervous system is in constant opposition to the sympathetic nervous system (see Table 6-1).

AUTONOMIC NERVOUS SYSTEM ANATOMY AND PHYSIOLOGY

The autonomic nervous system arises from the central nervous system. The nerves of the autonomic nervous system exit the central nervous system, and subsequently enter specialized structures called *autonomic ganglia*. In the autonomic ganglia the nerve fibers from the central nervous system interact with nerve fibers that extend from the ganglia to the various target organs. Autonomic nerve fibers that exit the central nervous system and terminate in the autonomic ganglia are called *pre-ganglionic nerves*. Autonomic nerve fibers that exit the ganglia and terminate in the various target tissues are called *post-ganglionic nerves*. The ganglia of the sympathetic nervous system are located close to the spinal cord, while the ganglia of the parasympathetic nervous system are located close to the target organs (see Figure 6-2).

No actual physical connection exists between two nerve cells or between a nerve cell and the organ it innervates. Instead, there is a space between nerve cells called a *synapse*. The space between a nerve cell and the target organ is called a *neuroeffector junction*. Specialized chemicals called *neurotransmitters* are used to conduct the nervous impulse between nerve cells, or between a nerve cell and its target organ. Neurotransmitters are released from pre-synaptic neurons and subsequently act on post-synaptic neurons or on the designated target organ. When released by the nerve ending, the neurotransmitter travels across the synapse and activates membrane receptors on the adjoining nerve or target tissue. The neurotransmitter is then either deactivated or taken back up into the pre-synaptic neuron. The

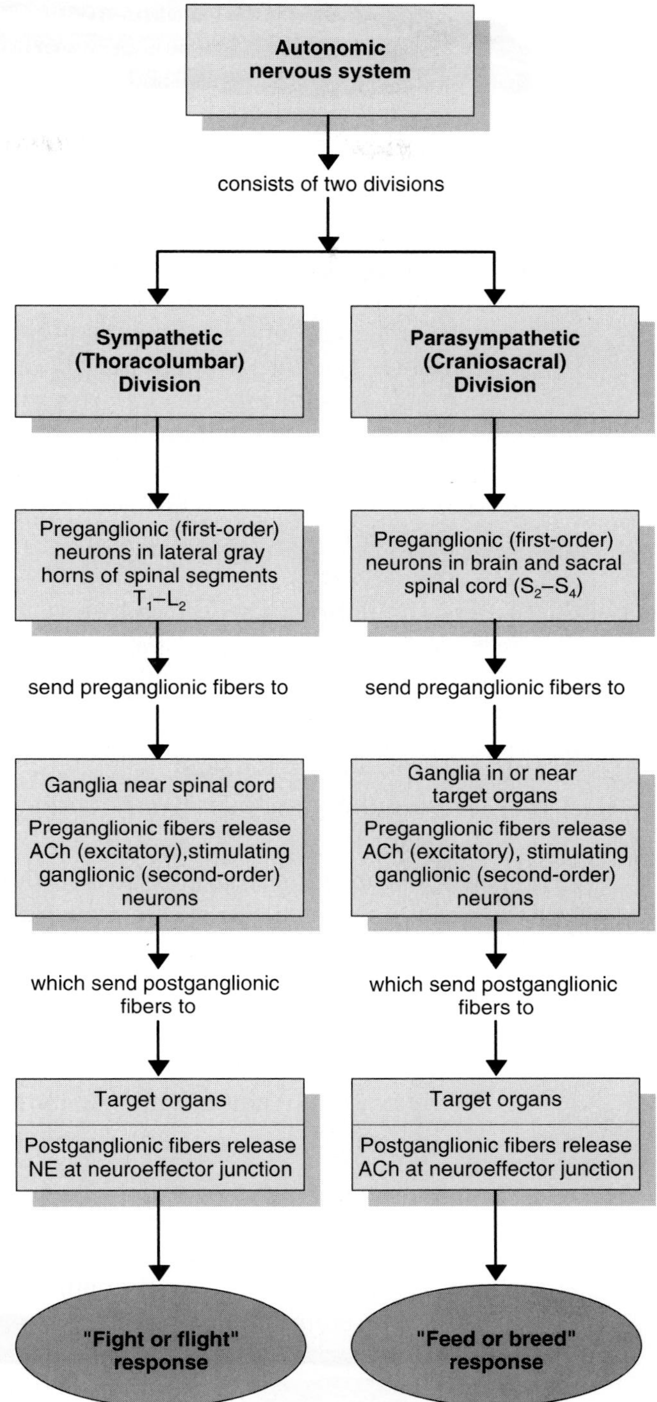

Figure 6-2 Components of the autonomic nervous system.

two neurotransmitters of the autonomic nervous system are *acetylcholine* and *norepinephrine*. Acetylcholine is utilized in the pre-ganglionic nerves of the sympathetic nervous system and in both the pre-ganglionic and post-ganglionic nerves of the parasympathetic nervous system. Norepinephrine is the post-ganglionic neurotransmitter of the sympathetic nervous system.

Synapses that use acetylcholine as the neurotransmitter are called *cholinergic* synapses. Synapses that use norepinephrine as the neurotransmitter are called *adrenergic* synapses.

THE SYMPATHETIC NERVOUS SYSTEM

The sympathetic nervous system arises from the thoracic and lumbar region of the spinal cord. Pre-ganglionic nerves leave the spinal cord through the spinal nerves and end in the sympathetic ganglia. There are two types of sympathetic ganglia: sympathetic chain ganglia and collateral ganglia (see Figure 6-3). In addition, special pre-ganglionic sympathetic nerve fibers innervate the adrenal medulla. Post-ganglionic nerves that exit the *sympathetic chain ganglia* extend to several peripheral target tissues of the sympathetic nervous system. When stimulated, these fibers have several effects including:

- stimulation of secretion by sweat glands,
- constriction of blood vessels in the skin,
- increase in blood flow to skeletal muscles,
- increase in heart rate and in the force of cardiac contractions,
- bronchodilation, and
- stimulation of energy production.

The *collateral ganglia* are located in the abdominal cavity. Nerves leaving the collateral ganglia innervate many of the organs of the abdomen. Stimulation of these fibers causes:

- reduction of blood flow to abdominal organs,
- decreased digestive activity,
- relaxation of smooth muscle in the wall of the urinary bladder, and
- release of glucose stores from the liver.

Sympathetic nervous system stimulation also results in direct stimulation of the *adrenal medulla*. The adrenal medulla in turn releases the hormones *norepinephrine* (noradrenalin) and *epinephrine* (adrenalin) into the circulatory system. Approximately 80 percent of the hormones released by the adrenal medulla are epinephrine with norepinephrine constituting the remaining 20 percent. Once released, these hormones are carried throughout the body where they cause their intended effects by acting on hormone receptors. The release of norepinephrine and epinephrine by the adrenal medulla stimulates tissues that are not innervated by sympathetic nerves. In addition, it prolongs the effects of direct sympathetic stimulation. All of these effects serve to prepare the body to deal with stressful and potentially dangerous situations.

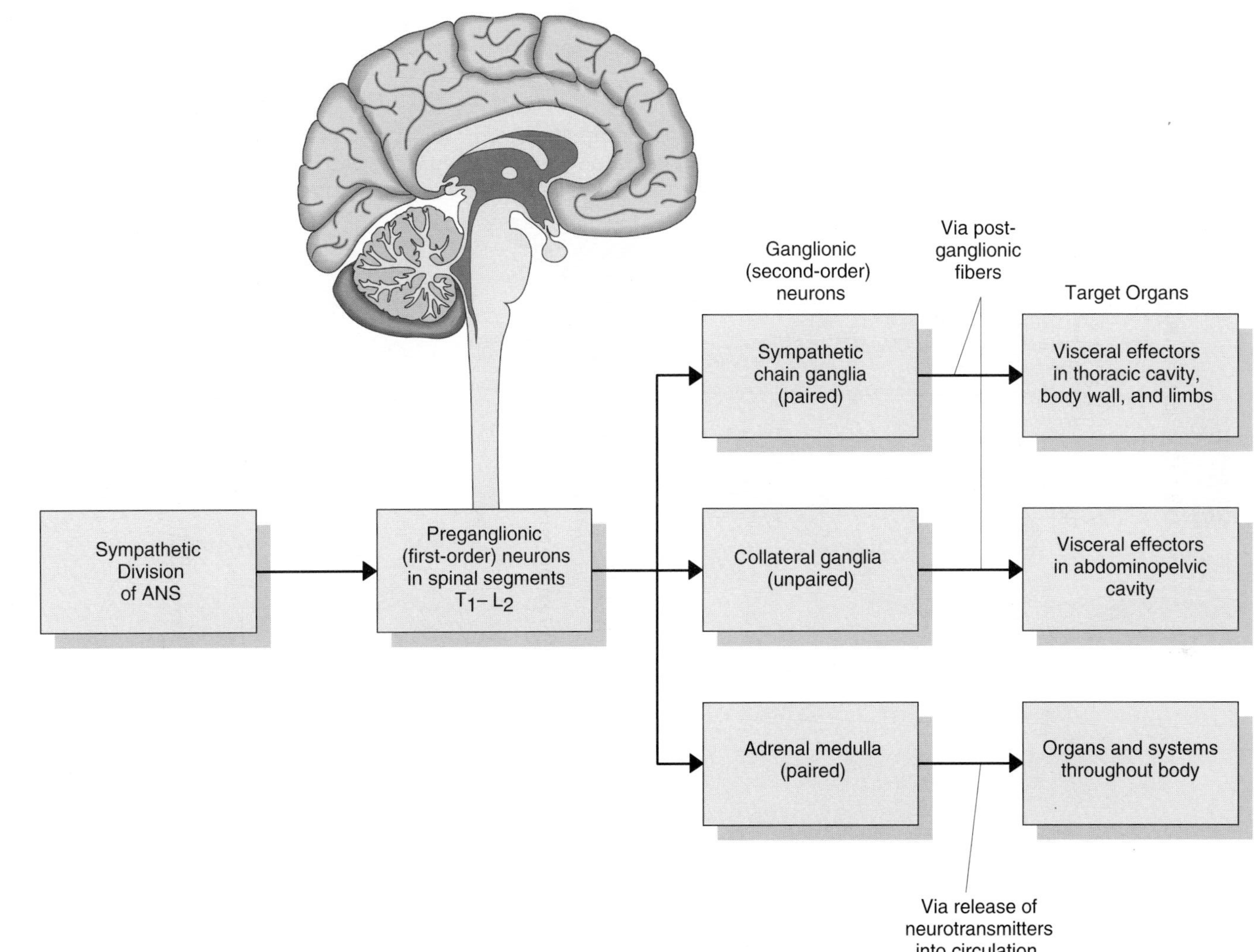

Figure 6-3 Organization of the sympathetic division of the autonomic nervous system.

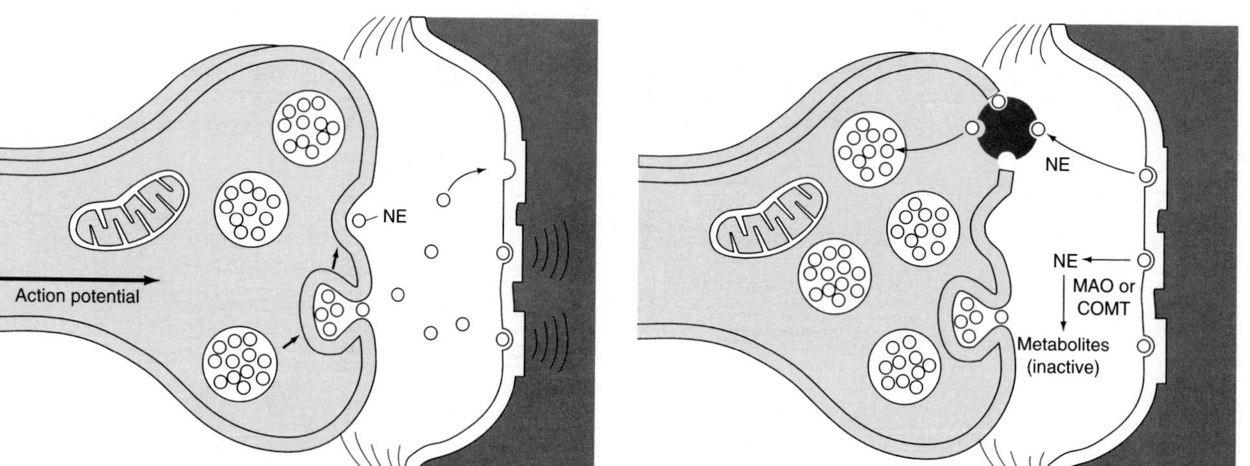

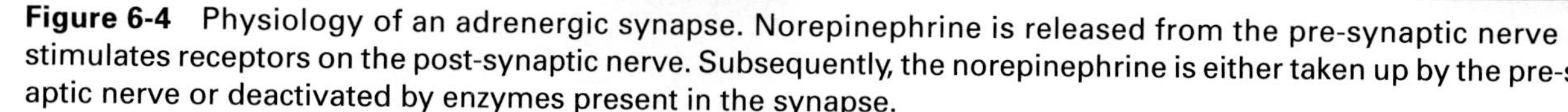

Figure 6-4 Physiology of an adrenergic synapse. Norepinephrine is released from the pre-synaptic nerve and stimulates receptors on the post-synaptic nerve. Subsequently, the norepinephrine is either taken up by the pre-synaptic nerve or deactivated by enzymes present in the synapse.

Adrenergic Receptors

Sympathetic stimulation ultimately results in the release of norepinephrine from post-ganglionic nerves. It subsequently crosses the synaptic cleft and interacts with adrenergic receptors. Shortly thereafter, the norepinephrine is taken up by the pre-synaptic neuron for re-use, or is broken down by enzymes present within the synapse (see Figure 6-4). Sympathetic stimulation also results in the release of epinephrine and norepinephrine from the adrenal medulla. Both epinephrine and norepinephrine also interact with specialized receptors on the membranes of the target organs. These receptors, called *adrenergic receptors*, are located throughout the body. Once stimulated by the appropriate hormone, they cause a response in the organ or organs they control.

The two known types of sympathetic receptors are the adrenergic receptors and the dopaminergic receptors. The *adrenergic receptors* are generally divided into four types. These four receptors are designated *alpha 1* (α_1), *alpha 2* (α_2), *beta 1* (β_1), and *beta 2* (β_2). The α_1 receptors cause peripheral vasoconstriction, mild bronchoconstriction, and stimulation of metabolism. The α_2 receptors are found on the *pre-synaptic* surfaces of sympathetic neuroeffector junctions. Stimulation of α_2 receptors is inhibitory. They serve to prevent over-release of norepinephrine in the synapse. When the level of norepinephrine in the synapse gets high enough, the α_2 receptors are stimulated and norepinephrine release is inhibited. Stimulation of β_1 receptors causes an increase in heart rate, cardiac contractile force, and an increase in cardiac automaticity and conduction. Stimulation of β_2 receptors causes vasodilation and bronchodilation (see Table 6-2). *Dopaminergic receptors*, although not fully understood, are believed to cause dilation of the renal, coronary, and cerebral arteries.

Medications that stimulate the sympathetic nervous system are referred to as *sympathomimetics*. Medications that inhibit the sympathetic nervous system are called *sympatholytics*. Some medications are pure α *agonists*, while others are pure α *antagonists*. Some medications are pure β agonists, while others are pure β antagonists. Medications such as

TABLE 6-2

Actions of the Adrenergic Receptors

Receptor	*Actions*
alpha 1 (α_1)	• Peripheral vasoconstriction • Increased contractile force (positive inotropic effect) • Decreased heart rate (negative chronotropic effect)
alpha 2 (α_2)	• Peripheral vasodilation (by limiting norepinephrine release)
beta 1 (β_1)	• Increased heart rate (positive chronotropic effect) • Increased contractile force (positive inotropic effect) • Increased automaticity (positive dromotropic effect)
beta 2 (β_2)	• Peripheral vasodilation • Bronchodilation • Uterine smooth muscle relaxation • Gastrointestinal smooth muscle relaxation
dopaminergic	• Renal vasodilation • Mesenteric vasodilation

epinephrine stimulate both alpha and beta receptors. Other medications, such as the bronchodilators, are termed β selective, since they act more on β_2 receptors than upon β_1.

THE PARASYMPATHETIC NERVOUS SYSTEM

The parasympathetic nervous system arises from the brainstem and the sacral segments of the spinal cord. The pre-ganglionic neurons are typically much longer than those of the sympathetic nervous system because the ganglia are located close to the target tissues. Parasympathetic nerve fibers that leave the brainstem travel within four of the cranial nerves including the oculomotor nerve (III), the facial nerve (VII), the glossopharyngeal nerve (IX), and the vagus nerve (X). These fibers synapse in the *parasympathetic ganglia* with short post-ganglionic fibers, which then continue to their target tissues. Post-synaptic fibers innervate much of the body including the intrinsic eye muscles, the salivary glands, the heart, the lungs, and most of the organs of the abdominal cavity. The sacral segment of the parasympathetic nervous system forms distinct pelvic nerves that innervate ganglia in the kidneys, bladder, sex organs, and the terminal portions of the large intestine (see Figure 6-5). Stimulation of the parasympathetic nervous system results in:

- pupillary constriction,
- secretion by digestive glands,
- increased smooth muscle activity along the digestive tract,
- bronchoconstriction, and
- reduction in heart rate and cardiac contractile force.

Through these and other functions, the processing of food, energy absorption, relaxation, and reproduction are facilitated.

All pre-ganglionic and post-ganglionic parasympathetic nerve fibers use *acetylcholine* as a neurotransmitter. Acetylcholine, when released by pre-synaptic neurons, crosses the synaptic cleft and activates receptors on the post-synaptic neuron or on the neuroeffector junction. Acetylcholine is also the neurotransmitter for the somatic nervous system and is present in the *neuromuscular junction*. Acetylcholine is very short-lived. Within a fraction of a second after its release, acetylcholine is deactivated by another chemical called *acetylcholinesterase. Acetic acid* and *choline*, which are produced when acetylcholine is deactivated, are taken back up by the pre-synaptic neuron (see Figure 6-6).

The emergency medication atropine is an antagonist to the parasympathetic nervous system and is used to increase heart rate. Atropine binds with acetylcholine receptors, thus preventing acetylcholine from exerting its effect. Medications like atropine, which block the actions of the parasympathetic nervous system, are referred to as *parasympatholytics* or anticholinergics. Medications that stimulate the parasympathetic nervous system are referred to as *parasympathomimetics*.

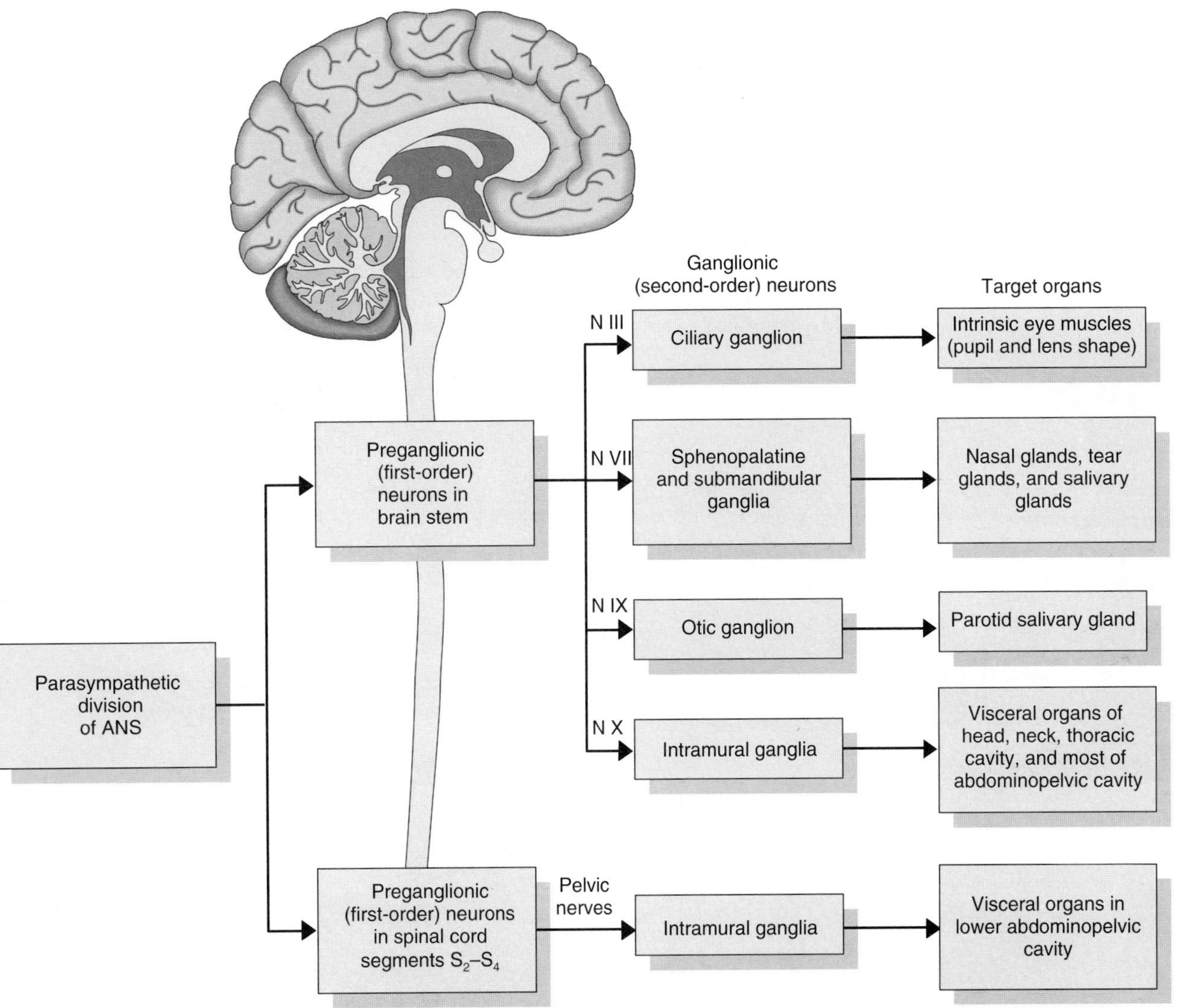

Figure 6-5 Organization of the parasympathetic division of the autonomic nervous system.

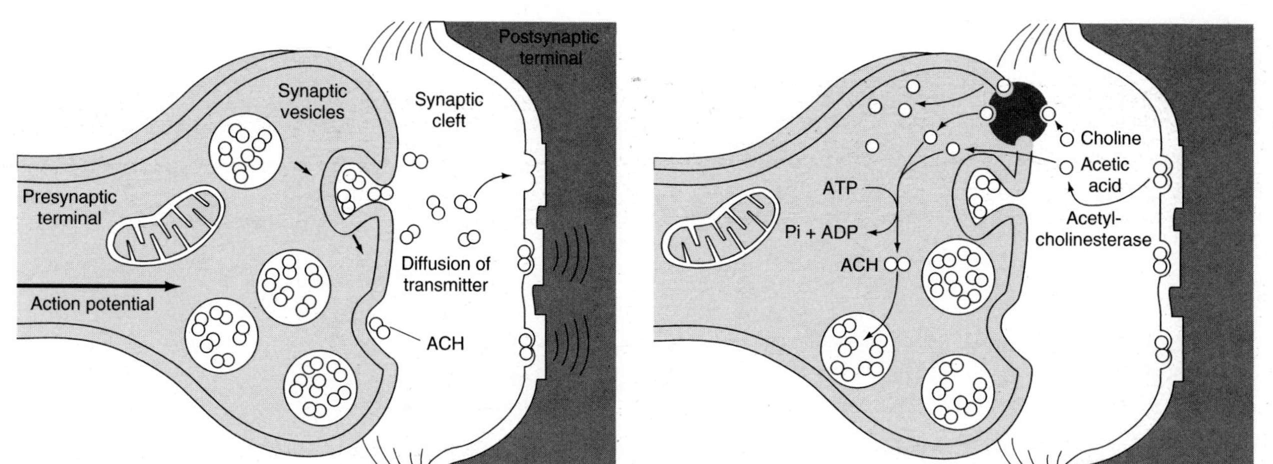

Figure 6-6 Physiology of a cholinergic synapse. Acetylcholine is released from the pre-synaptic nerve and stimulates receptors on the post-synaptic nerve. Subsequently, the acetylcholine is broken down by acetylcholinesterase and the products are taken up by the pre-synaptic nerve fiber.

SUMMARY

The autonomic nervous system is a part of the peripheral nervous system and is responsible for control of involuntary or visceral bodily functions. It maintains the body's internal environment by controlling crucial cardiovascular, respiratory, digestive, urinary, and reproductive functions. It also plays a key role in the body's response to stress.

Since many of the medications used in prehospital care act directly or indirectly on the autonomic nervous system, it is essential that prehospital personnel have a good understanding of the structure and function of the autonomic nervous system.

KEY WORDS AND PHRASES

acetylcholine. Chemical neurotransmitter found in all autonomic preganglionic synapses and in parasympathetic post-ganglionic synapses.

adrenal medulla. An endocrine gland, located atop the kidney, that manufactures and secretes epinephrine and norepinephrine.

adrenergic. Related to or pertaining to the sympathetic nervous system.

alpha 1 adrenergic receptor. A type of adrenergic receptor that, when stimulated, causes peripheral vasoconstriction, mild bronchoconstriction, and stimulation of metabolism.

alpha 2 adrenergic receptor. A type of adrenergic receptor that, when stimulated, inhibits parts of the sympathetic nervous system. This serves to prevent the over-release of norepinephrine in the synapse.

autonomic nervous system (ANS). Part of the peripheral nervous system responsible for control of involuntary or visceral bodily functions.

beta 1 adrenergic receptor. A type of adrenergic receptor that, when stimulated, causes an increase in heart rate, cardiac contractile force, and cardiac automaticity and conduction.

beta 2 adrenergic receptor. A type of adrenergic receptor that, when stimulated, causes vasodilation and bronchodilation.

bronchodilator. A drug that helps to improve breathing by relaxing the smooth muscle of the bronchioles, causing bronchodilation.

central nervous system (CNS). The central portion of the nervous system consisting of the brain and spinal cord.

cholinergic. Related to or pertaining to the parasympathetic nervous system.

chronotrope. A drug or other substance that affects heart rate.

dromotrope. A drug or other substance that affects nerve conduction.

epinephrine. A naturally occurring hormone that stimulates the adrenal glands, increases cardiac output, and causes bronchodilation.

ganglia. A mass of nerve cells.

inotrope. A drug or other substance that affects the strength of the cardiac contraction.

neurotransmitter. A substance that is released from the axon terminal of a presynaptic neuron. On excitation it travels across the synaptic cleft to either excite or inhibit the target cell. Examples include acetylcholine, norepinephrine, and dopamine.

norepinephrine. A naturally occurring hormone. It also serves as a sympathetic neurotransmitter. It is found in most post-ganglionic synapses.

parasympathetic nervous system. The division of the autonomic nervous system that is responsible for controlling vegetative functions.

peripheral nervous system. The portion of the nervous system outside the brain and spinal cord. It is composed of the cranial nerves and peripheral nerves.

somatic nervous system (SNS). The portion of the nervous system that controls voluntary "motor" functions such as movement.

sympathetic nervous system. The division of the autonomic nervous system that prepares the body for stressful situations.

sympathomimetic. A drug or other substance that causes effects like those of the sympathetic nervous system (also called adrenergic).

chapter 7

Drugs Used in the Treatment of Cardiovascular Emergencies

OBJECTIVES

1. Describe and list the indications, contraindications, and dosages for the sympathomimetics epinephrine, norepinephrine, dopamine, isoproterenol, dobutamine, metaraminol, and amrinone.
2. Explain the class of drugs known as sympathetic blockers.
3. Describe and list the indications, contraindications, and dosages for the sympathetic blockers propranolol, metoprolol, labetalol, and esmolol.
4. Discuss the use of antiarrhythmic medications.
5. Describe and list the indications, contraindications, and dosages for the antiarrythmics lidocaine, procainamide, bretylium tosylate, adenosine, verapamil, diltiazem, phenytoin, edrophonium chloride, and magnesium sulfate.
6. Explain the role of the parasympatholytic atropine and list the indications, contraindications, and dosages for its use.
7. Describe digitalis and list the indications, contraindications, and dosages for its use.
8. Discuss the use of thrombolytics and aspirin in the treatment of myocardial infarction.
9. Describe and list the indications, contraindications, and dosages for aspirin and the thrombolytic agents streptokinase, anistreplase, and tissue plasminogen activator.

10. List the indications, contraindications, and dosages for sodium bicarbonate.
11. Explain the indications, contraindications, and dosages for morphine and nitrous oxide in the treatment of cardiac chest pain.
12. Discuss the use of diuretics in the management of congestive heart failure.
13. List the indications, contraindications, and dosages for the diuretics furosemide and bumetanide.
14. Describe the action of nitroglycerin in cardiac chest pain.
15. List the indications, contraindications, and dosages for the antianginal agents nitroglycerin, nitroglycerin spray, and nitroglycerin paste.
16. Define and explain a "hypertensive crisis."
17. List the indications, contraindications, and dosages for the antihypertensives nifedipine, sodium nitroprusside, diazoxide, and hydralazine.
18. List the indications, contraindications, and dosages for calcium chloride.

INTRODUCTION

Most prehospital emergency drugs are used in the treatment of cardiac emergencies. These drugs, because of the nature of their actions, may be accompanied by many side effects.

Some general classifications follow for our discussion of the emergency cardiovascular drugs:

Oxygen

Oxygen

Sympathomimetics

Epinephrine
Norepinephrine (Levophed)
Isoproterenol (Isuprel)
Dopamine (Intropin)
Dobutamine (Dobutrex)
Metaraminol (Aramine)
Amrinone (Inocor)

Sympathetic Blockers

Propranolol (Inderal)
Metoprolol (Lopressor)
Labetalol (Trandate, Normodyne)
Esmolol (Brevibloc)

Antiarrhythmics

Lidocaine (Xylocaine)
Procainamide (Pronestyl)
Bretylium tosylate (Bretylol)
Adenosine (Adenocard)

Verapamil (Isoptin, Calan)
Diltiazem (Cardizem)
Phenytoin (Dilantin)
Edrophonium chloride (Tensilon)
Magnesium sulfate
Propranolol (Inderal)

Parasympatholytics
Atropine sulfate

Cardiac Glycosides
Digoxin (Lanoxin)

Platelet Aggregation Inhibitors
Aspirin

Thrombolytics
Streptokinase (Streptase)
Anistreplase (Eminase)
Alteplase, Tissue Plasminogen Activator (tPA) (Activase)

Alkalinizing Agents
Sodium bicarbonate

Analgesics
Morphine sulfate
Nitrous oxide (Nitronox)

Diuretics
Furosemide (Lasix)
Bumetanide (Bumex)

Antianginal Agents
Nitroglycerin (Nitrostat)
Nitroglycerin paste (Nitro-Bid Ointment)
Nitroglycerin spray (Nitrolingual Spray)

Antihypertensives
Nifedipine (Procardia)
Sodium nitroprusside (Nipride)
Hydralazine (Apresoline)
Diazoxide (Hyperstat)

Other Cardiovascular Drugs
Calcium chloride

OXYGEN

Oxygen is one of the most important drugs used in prehospital care. It is required by the body's cells to facilitate the breakdown of glucose into usable energy forms. Without oxygen, the breakdown of glucose is ineffective and incomplete. This breakdown without oxygen is termed *anaerobic metabolism*. Anaerobic metabolism yields *lactic acid*, a strong acid, as its end product. This acid, in conjunction with an increased carbon dioxide level, leads to systemic acidosis.

Oxygen is an odorless, tasteless, colorless gas that vigorously supports combustion. It is present in room air at a concentration of approximately 21%. This concentration is adequate for our daily activities. In injury and illness, however, the body needs increased levels of oxygen to maintain homeostasis.

Oxygen

Class: Gas

Description

Oxygen is an odorless, tasteless, colorless gas necessary for life.

Mechanism of Action

Oxygen enters the body through the respiratory system and is transported to the cells by hemoglobin, found in the red cells. Oxygen is required for the efficient breakdown of glucose into a usable energy form. Its onset of action following administration is immediate. The administration of enriched oxygen increases the oxygen concentration in the alveoli, which subsequently increases the oxygen saturation of available hemoglobin.

Indication

- Hypoxia. Oxygen is indicated whenever hypoxia is suspected or possible. This includes all forms of trauma, medical emergencies, chest pain that may be due to cardiac ischemia, any respiratory difficulty, during labor and delivery, and in any critical patient.

Contraindications

There are no contraindications to oxygen. NEVER DEPRIVE THE HYPOXIC PATIENT OF OXYGEN FOR FEAR OF RESPIRATORY DEPRESSION.

Precautions

Oxygen should be used cautiously in patients with chronic obstructive pulmonary disease (COPD). In these patients respirations are often regulated by the level of oxygen in the blood (hypoxic drive) instead of carbon dioxide. In some cases COPD patients may suffer respiratory depression if high concentrations of oxygen are delivered.

The administration of high concentrations of oxygen to neonates for a prolonged period of time can damage the infant's eyes (retrolental fibroplasia). Although this is rarely a problem in prehospital care, it is a consideration in long distance and prolonged transport.

Oxygen delivered at a flow rate of 6 liters per minute or greater should be humidified to prevent drying of the mucous membranes of the upper respiratory system.

When possible, oxygen administration should be monitored by use of pulse oximetry. Pulse oximetry is a non-invasive device that accurately measures the oxygen saturation of hemoglobin. It is relatively inexpensive, easy to apply, and quite accurate in detecting oxygen delivery problems.

Side Effects

There are few, if any, side effects associated with oxygen administration. Prolonged administration of high-flow, non-humidified oxygen may result in drying of the mucous membranes resulting in irritation and possibly nose bleeds.

Interactions

There are no interactions associated with oxygen administration. However, oxygen may increase the toxicity of certain herbicides (i.e., paraquat, diaquat) in patients who have ingested these poisons. These chemicals are sometimes sprayed on illicit agricultural products such as marijuana. Poisoning by these agents is uncommon.

Dosage

The dosage of oxygen is based on the patient's underlying problems. In the prehospital setting oxygen should be administered at the highest concentration available (see Table 7-1). Pulse oximetry, if available, should be used to guide care. General guidelines follow:

- Cardiac arrest and other critical patients—100% oxygen concentration
- Chronic obstructive pulmonary disease—35% oxygen concentration (increase as needed)

How Supplied

Oxygen is supplied in pressurized cylinders of varying size (see Table 7-2). Liquid oxygen is becoming more common in prehospital care. The sizes and types of liquid oxygen containers vary.

TABLE 7-1

Oxygen Delivery by Device

Oxygen Delivery Device	*Flow Rate (L/min)*	*Percentage Delivered*
Nasal cannula	1–6	24–44
Simple face mask	8–10	40–60
Venturi mask	4–12	24–50
Partial rebreathing mask	6–10	35–60
Nonrebreathing mask	6–10	60–95
Bag-Valve-Mask with reservoir	10–15	40–90
Demand valve	10–15	100

TABLE 7-2

Capacity of Common Oxygen Cylinders

Cylinder Name	*Volume (Liters)*
D	400
E	660
M	3,000

SYMPATHOMIMETICS

The term *sympathomimetic* means to mimic the actions of the sympathetic nervous system. Drugs in this group do exactly that. They will either act directly on receptors of the sympathetic nervous system or will act indirectly by stimulating the release of *endogenous* catecholamines. *Catecholamine* is the name used to describe several drugs that are chemically similar. These drugs are epinephrine, norepinephrine (Levophed), dopamine (Intropin), isoproterenol (Isuprel), and dobutamine (Dobutrex). All of these agents, except isoproterenol and dobutamine, can be found naturally in the body. Isoproterenol and dobutamine are synthetic catecholamines. To understand and appreciate the actions and roles of the sympathomimetics fully, it is essential to first review the sympathetic nervous system.

Sympathetic Nervous System

The *sympathetic nervous system* is sometimes called the "fight or flight" system. It is this part of the nervous system that prepares the body to deal with various stresses, whether real or imagined. Sometimes it is referred to as the *adrenergic system*. Both it, and the other aspect of the autonomic nervous system, the parasympathetic, functionally oppose each other to maintain *homeostasis*. The *parasympathetic system* is sometimes called the *cholinergic system*.

As indicated by Table 7-3, the sympathetic nervous system tends to stimulate those organs needed to deal with stressful situations. It also tends to inhibit the use of organs not needed, like the digestive tract.

The sympathetic nervous system uses the hormone *norepinephrine* to transmit impulses from the nerve to the effector cell. Chemicals that propagate the nervous impulse, like norepinephrine, are called *neurotransmitters*. In emergency situations the norepinephrine released by the nerve endings may be augmented with epinephrine and norepinephrine secreted from the adrenal medulla. Like the adrenergic nerves, the adrenal medulla secretes norepinephrine. About 20 percent of the catecholamines secreted by the adrenals are in the form of norepinephrine. The remaining 80 percent are in the form of epinephrine (adrenalin).

When released, norepinephrine will act on specialized chemical receptors. These receptors are located at various points throughout the body. Once stimulated by the appropriate catecholamine, they will cause a response in the organ or organs they control. There are two types of receptors, the *adrenergic receptors* and the *dopaminergic receptors*. The adren-

TABLE 7-3

Comparison of Sympathetic and Parasympathetic Actions

Organ	*Sympathetic Stimulation*	*Parasympathetic Stimulation*
Heart	Increased rate	Decreased rate
	Increased contractile force	Decreased contractile force
Lungs	Bronchodilatation	Bronchoconstriction
Kidneys	Decreased output	No change
Systemic Blood Vessels		
Abdominal	Constricted	None
Muscle	Constricted (α)	None
	Dilated (β)	None
Skin	Constricted	None
Liver	Glucose release	Slight glycogen synthesis
Blood Glucose	Increased	None
Pupils	Dilated	Constricted
Sweat Glands	Copious sweating	None
Basal Metabolism	Increased up to 100%	None
Skeletal Muscle	Increased strength	None

ergic receptors are further divided into four different types. These four types of receptors are designated *alpha 1* (α_1), *alpha 2* (α_2), *beta 1* (β_1), and *beta 2* (β_2). The α_1 receptors cause peripheral vasoconstriction and occasionally mild bronchoconstriction. The α_2 receptors, when stimulated, inhibit the release of norepinephrine. This effect is antagonistic to the actions of α_1 receptors and, over time, can cause peripheral vasodilation. The β_1 receptors, once stimulated, will cause an increase in cardiac rate, cardiac force, and cardiac automaticity and conduction. The β_2 receptors will cause vasodilation and bronchodilation. Dopaminergic receptors, though not totally understood, are believed to cause dilatation of the renal, coronary, and cerebral arteries. See Chapter 6 for a more detailed discussion of the autonomic nervous system.

Catecholamines

Certain drugs will stimulate certain receptors to one degree or another. Norepinephrine, for example, has an effect on both α and β receptors. However, its effects on α receptors is considerably stronger than on the β receptors. Because of this, norepinephrine is primarily regarded as an α-receptor-stimulating agent. Epinephrine, like norepinephrine, acts on both α and β receptors. However, unlike norepinephrine, epinephrine has a much greater effect on β receptors and is considered a β-receptor-stimulating agent. Isoproterenol, the synthetic catecholamine occasionally used in emergency medicine, acts entirely on β receptors with no α effects noted. Dopamine acts on both α and β receptors depending on the dosage. In addition to this, when used in certain doses, it acts on the dopaminergic receptors. This dopaminergic effect is quite useful because it tends to keep blood flowing to the renal arteries, even in emergency situations. One of the long-term major complications of severe medical emergencies, like cardiac arrest, is renal failure. Using agents like dopamine, which will maintain renal perfusion, will help in the long-term survival of the patient.

Drugs that cause an increase in the cardiac rate are called *positive chronotropic agents*. Drugs that cause an increase in cardiac force are referred to as *positive inotropic agents*.

The primary use of the sympathomimetics in emergency medicine is to increase the blood pressure in cardiogenic shock. These drugs raise the blood pressure by one of two different methods. Drugs that stimulate α receptors elevate blood pressure merely by peripheral vasoconstriction. Vasoconstriction reduces the size of the vascular pool, thus increasing the blood pressure. Drugs that act on β receptors elevate blood pressure by causing an increase in the cardiac output. Cardiac output can be defined as follows:

$$\text{Cardiac Output} = \text{Stroke Volume} \times \text{Heart Rate}$$

Thus:

$$\text{Blood Pressure} = \text{Cardiac Output} \times \text{Peripheral Resistance}$$

The β-receptor-stimulating drugs, like epinephrine and dopamine, cause both an increase in heart rate (positive chronotropic) and stroke volume (positive inotropic). The different receptor effects are summarized in Table 7-4. Table 7-5 lists many of the sympathomimetic drugs used in emergency care, including their adrenergic effects and arrhythmia potential.

TABLE 7-4

Comparison of Effects of α and β Adrenergic Receptor Activity on Selected Organs

Organ	*α-Adrenergic Receptors*	*β-Adrenergic Receptors*
Heart	No cardiac effect	Increased heart rate (β_1) Increased contractile force (β_1) Increased automaticity (β_1)
Systemic Blood Vessels	Vasoconstriction	Vasodilatation (β_2)
Lungs	Mild bronchoconstriction	Bronchodilatation (β_2)

TABLE 7-5

Listing of Sympathomimetic Drugs with Adrenergic Actions

	Adrenergic Effects		
Drug	*α*	*β*	*Arrhythmia Potential*
Epinephrine			
Low dose	+	++	+++
High dose	++	+++	+++
Norepinephrine			
Low dose	++	+	++
High dose	+++	++	++
Dopamine			
Low dose	+	+	++
High dose	+++	++	++
Isoproterenol	0	+++	+++
Dobutamine	0	+++	+
Amrinone	0	0	+

Epinephrine 1:10,000

Class: Sympathetic Agonist

Description

Epinephrine is a naturally occurring catecholamine. It is a potent α and β adrenergic stimulant; however, its effect on β receptors is more profound.

Mechanism of Action

Epinephrine acts directly on α and β adrenergic receptors. Its effect on β receptors is much more profound than its effect on α receptors. The effects of epinephrine include:

- Increased heart rate
- Increased cardiac contractile force
- Increased electrical activity in the myocardium
- Increased systemic vascular resistance
- Increased blood pressure
- Increased automaticity

Epinephrine can stimulate spontaneous firing of myocardial conductive cells. In the emergency setting it is used to convert fine ventricular fibrillation to coarse ventricular fibrillation. This change significantly increases the chances of successful electrical defibrillation. In asystole it is used to initiate electrical activity in the myocardium. Once initiated, electrical defibrillation may be attempted.

Epinephrine's effects usually appear within 90 seconds of administration, and they are usually of short duration. Therefore, it must be administered every 3–5 minutes to maintain therapeutic levels.

Indications

- Cardiac arrest (asystole, ventricular fibrillation, pulseless ventricular tachycardia, pulseless electrical activity)
- Severe anaphylaxis
- Severe reactive airway disease

Contraindications

Epinephrine 1:10,000 is contraindicated in patients who do not require extensive cardiopulmonary resuscitative efforts. With simple allergic reactions and asthma, the 1:1,000 dilution should be used and is administered subcutaneously.

Precautions

Epinephrine, like all catecholamines, should be protected from light. It can be deactivated by alkaline solutions such as sodium bicarbonate. Because of this, it is essential that the IV line is adequately flushed between the administration of epinephrine and sodium bicarbonate.

Side Effects

Epinephrine can cause palpitations, anxiety, tremulousness, headache, dizziness, nausea, and vomiting. Because of its strong inotropic and chronotropic properties, epinephrine increases myocardial oxygen demand. Even in low doses it can cause myocardial ischemia. When administering epinephrine in the emergency setting, these effects should be kept in mind. Like most of the other drugs used in emergency medicine, epinephrine is only effective when the myocardium is adequately oxygenated.

Interactions

Epinephrine is pH dependent and can be deactivated when administered with highly alkaline solutions such as sodium bicarbonate. The effects of epinephrine can be intensified in patients who are taking anti-depressants.

Dosage

Epinephrine 1:10,000 can be administered intravenously, intraosseously, or endotracheally. Common doses include:

- ***Cardiac Arrest (Adults)***. The dose of epinephrine in cardiac arrest is 0.5 to 1.0 milligram of a 1:10,000 solution intravenously. This can be repeated every 3–5 minutes as required. Higher dosages may be ordered by medical control and are potentially helpful in the cardiac arrest setting. If an IV cannot be started, epinephrine can be administered endotracheally. The endotracheal dose should be increased at least 2 to 2.5 times the intravenous dose.
- ***Cardiac Arrest (Children).*** The initial dose of epinephrine in pediatric cardiac arrest is 0.01 mg/kg of a 1:10,000 solution intravenously (0.1 ml/kg). Second and subsequent doses should be 0.1 mg/kg of a 1:1,000 solution intravenously (0.1 ml/kg). The second and subsequent dose is ten times the initial dose. The total volume of drug administered remains the same, as epinephrine 1:1,000 is used instead of epinephrine 1:10,000.
- ***Severe Anaphylaxis/Severe Asthma (Adults)***. Intravenous epinephrine should only be used for life-threatening, severe anaphylaxis and severe asthma. Less severe cases should be treated with epinephrine 1:1,000 subcutaneously or with another β agonist. In severe anaphylaxis/asthma the initial dose should be 0.3–0.5 milligram intravenously. The dose may be repeated every 5–15 minutes as required. An epinephrine drip may be required in severe cases.

- ***Severe Anaphylaxis/Severe Asthma (Children)***. Intravenous epinephrine should only be used for life-threatening, severe anaphylaxis and severe asthma. Less severe cases should be treated with epinephrine 1:1,000 subcutaneously or with another β agonist. In severe anaphylaxis/asthma the initial dose should be 0.01 mg/kg intravenously. The dose may be repeated every 5–15 minutes as required. An epinephrine drip may be required in severe cases.

How Supplied

Epinephrine 1:10,000 comes in prefilled syringes containing 1 milligram of the drug in 10 milliliters of solvent.

Norepinephrine (Levophed)

Class: Sympathetic Agonist

Description

Norepinephrine is a naturally occurring catecholamine. It acts on both α and β beta adrenergic receptors. However, its action on α receptors is more profound.

Mechanism of Action

Because of its action on α receptors, norepinephrine is a potent peripheral vasoconstrictor. This vasoconstriction serves to increase blood pressure in cardiogenic shock and other hypotensive emergencies. Because norepinephrine also tends to constrict the renal and mesenteric blood vessels, it is reserved for emergencies where dopamine may not be effective. As a rule, dopamine, which maintains renal and mesenteric perfusion, is the preferred vasopressor for treating cardiogenic shock.

Indications

- Hypotension (systolic blood pressure <70 mmHg) refractory to other sympathomimetics
- Neurogenic shock

Contraindications

Norepinephrine should not be given to patients who are hypotensive from hypovolemia.

Precautions

Because of the powerful effects of norepinephrine, it is essential to measure the blood pressure every 5 to 10 minutes to prevent dangerously high blood pressures. Norepinephrine should be given through the largest vein readily available because it may cause local tissue necrosis if it extravasates. Phentolamine (Regitine) can be diluted in saline and infiltrated into the area of extravasation to help minimize necrosis and sloughing.

Like the other sympathomimetics, norepinephrine can increase myocardial oxygen demand. It should be used with caution in persons suffering from cardiac ischemia.

Side Effects

Norepinephrine can cause anxiety, tremulousness, headache, dizziness, nausea, and vomiting. It can also cause bradycardia as a reflex response to increased peripheral vasoconstriction. Because of its inotropic and chronotropic properties, norepinephrine increases myocardial oxygen demand. Even in low doses it can cause myocardial ischemia. When administering norepinephrine in the emergency setting, these effects should be kept in mind.

Interactions

Norepinephrine can be deactivated by alkaline solutions such as sodium bicarbonate. Concomitant administration with beta blockers can result in markedly elevated blood pressure.

Dosage

The current dosage recommended by the American Heart Association for norepinephrine is 0.5 to 30 micrograms per minute. Higher doses may be required to maintain adequate blood pressure. The best dilution is attained by placing 8 milligrams in 500 milliliters of D_5W. This will give a concentration of 16 micrograms per milliliter. The same concentration can be attained by placing 4 milligrams in 250 milliliters of D_5W (see Figure 7-1).

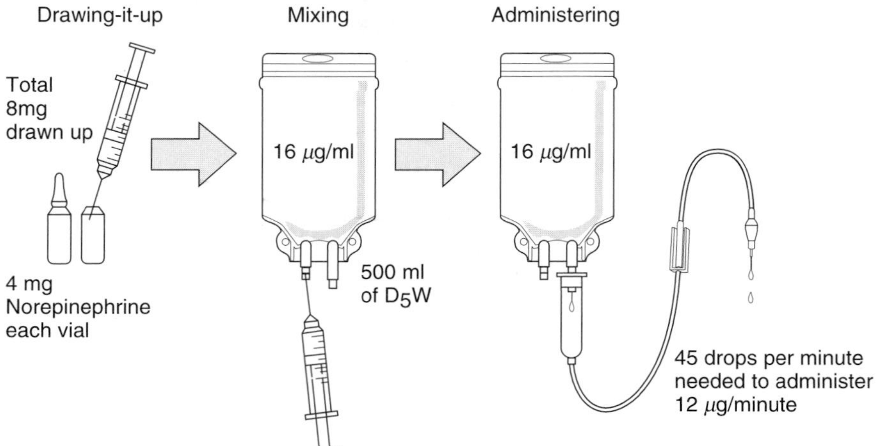

Figure 7-1 Preparation of norepinephrine infusion.

Because of its potency, norepinephrine is given only in extremely diluted IV infusions. To control its administration, it should be "piggy-backed" into an already established IV line.

How Supplied

Norepinephrine is supplied in 4-milliliter ampules containing 4 milligrams of the drug.

Isoproterenol (Isuprel)

Class: Sympathetic Agonist

Description

Isoproterenol is a synthetic catecholamine. It primarily acts on β adrenergic receptors.

Mechanism of Action

Isoproterenol is a potent, synthetic catecholamine that acts almost exclusively on β receptors. Because it has no significant α-receptor-stimulating capabilities, its actions are primarily on the heart and lungs. In cardiac emergencies it is used to increase heart rate in bradycardias that are refractory to atropine. With the advent of transcutaneous pacing, isoproterenol has fallen into relative disuse.

Indications

- Bradycardias refractory to atropine (when transcutaneous pacing is unavailable)
- Bradycardias resulting from high-degree heart blocks (that is, second-degree Mobitz II and third-degree blocks) when transcutaneous pacing is unavailable
- Severe status asthmaticus

Contraindications

Isoproterenol is not used to increase blood pressure in cardiogenic shock. It should only be used in shock owing to bradycardias. Other sympathomimetics, like dopamine and norepinephrine, should be used in cases of cardiogenic shock.

Precautions

When administering isoproterenol, the patient must be monitored for signs of ventricular irritability. These may take the form of premature ventricular contractions, ventricular tachycardia, or even ventricular fibrillation. Lidocaine should be readily available whenever administering isoproterenol.

It is important to be careful when administering isoproterenol. Like epinephrine, it significantly increases myocardial oxygen demand. The increase in myocardial oxygen uptake may increase myocardial infarction size. In patients who have not suffered a myocardial infarction, isoproterenol may cause myocardial ischemia. External pacing, if available, should be used instead of isoproterenol.

Side Effects

Isoproterenol can cause nervousness, headache, tremor, dysrhythmias, hypertension, angina, nausea, and vomiting. Many of these side effects are dose-related.

Interactions

Isoproterenol can be deactivated by alkaline solutions such as sodium bicarbonate. It should be used with caution in patients with digitalis toxicity as it may aggravate tachydysrhythmias.

Dosage

One milligram of isoproterenol should be diluted in 500 milliliters of D_5W. This will give a concentration of 2 micrograms per milliliter. It should be titrated until the desired heart rate is attained or until signs of ventricular irritability, such as premature ventricular contractions, occur. The recommended infusion rate is 2 to 10 micrograms per minute (see Figure 7-2).

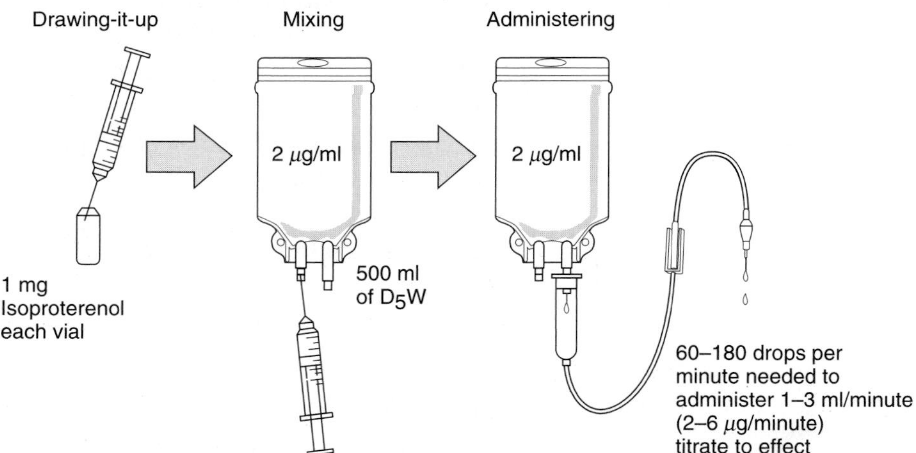

Figure 7-2 Preparation of isoproterenol infusion.

Because of its potency, isoproterenol should only be given by IV infusion. An established IV line, into which the isoproterenol is piggybacked, should be maintained.

How Supplied

Isoproterenol is supplied in ampules containing 1 milligram in either 1 milliliter or 5 milliliters of solvent. Prefilled syringes, designed especially for IV infusion preparation, are available.

Dopamine (Intropin)

Class: Sympathetic Agonist

Description

Dopamine is a naturally occurring catecholamine. It is a chemical precursor of norepinephrine. It acts on α, β_1, and dopaminergic adrenergic receptors. Its effect on α receptors is dose-dependent.

Mechanism of Action

Dopamine is one of the most frequently used agents in the treatment of hypotension associated with cardiogenic shock. It is chemically related to both epinephrine and norepinephrine and increases blood pressure by acting on both α and β_1 adrenergic receptors. Dopamine's effect on β_1 receptors causes a positive inotropic effect on the heart. It does not increase myocardial oxygen demand as much as isoproterenol and epinephrine and does not have the same powerful chronotropic effects. Dopamine also acts on α adrenergic receptors causing peripheral vasoconstriction. Unlike norepinephrine, when used in therapeutic dosages dopamine maintains renal and mesenteric blood flow because of its effect on the dopaminergic receptors. For these reasons, dopamine is the most commonly used vasopressor. Dopamine will increase both the systolic blood pressure and the pulse pressure (the difference between the systolic and diastolic blood pressures), but, as a rule, there is usually less effect on the diastolic pressure.

Indications

- Hemodynamically significant hypotension (systolic blood pressure of 70–100 mmHg) not resulting from hypovolemia
- Cardiogenic shock

Contraindications

Dopamine should not be used as the sole agent in the management of hypovolemic shock unless fluid resuscitation is well under way. Dopamine should not be used in patients with known pheochromocytoma (a tumor of the adrenal gland).

Precautions

Dopamine will increase the heart rate and can induce or worsen supraventricular and ventricular arrhythmias. Whenever the dosage of dopamine surpasses 20 micrograms/kilogram/minute, its α effects predominate and it functions very much like norepinephrine. Dopamine, like the other catecholamines, should not be administered in the presence of tachyarrhythmias or ventricular fibrillation.

Side Effects

Dopamine can cause nervousness, headache, dysrhythmias, palpitations, chest pain, dyspnea, nausea, and vomiting. Many of these side effects are dose-related.

Interactions

Like all of the catecholamines, dopamine can be deactivated by alkaline solutions such as sodium bicarbonate. If the patient is taking monoamine oxidase inhibitors (a type of antidepressant), the dose should then be reduced. Dopamine may cause hypotension when used concomitantly with phenytoin (Dilantin).

Dosage

The standard method of preparing a dopamine infusion is to place 800 milligrams in 500 milliliters of D_5W. This dilution can be attained by adding 400 milligrams to 250 milliliters of D_5W. This gives a concentration of 1,600 micrograms per milliliter. The effects of dopamine are dose-dependent. Table 7-6 illustrates effects based on common dosages.

The initial infusion rate is from 2 to 5 micrograms per kilogram per minute. This may be increased until blood pressure improves (see Figure 7-3). Dopamine is administered only by IV drip, which should be piggybacked into an already established IV infusion.

How Supplied

Dopamine comes in prefilled syringes, ampules, and pre-mixed bags. The standard preparation is 200 milligrams in 5 milliliters of solvent; 400-milligram preparations in 5 milliliters of solvent are also available (see Table 7-7).

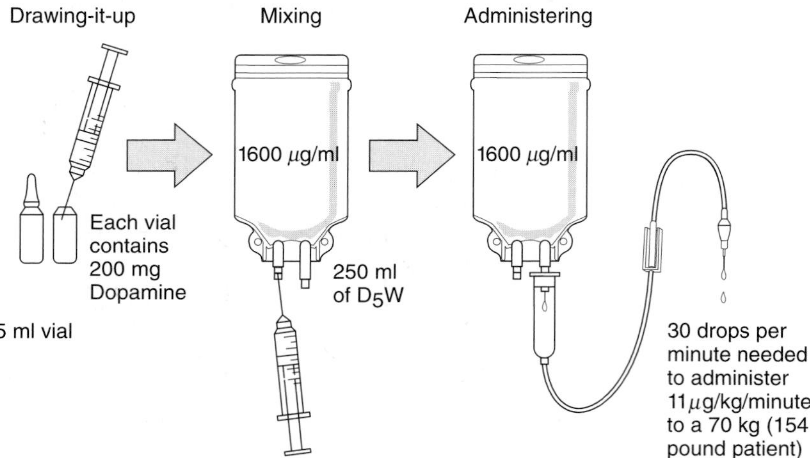

Figure 7-3 Preparation of dopamine infusion.

TABLE 7-6

Dopamine Hydrochloride (Intropin®) Dosage Phenomena

Physiological Effect	*2–5 mcg/kg/min*	*5–20 mcg/kg/min*	*More Than 20 mcg/kg/min*
Cardiac Output	No change	Increase	Increase
Stroke Volume	No change	Increase	Increase
Heart Rate	No change	There is an initial increase followed by a decrease toward normal rates as infusion continues	
Myocardial Contractility	No change	Increase	Increase
Potential for Excessive Myocardial Oxygen Demands	Low[a] Coronary blood flow increased	Low[a] Coronary blood flow increased	Data unavailable
Potential for Tachyarrhythmias	Low[a]	Low[a]	Moderate
Total Systemic Vascular Resistance	Slight decrease to no change	No change to slight increase	Increase
Renal Blood Flow	Increase	Increase	Decrease[b]
Urine Output	Increase	Increase	Decrease[b]

[a]Low but needs monitoring.

[b]Relative to peak values achieved at lower dosages.

TABLE 7-7

Dopamine Hydrochloride (Intropin®) Dosage Chart

For a concentration of 1600 μg dopamine hydrochloride/ml (800 mg Intropin per 500 ml—or—400 mg Intropin per 250 ml)

Body Wt lbs	77	88	99	110	121	132	143	154	165	176	187	198	209	220	231	242
kgs	35	40	45	50	55	60	65	70	75	80	85	90	95	100	105	110
Flow Rate in Drops[a] per Minute																
5	3.8	3.4	2.9	2.6	2.4	2.2	2.0	1.9	1.8	1.6	1.55	1.5	1.4	1.3	1.25	1.2
10	7.6	6.7	5.9	5.3	4.9	4.5	4.1	3.8	3.6	3.3	3.1	3.0	2.8	2.7	2.5	2.4
15	11	10	8.9	8.0	7.3	6.6	6.1	5.7	5.3	5.0	4.7	4.4	4.2	4.0	3.8	3.6
20	15	13	12	11	9.7	8.9	8.2	7.6	7.1	6.7	6.3	5.9	5.6	5.3	5.1	4.9
25	19	17	15	13	12	11	10	9.5	8.9	8.4	7.8	7.4	7.0	6.6	6.3	6.0
30	23	20	18	16	15	13	12	11	11	10	9.4	8.9	8.4	8.0	7.6	7.3
35	27	23	21	19	17	16	14	13	12	12	11	10	9.8	9.3	8.9	8.5
40	31	27	24	21	19	18	16	15	14	13	13	12	11	11	10	9.7
45	34	30	27	24	22	20	18	17	16	15	14	13	13	12	11	11
50	38	33	30	27	24	22	21	19	18	17	16	15	14	13	13	12
55	42	37	33	29	27	24	23	21	20	18	17	16	15	15	14	13
60	46	40	36	32	29	27	25	23	21	20	19	18	17	16	15	15
70	53	47	42	37	34	31	29	27	25	23	22	21	20	19	18	17
80	61	53	47	43	39	36	33	31	28	27	25	24	23	21	20	19
90	69	60	53	48	44	40	37	34	32	30	28	27	25	24	23	22
100	76	67	59	53	49	45	41	38	36	33	31	30	28	27	25	24

Dosage = mcg Dopamine hydrochloride/kg/min

[a]Based on a microdrip calibration of 60 drops equal to 1.0 milliliter.

Note: All dosages of 10 μg/kg/min and greater have been rounded off to the nearest μg/kg/min.

Dobutamine (Dobutrex)

Class: Sympathetic Agonist

Description

Dobutamine is a synthetic catecholamine. It acts primarily on β_1 receptors but is less of a β agonist than isoproterenol.

Mechanism of Action

Dobutamine increases the force of the systolic contraction (positive inotropic effect) with little chronotropic activity. For these reasons, it is useful in the management of congestive heart failure when an increase in heart rate is not desired.

Indication

- Short-term management of congestive heart failure when an increased cardiac output, without an increase in cardiac rate, is desired

Contraindications

Dobutamine should not be used as the sole agent in hypovolemic shock unless fluid resuscitation is well under way. To increase cardiac output in severe emergencies, like cardiogenic shock, dopamine is the preferred agent.

Precautions

Tachycardia and an increase in the systolic blood pressure are common following the administration of dobutamine. Increases in heart rate of more than 10 percent may induce or exacerbate myocardial ischemia. Premature ventricular contractions (PVCs) can occur in conjunction with dobutamine administration. Lidocaine should be readily available. As with any sympathomimetic, blood pressure should be monitored.

Side Effects

Dobutamine can cause nervousness, headache, hypertension, dysrhythmias, palpitations, chest pain, dyspnea, nausea, and vomiting. Many of these side effects are dose-related.

Interactions

Dobutamine may be ineffective when administered to patients on beta blockers as these medications can block the β receptors on which dobutamine acts. Patients taking tricyclic antidepressants are at increased risk of hypertension with dobutamine administration.

Dosage

The desired dosage range for dobutamine is between 2 and 20 micrograms per kilogram per minute. Dobutamine should be administered according to the patient's response (see Figure 7-4).

Dobutamine should be diluted in either 500 milliliters or 1 liter of D_5W and administered via IV infusion..

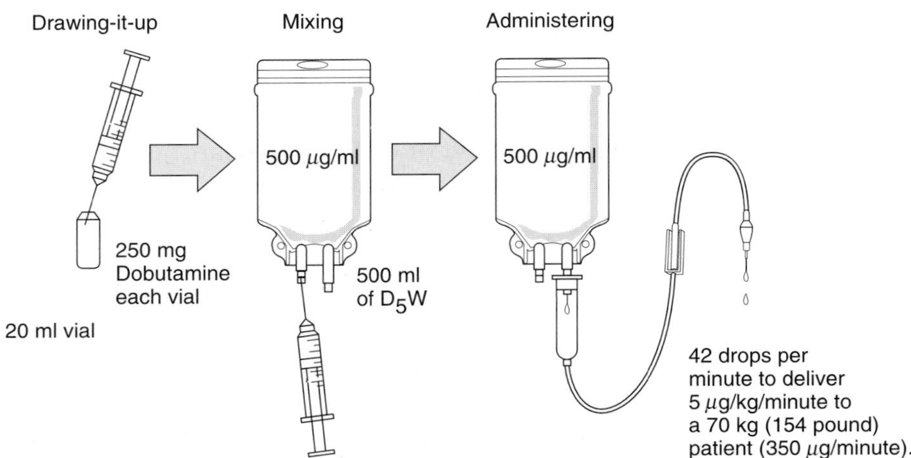

Figure 7-4 Preparation of dobutamine infusion.

How Supplied

Dobutamine is supplied in 20-milliliter ampules containing 250 milligrams of the drug. 250 milligrams is usually placed in 500 milliliters of solvent to give a concentration of 0.5 milligram (500 micrograms) per milliliter

Metaraminol (Aramine)

Class: Sympathetic Agonist

Description

Metaraminol is a sympathetic agonist with effects similar to norepinephrine. It is much less potent than norepinephrine but has a more prolonged action.

Mechanism of Action

Although metaraminol is not a catecholamine, it is used in the treatment of hypotensive states. It is both an α and β agonist. Its vasopressor properties are primarily derived from its action on endogenous catecholamines. It causes the release of norepinephrine from sympathetic nerve endings. In recent years metaraminol has fallen into disuse, with dopamine being the preferred agent.

Indication

- Hemodynamically significant hypotension not due to hypovolemia

Contraindications

Metaraminol should not be used in hypovolemia unless fluid resuscitation is well under way.

Precautions

Rapid administration can cause hypertension. Ventricular ectopic activity, especially PVCs, has been known to occur with the administration of metaraminol. Lidocaine should be readily available.

Side Effects

Metaraminol can cause anxiety, tremulousness, headache, dizziness, nausea, and vomiting. It can also cause bradycardia as a reflex response to increased peripheral vasoconstriction.

Interactions

Metaraminol can be deactivated by alkaline solutions such as sodium bicarbonate. Concomitant administration with beta blockers can result in markedly elevated blood pressure. Caution should be used when administering metaraminol to patients on digitalis.

Dosage

Two hundred milligrams of metaraminol should be placed into 500 milligrams of D_5W. This will give a dilution of 0.4 milligrams per milliliter. The infusion rate should be titrated according to the blood pressure response. An IV infusion should already be established into which the metaraminol should be piggybacked.

Metaraminol can be administered intramuscularly when an IV cannot be established. The initial adult dose should be 5–10 mg IM.

Many agents, such as dopamine, are far superior to metaraminol and should be used initially.

How Supplied

Metaraminol comes in a concentration of 10 milligrams per milliliter. Ampules contain either 1 or 10 milliliters. Thus, each ampule will contain 10 and 100 milligrams, respectively.

Amrinone (Inocor)

Class: Inotrope (phosphodiesterase inhibitor)

Description

Amrinone is a rapidly-acting inotropic agent. It is a phosphodiesterase inhibitor and does not act on adrenergic receptors.

Mechanism of Action

Amrinone, like the other medications previously presented, increases cardiac output promptly following intravenous administration. It is a positive inotrope and does possess some vasodilatory properties. Unlike the other medications, however, it does not stimulate either α- or β-adrenergic receptors. The exact mechanism by which amrinone increases blood pressure is not well understood. It does not increase cardiac output in the same manner as the digitalis preparations. Clinically, amrinone resembles dobutamine in its effects. Because amrinone does not stimulate β-adrenergic receptors, it may be effective in cases of congestive heart failure that do not respond to dobutamine or one of the other inotropic agents.

Indication

- Short-term management of severe congestive heart failure refractory to diuretics, vasodilators, and conventional inotropic agents

Contraindications

Amrinone should not be administered to patients with a known hypersensitivity to the drug or to the bisulfite class of chemicals.

Precautions

Amrinone should not be used in cases of congestive heart failure occurring immediately after myocardial infarction. Like dobutamine, amrinone may increase myocardial ischemia. As with the other inotropic agents, the blood pressure, pulse, and electrocardiogram (EKG) should be constantly monitored.

Amrinone should not be diluted in solutions containing dextrose (that is, D_5W). Amrinone should be diluted with 0.9% sodium chloride (normal saline) or 0.45% sodium chloride (1/2 normal saline).

Side Effects

Amrinone can cause arrhythmias, hypotension, nausea, vomiting, abdominal pain, and decreased platelets (thrombocytopenia).

Interactions

Furosemide (Lasix) should not be administered into an intravenous line delivering amrinone. A chemical reaction occurs between these two drugs resulting in the formation of a precipitate in the intravenous line. Amrinone should not be diluted in solutions containing dextrose.

Dosage

Therapy should be initiated with an IV bolus of 0.75 milligrams per kilogram given slowly during a 2- to 5-minute interval (see Figure 7-5). This should be followed by a maintenance infusion of 2 to 15 micrograms per kilogram per minute. This infusion can be prepared by placing one ampule (100 milli-

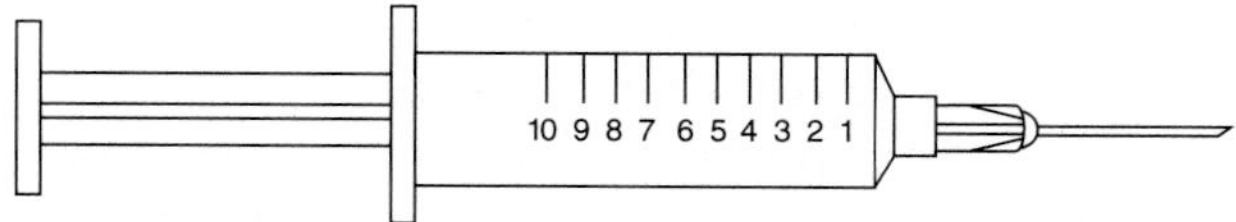

Figure 7-5 Loading bolus of amrinone.

grams) in 500 milliliters of normal saline solution. This will give a concentration of 0.2 milligram per milliliter (200 micrograms per milliliter) (see Figure 7-6).

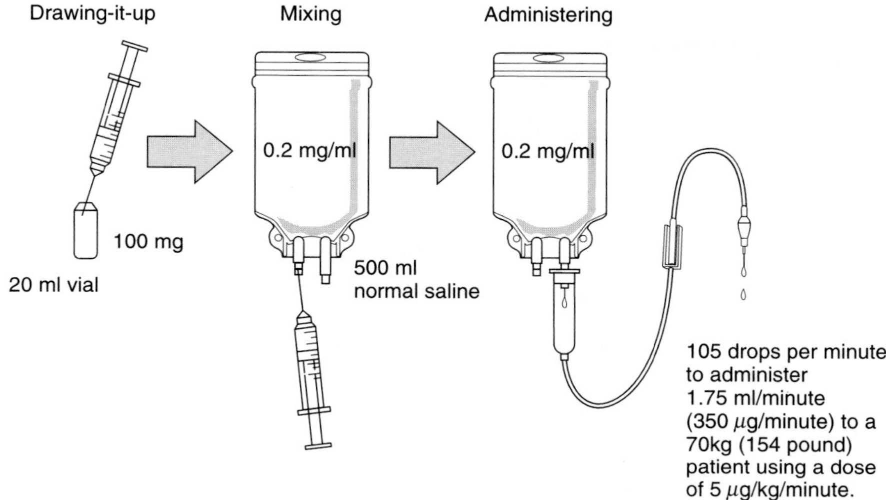

Figure 7-6 Preparation of amrinone infusion.

An additional bolus of 0.75 milligram per kilogram given slowly over 2 to 3 minutes can be given 30 minutes later if required.

The overall rate of amrinone administration must be carefully adjusted and based on the patient's clinical response.

Amrinone should only be administered by the IV route, either as a bolus or infusion, as described earlier.

How Supplied

Amrinone is supplied in 20-milliliter ampules containing 5 milligrams per milliliter.

SYMPATHETIC BLOCKERS

Sympathetic blockers are a unique class of drugs that antagonize adrenergic receptor sites. Certain drugs will block only α receptors, whereas others block only β receptors. Some of the β blockers are so selective that they block only β_1 or β_2 receptors. The drugs that block the β receptors are receiving the most use. They are useful in the treatment of hypertension, cardiac arrhythmias, and angina pectoris. The most popular sympathetic blocker is propranolol (Inderal), a nonselective beta blocker that is both a β_1 and β_2 antagonist. Although used selectively in emergency medicine, propranolol does play a role in the treatment of certain cardiac arrhythmias.

It is thought that some ventricular arrhythmias, such as ventricular tachycardia and recurrent ventricular fibrillation, can be caused by excessive β stimulation. Administration of propranolol may inhibit these arrhythmias. Propranolol should not be used in combination with verapamil. The concomitant blocking of slow calcium channels by verapamil, and the β receptor antagonism caused by propranolol, may result in asystole. (Verapamil will be discussed in detail on pages 150–151.)

Propranolol (Inderal)

Class: Non-selective Beta Blocker

Description

Propranolol is a non-selective β antagonist. It inhibits the effects of circulating catecholamines.

Mechanism of Action

Propranolol non-selectively blocks both β_1 and β_2 adrenergic receptors. It causes a reduction in heart rate (negative chronotropic effect), cardiac contractile force (negative inotropic effect), blood pressure, and myocardial oxygen demand. It is useful in treating recurrent ventricular tachycardia and recurrent ventricular fibrillation that does not respond to lidocaine. It may also be of value in the treatment of tachyarrhythmias resulting from digitalis toxicity and selected supraventricular tachycardias.

Indications

- Ventricular tachycardia refractory to lidocaine and bretylium
- Recurrent ventricular fibrillation refractory to lidocaine and bretylium
- Selected supraventricular tachyarrhythmias

Contraindications

Propranolol is contraindicated in patients with bradycardia, a history of asthma, chronic obstructive pulmonary disease (COPD), and congestive heart failure.

Precautions

Because propranolol may decrease heart rate, atropine should be readily available. In bradycardia refractory to atropine, transcutaneous pacing should be utilized. Propranolol should be used with caution in diabetics as it may mask the signs and symptoms of hypoglycemia. Glucagon can be used in the management of severe beta blocker overdose. It helps to maintain the heart rate and blood pressure.

Side Effects

Propranolol may cause bradycardia, hypotension, lethargy, congestive heart failure, dyspnea, wheezing, and weakness.

Interactions

Propranolol should not be administered to patients who have received intravenous verapamil. It should be used with caution in patients on antihypertensive agents.

Dosage

Propranolol may produce significant, even life-threatening, side effects. When administered intravenously, care must be taken to dilute 1 milligram in 10 milliliters of D_5W. The standard dosage is 1 to 3 milligrams, diluted in 10 to 30 milliliters of D_5W. Propranolol should be administered *slowly* (over 2–5 minutes). Propranolol should not be administered faster than 1 mg/minute. Throughout administration, careful blood pressure monitoring is required. Like all drugs acting on the heart, it should only be administered to patients who are on cardiac monitors. The dosage may be repeated, again under careful monitoring, until a maximum of 3 to 5 milligrams has been administered.

Propranolol should be administered intravenously in the treatment of life-threatening tachyarrhythmias.

How Supplied

The standard preparation of propranolol comes in 1 milliliter vials containing 1 milligram of the drug.

Metoprolol (Lopressor)

Class: Selective Beta Blocker

Description

Metoprolol is a β antagonist that blocks both β_1 and β_2 adrenergic receptors. Unlike propranolol, however, metoprolol is selective for β_1 adrenergic receptors.

Mechanism of Action

Metoprolol causes a reduction in heart rate, systolic blood pressure, and cardiac output following administration. This is due to its selective effects on β_1 adrenergic receptors. In addition, metoprolol appears to inhibit tachycardia, especially in the period following an acute myocardial infarction. Because of these effects, metoprolol is thought to be protective of the heart and is used to reduce potential complications in selected patients who have suffered an acute myocardial infarction. Metoprolol has proved effective in reducing the incidence of ventricular fibrillation and chest pain in these patients, thus reducing overall patient mortality in the post-myocardial infarction period.

Indication

- Patients with suspected or definite acute myocardial infarction who are hemodynamically stable

Contraindications

Metoprolol is contraindicated in any patient with a heart rate of less than 45 beats per minute, a systolic blood pressure less than 100 millimeters of mercury, or congestive heart failure. In addition, metoprolol is contraindicated in patients with first-degree heart block with a PR interval greater than 0.24 second, a second-degree heart block (either Mobitz I or Mobitz II), or third-degree block. It is also contraindicated in any patient showing either early or late signs of shock.

Metoprolol should not be administered to any patient with a history of asthma or bronchospastic disease in the prehospital setting.

Precautions

The blood pressure, pulse rate, EKG, and respiratory status should be continuously monitored during metoprolol therapy. Prehospital personnel should be alert for signs and symptoms of congestive heart failure, bradycardia, shock, heart block, or bronchospasm when administering metoprolol. The presence of any of these signs or symptoms is an indication for discontinuing the medication.

Side Effects

Metoprolol may cause bradycardia, hypotension, lethargy, congestive heart failure, dyspnea, wheezing, and weakness.

Interactions

Metoprolol should not be administered to patients who have received intravenous verapamil. It should be administered with caution to patients on antihypertensive agents.

Dosage

When administered following an acute myocardial infarction, an initial bolus of 5 milligrams metoprolol should be given by slow IV injection. If the vital signs remain stable, a second 5-milligram bolus should be given 2 minutes after the first. Finally, if the first two boluses are well tolerated, a third 5-milligram bolus should be administered 2 minutes after the second bolus. The total dose should not exceed 15 milligrams. As mentioned previously, the vital signs and EKG should be constantly monitored.

Metoprolol should only be administered by slow IV injection in the manner described earlier.

How Supplied

Metoprolol (Lopressor) is supplied in ampules and prefilled syringes containing 5 milligrams of the drug in 5 milliliters of solvent.

Labetalol (Trandate, Normodyne)

Class: Non-selective Beta Blocker

Description

Labetalol is a non-selective β blocker and a selective α_1 blocker.

Mechanism of Action

Labetalol differs considerably in its action from the β blockers previously presented. Like propranolol, labetalol is a non-selective β adrenergic antagonist showing no preference for either β_1 or β_2 receptors. However, unlike the other β blockers, labetalol also blocks α_1 adrenergic receptors. Blockage of α_1 receptors inhibits peripheral vasoconstriction, thus causing peripheral vasodilatation. Because of these properties, labetalol is a potent agent for lowering blood pressure in cases of hypertensive crisis. It does this by decreasing cardiac output through its β_1 blocking properties and by causing peripheral vasodilatation through its α_1 blocking properties.

Indication

- Labetalol is indicated for the acute management of hypertensive crisis.

Contraindications

Labetalol is contraindicated in patients with bronchial asthma, congestive heart failure, heart block, bradycardia, or cardiogenic shock.

Precautions

As with all β blockers the blood pressure, pulse rate, EKG, and respiratory status should be continuously monitored. Prehospital personnel should be alert for signs and symptoms of congestive heart failure, bradycardia, shock, heart block, or bronchospasm when administering labetalol. The appearance of any of these signs or symptoms is an indication for discontinuing the drug.

Because of the effects of labetalol on β_1 receptors, postural hypotension might occur and should be anticipated. The patient should be supine at all times during drug administration.

Side Effects

Labetalol may cause bradycardia, hypotension, lethargy, congestive heart failure, dyspnea, wheezing, and weakness.

Interactions

Labetalol should not be administered to patients who have received intravenous verapamil. It should be administered with caution to patients on antihypertensive agents.

Dosage

The following are two accepted methods of administering labetalol in the treatment of hypertensive crisis:

1. Twenty milligrams of labetalol can be administered by slow IV injection over 2 minutes. Immediately before the injection and at 5 and 10 minutes after the injection, the supine blood pressure should be recorded. Additional injections of 40 milligrams can be given every 10 minutes until a desired supine blood pressure is achieved or 300 milligrams of the drug has been given (see Figure 7-7).

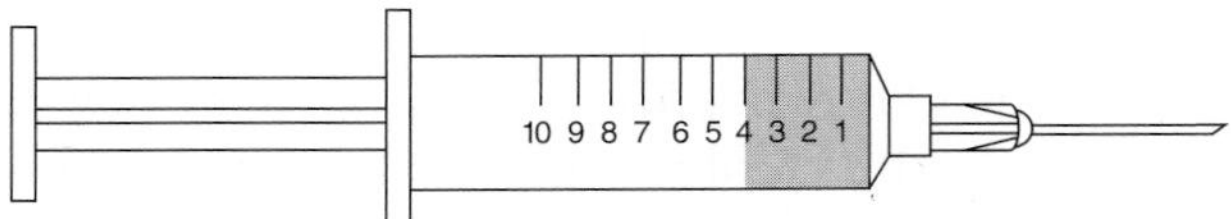

Figure 7-7 Bolus administration of labetalol.

2. Two ampules (200 milligrams) of labetalol can be added to 250 milliliters of D_5W. This gives a concentration of 0.8 milligram per milliliter. This solution should be administered at a rate of 2 milligrams per minute (2.5 milliliters per minute). The blood pressure should be continuously monitored (see Figure 7-8).

Labetalol should be administered by slow IV injection or infusion as described above.

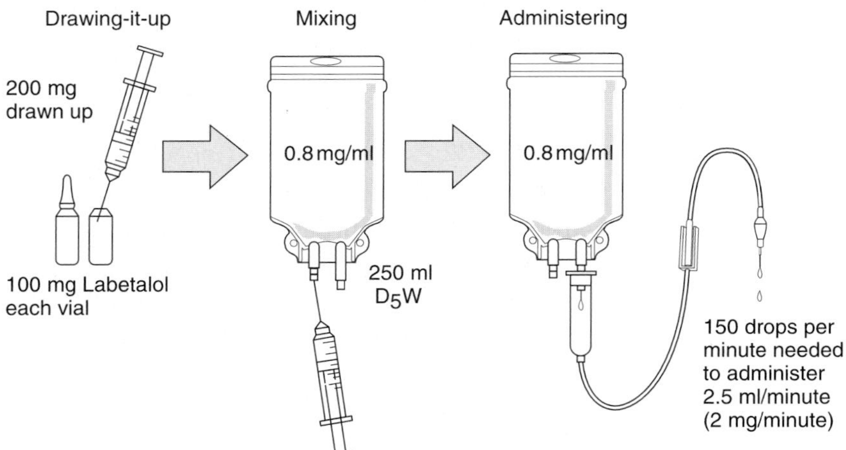

Figure 7-8 Preparation of labetalol infusion.

How Supplied

Labetalol (Trandate, Normodyne) is supplied in ampules containing 100 milligrams in 20 milliliters of solvent (5 milligrams per milliliter).

Esmolol (Brevibloc)

Class: Selective Beta Blocker

Description

Esmolol is a β_1 selective (cardioselective) β blocker with a very short half-life.

Mechanism of Action

Esmolol is a selective β_1 blocker. It has a very rapid onset and a short duration of action (9 minutes). Esmolol is used to slow rapid heart rates in patients with supraventricular tachycardia including atrial flutter and atrial fibrillation. Patients with extremely rapid heart rates can develop congestive heart failure or angina because the rapid heart rate may prevent adequate filling of the ventricles. The duration of action of esmolol is so brief that it should be administered by intravenous infusion.

Indication

- Supraventricular tachycardia (including atrial fibrillation and atrial flutter) accompanied by a rapid ventricular rate

Contraindications

Esmolol should not be used in patients with sinus bradycardia, heart block greater than first degree, cardiogenic shock, or overt congestive heart failure.

Precautions

A significant number of patients receiving esmolol may experience hypotension (systolic less than 90 millimeters of mercury). Hypotension can occur at any dose but primarily is dose-related. If hypotension develops, the dosage should be reduced.

Patients with congestive heart failure may have worsening of their symptoms with esmolol. Because esmolol can potentially depress cardiac contractility, it should be used with extreme caution in patients prone to congestive heart failure.

Patients with bronchospastic disease (asthma, COPD) should not receive β blockers, including esmolol, unless the medical control physician deems the benefits outweigh the risks.

Side Effects

Esmolol may cause bradycardia, dizziness, hypotension, lethargy, congestive heart failure, dyspnea, wheezing, and weakness.

Interactions

Esmolol should not be administered to patients who have received intravenous verapamil. It should be administered with caution to patients on antihypertensive agents. Morphine can increase the blood levels of esmolol, requiring a reduction in dosage. Esmolol should not be used in cases of supraventricular tachycardia caused by epinephrine, dopamine, and norepinephrine.

Dosage

Esmolol therapy is started by administering a loading dose of 500 micrograms per kilogram per minute for 1 minute. After 1 minute this should be reduced to a maintenance dose of 50 micrograms per kilogram per minute for 4 minutes. If an adequate therapeutic effect is not seen, repeat the loading dose for 1 minute, and then increase the maintenance dose to 100 micrograms per kilogram per minute. The dose can be titrated at 4-minute intervals by repeating the loading dose for 1 minute and increasing the maintenance dose by 50 micrograms per kilogram per minute at 4-minute intervals until the desired effect is obtained. The maintenance dose should not exceed 200 micrograms per kilogram per minute. In the event of an adverse reaction, the dose of esmolol can be reduced or discontinued immediately (see Figure 7-9).

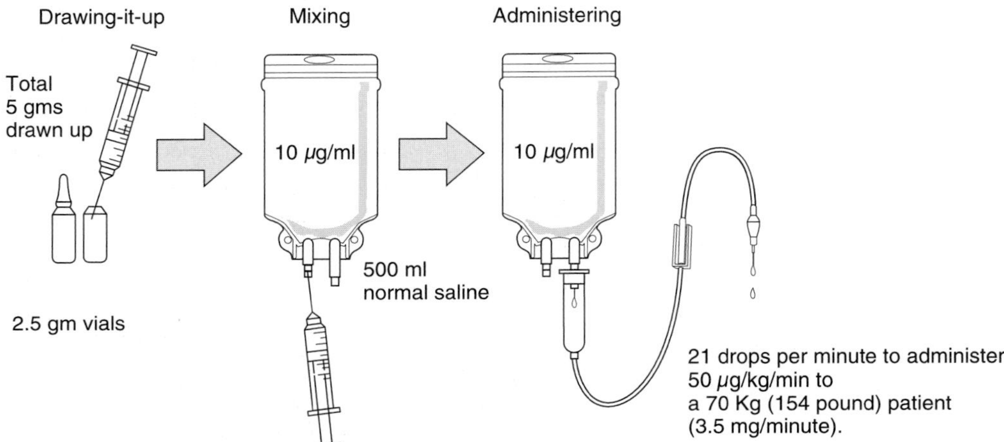

Figure 7-9 Administration of esmolol (Brevibloc).

The esmolol infusion is prepared by placing two 2.5-gram ampules of esmolol in 500 milliliters of 5% dextrose, normal saline, or lactated Ringer's. An alternative method is to place one 2.5-gram ampule in 250 milliliters of fluid. Either will provide a 10-milligrams per milliliter concentration.

Esmolol should be administered intravenously.

How Supplied

Esmolol is supplied in 100-milligram vials containing 100 milligrams in 10 milliliters (10 milligrams per milliliter) for loading-dose administration. It is also supplied in 2.5-gram vials for preparation of the infusion.

The 2.5-gram vials are for preparation of the infusion only, not for intravenous injection.

ANTIARRHYTHMICS

Many different drugs are useful in the treatment and prevention of cardiac arrhythmias. Some drugs are useful in the treatment of atrial arrhythmias, whereas others are useful in the treatment of ventricular arrhythmias. As a result, it is essential to distinguish between these two types of arrhythmias. The common antiarrhythmic drugs are classified based on their action (see Table 7-8).

The most common antiarrhythmic drugs used in emergency medicine include the following:

Lidocaine (Xylocaine). Lidocaine is the drug of choice in the treatment of ventricular tachycardia and malignant premature ventricular contractions.

Procainamide (Pronestyl). Procainamide, like lidocaine, is useful in the suppression of ventricular arrhythmias. It is generally not a first-line drug, and its use is reserved for arrhythmias that do not respond to lidocaine.

Bretylium Tosylate (Bretylol). Bretylium is used in the treatment of ventricular fibrillation that is refractory to lidocaine.

Adenosine (Adenocard). Adenosine is a naturally occurring nucleoside useful in the treatment of supraventricular tachycardias.

Verapamil (Isoptin). Verapamil is a slow channel calcium blocker. It is a first-line drug used in the treatment of paroxysmal supraventricular tachycardia and other atrial arrhythmias.

TABLE 7-8

Classification of Antiarrhythmic Agents

Class	*Drugs*
I	A. Procainamide (Pronestyl®) Disopyramide (Norpace®) Quinidine (Quiniglute®)
	B. Lidocaine (Xylocaine®) Phenytoin (Dilantin®) Mexilitine (Mexitil®) Tocainide (Tonocard®)
	C. Flecanide (Tambocor®) Encainide (Enkaid®)
II	Propranolol (Inderal®) Atenolol (Tenormin®) Labetolol (Trandate®, Normodyne®) Metoprolol (Lopressor®) Esmolol (Brevibloc®)
III	Bretylium (Bretylol®) Amiodarone (Cordarone®)
IV	Verapamil (Isoptin®, Calan®) Diltiazem (Cardizem®) Nefedipine (Procardia®) Nicardipine (Cardene®)

Diltiazem (Cardizem). Diltiazem is a calcium channel blocker and is used to slow the rapid ventricular rate that often accompanies atrial flutter and atrial fibrillation.

Phenytoin (Dilantin). Phenytoin is infrequently used in the emergency setting as an antiarrhythmic agent. It has proven effectiveness, however, in the management of life-threatening arrhythmias resulting from digitalis toxicity.

Edrophonium Chloride (Tensilon). Edrophonium chloride is an anticholinesterase agent that has proven effectiveness in terminating paroxysmal supraventricular tachycardias that do not respond to vagal maneuvers. Its usage is rapidly declining with verapamil and adenosine being preferred.

Magnesium Sulfate. Magnesium is a cofactor in many of the chemical and enzyme reactions that occur in the body. Magnesium deficiency is associated with a high frequency of cardiac arrhythmias and sudden death. Pharmacologically, it functions like a physiological calcium channel blocker.

Propranolol (Inderal). Propranolol, discussed in the previous section, plays a role in the treatment of supraventricular arrhythmias. Students are encouraged to review the section on propranolol and integrate it with the drugs mentioned here.

Lidocaine (Xylocaine)

Class: Antiarrhythmic

Description

Lidocaine is an amide-type local anesthetic. It is frequently used to treat life-threatening ventricular dysrhythmias.

Mechanism of Action

Lidocaine is probably the most frequently used antiarrhythmic agent in the treatment of life-threatening cardiac emergencies. Moreover, it has been shown to be effective in suppressing premature ventricular contractions, in treating ventricular tachycardia and some cases of ventricular fibrillation, and in increasing the fibrillation threshold in acute myocardial infarction.

Lidocaine depresses depolarization and automaticity in the ventricles. It has very little effect on atrial tissues. In therapeutic doses it does not slow AV conduction and does not depress myocardial contractility. The most common cause of ventricular arrhythmias is acute myocardial infarction. Lidocaine suppresses ventricular ectopy in the setting of myocardial infarction and increases the ventricular fibrillation threshold. This prevents PVCs from inducing ventricular fibrillation. After acute myocardial infarction, the ventricular fibrillation threshold is often significantly reduced. Moreover, because electrical defibrillation tends to cause ventricular irritability, patients who have been successfully defibrillated should be treated with lidocaine.

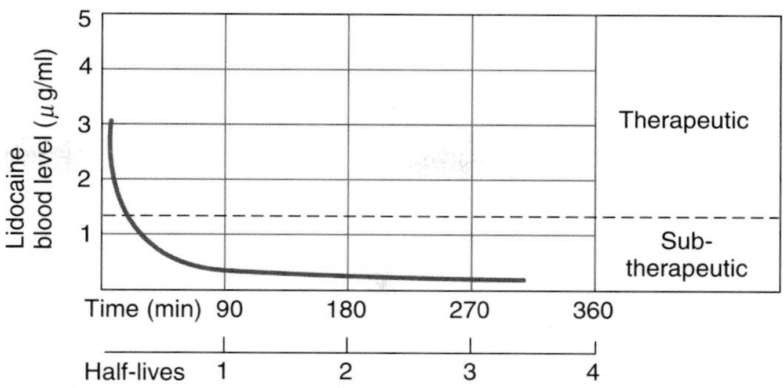

Figure 7-10 Blood levels of lidocaine following bolus without drip.

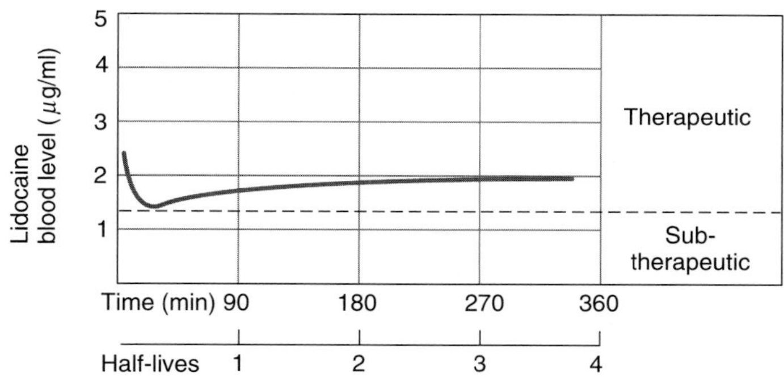

Figure 7-11 Blood levels of lidocaine following bolus with drip.

Lidocaine is most apt to suppress ventricular arrhythmias only when the level of the drug in the blood is between 1.5 and 6.0 micrograms per milliliter of blood. A 75-milligram to 100-milligram bolus of lidocaine will maintain adequate blood levels for only 20 minutes (see Figure 7-10). Therefore, once an arrhythmia is suppressed, the lidocaine bolus should be followed by a 2- to 4-milligrams per minute infusion to assure therapeutic blood levels (see Figure 7-11). It is important to distinguish patterns of premature ventricular contractions that are likely to lead to serious arrhythmias. Premature ventricular contractions that may lead to life-threatening arrhythmias are called "malignant premature ventricular contractions." These include the following:

- More than six unifocal PVCs per minute
- PVCs that appear to be coming from more than one ectopic focus (for example, multifocal PVCs)
- PVCs that occur in couplets (two PVCs together without a normal QRS complex in between)
- Runs of more than two PVCs, or ventricular tachycardia PVCs falling in the vulnerable period of the preceding normal complex (R on T phenomena)

The aforementioned premature ventricular contractions, as well as ventricular tachycardia and ventricular fibrillation, must be treated vigorously with lidocaine.

Indications

- Ventricular tachycardia
- Ventricular fibrillation
- Malignant premature ventricular contractions

Contraindications

Lidocaine is usually contraindicated in second-degree Mobitz II and third-degree blocks. Lidocaine slows conduction of the electrical impulse from the atria to the ventricles. Decreased ventricular rates may accompany high-grade heart block, resulting in escape beats that are premature ventricular contractions. Whenever premature ventricular contractions occur in conjunction with bradycardia (heart rate less than 60), the bradycardia should be treated first. The drug of choice is atropine sulfate followed by external pacing if atropine is not effective. If PVCs are still present after increasing the rate, lidocaine should be administered.

Precautions

Central nervous system depression may occur when the dosage exceeds 300 milligrams per hour. Symptoms of central nervous system depression include a decreased level of consciousness, irritability, confusion, muscle twitching, and, eventually, seizures. Exceedingly high doses can result in coma and death.

Routine prophylactic lidocaine therapy in patients with acute myocardial infarction is no longer recommended. However, it may be used in conjunction with thrombolytic therapy to suppress expected reperfusion dysrhythmias.

Side Effects

Lidocaine may cause drowsiness, seizures, confusion, hypotension, bradycardia, heart blocks, nausea, vomiting, and respiratory and cardiac arrest.

Interactions

Lidocaine should be used with caution when administering concomitantly with procainamide, phenytoin, quinidine, and β blockers as drug toxicity may result.

Dosage

- ***Refractory Ventricular Fibrillation and Pulseless Ventricular Tachycardia***. The initial dose of lidocaine should be 1.0–1.5 milligram per kilogram body weight. Lidocaine can be repeated every 3–5 minutes at a dose of 0.5–0.75 mg/kg to a maximum of 3.0 mg/kg. A single bolus dose of 1.5 mg/kg in cardiac arrest is generally acceptable as plasma lidocaine levels will remain therapeutic be-

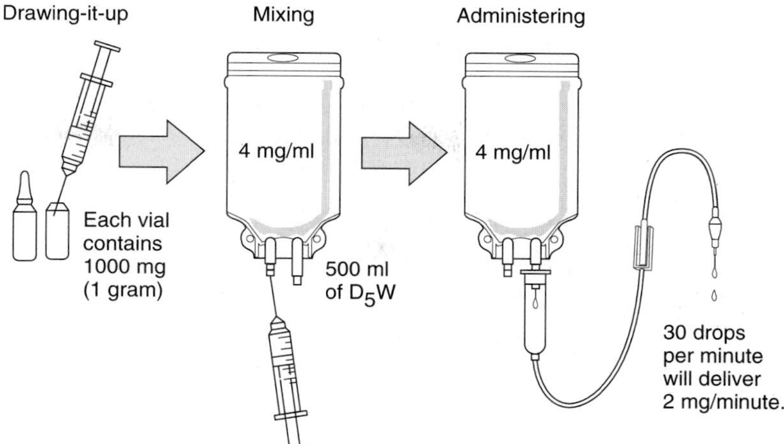

Figure 7-12 Preparation of lidocaine infusion.

cause of reduced drug elimination during CPR. Only bolus therapy should be used during CPR. Once a patient has been resuscitated, IV infusion therapy can be started to maintain therapeutic blood levels of the drug.

- ***Ventricular Tachycardia with a Pulse and Malignant PVCs.*** The initial dose of lidocaine should be 1.0–1.5 milligram per kilogram. Repeat boluses of 0.5–0.75 mg/kg can be repeated every 5–10 minutes as required to a maximum dose of 3.0 mg/kg. Once the arrhythmia has been suppressed, a lidocaine drip should be initiated at 2–4 mg/minute.

The dosage of lidocaine should be reduced 50% in patients over 70 years of age and in patients with liver disease, heart failure, bradycardias, or conduction disturbances.

Lidocaine is generally given in an IV bolus followed by an infusion (see Figure 7-12). It can also be given endotracheally, however, when an IV line cannot be established. The dose should be increased 2 to 2.5 times the intravenous dose when administering it endotracheally. A preparation of lidocaine is also available that can be given intramuscularly for ventricular arrhythmias. This should be reserved for times when an IV line cannot be established and the patient is not intubated.

How Supplied

Lidocaine is supplied in the following dosages: Prefilled syringes—100 milligrams in 5 milliliters of solvent 1- and 2-gram additive syringes; ampules—100 milligrams in 5 milliliters of solvent 1- and 2-gram vials (in 30 milliliters of solvent); and premixed bags containing 1 to 2 grams in 500 milliliters of 5% dextrose.

CASE PRESENTATION

EMS is dispatched to a residence for a man with chest pain. The patient is conscious, breathing, and has a history of angina. Upon arrival paramedics are directed to a 60-year-old male (weight 80 kg) sitting on a chair in the kitchen. The patient is pale, cool, and diaphoretic.

On Examination

CNS: The patient is conscious, alert, and oriented × 4

Resp: Respirations are 22 and shallow, lung sounds clear bilaterally, trachea is midline, no signs of trauma

CVS: Carotid and radial pulses are weak and irregular; skin is pale, cool, and diaphoretic

ABD: Soft and non-tender

Vitals:

Pulse: 104/min, irregular, weak

Resp: 22/min, shallow

BP: 136/82

SpO_2: 90%

ECG: Regular sinus rhythm with unifocal PVCs at 8/min

HX:
- **P** no provoking factors
- **Q** squeezing pain
- **R** radiating to back
- **S** 7/10, worst pain ever
- **T** started suddenly 1 hour ago

Past Hx: The patient's wife states that her husband has had several episodes of chest pain brought on by exertion over the past week. He was diagnosed with angina 6 years ago. He has nitro spray, which he has used 4 times today. The patient takes nitro spray, Inderal, Synthroid, and Tylenol #3 for headaches.

Treatment

Oxygen was administered by non-rebreather at 12 l/min. An IV was started with an 18 gauge catheter in the left arm and run TKO. The paramedics noticed a change on the ECG monitor to ventricular trigeminy. The patient was not given nitro since he had already taken four nitro with no relief and the nitro was not expired. 2.5 mg of morphine was administered. Lidocaine 120 mg was given IV push. Transport to the hospital was initiated. After 5 minutes there was no change in the rhythm. Another bolus of 60 mg was given, and the drip was increased to 3 mg/min. The patient converted to a sinus rhythm with occasional unifocal PVCs. The pain was rated at 6/10 and another 2.5 mg of morphine was given.

Procainamide (Pronestyl)

Class: Antiarrhythmic

Description

Procainamide is an ester-type local anesthetic. It is frequently used to treat life-threatening ventricular dysrhythmias refractory to lidocaine.

Mechanism of Action

Procainamide is effective in suppressing ventricular ectopy. It may be effective in cases where lidocaine has not suppressed life-threatening ventricular arrhythmias. Procainamide reduces the automaticity of the various pacemaker sites in the heart. Procainamide slows intraventricular conduction to much greater degree than lidocaine.

Indications

- Persistent cardiac arrest due to ventricular fibrillation and refractory to lidocaine
- Premature ventricular contractions refractory to lidocaine
- Ventricular tachycardia refractory to lidocaine

Contraindications

Procainamide should not be administered to patients with severe conduction system disturbances, especially second- and third-degree heart blocks.

Precautions

Procainamide must not be administered to patients demonstrating PVCs in conjunction with a bradycardia. The heart rate should be first increased with atropine or transcutaneous pacing. Only after increasing the heart rate can the PVCs be treated with lidocaine or procainamide if they persist.

Hypotension is common with intravenous infusion. Constant blood pressure monitoring is essential.

Side Effects

Procainamide may cause drowsiness, seizures, confusion, hypotension, bradycardia, heart blocks, nausea, vomiting, and respiratory and cardiac arrest.

Interactions

The hypotensive effects of procainamide may be increased if administered with antihypertensive drugs. The chance of neurological toxicity by both lidocaine and procainamide increases when the medications are administered together.

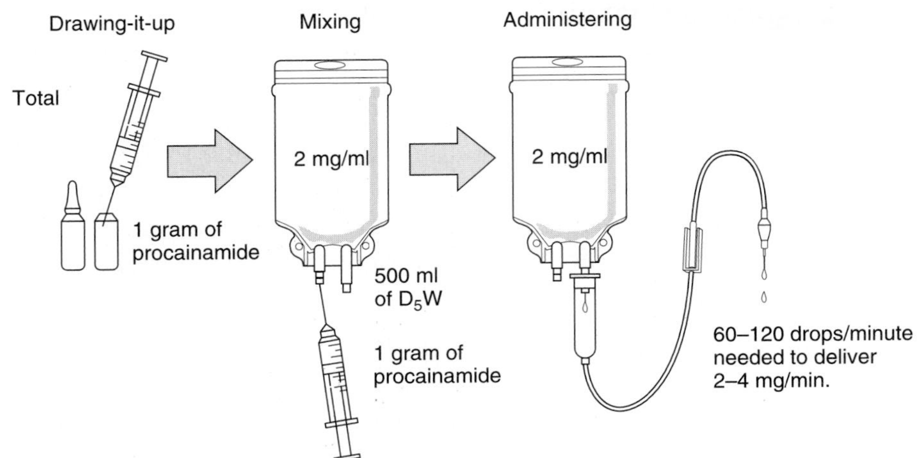

Figure 7-13 Preparation of procainamide infusion.

Dosage

In treating PVCs or ventricular tachycardia, 100 milligrams should be administered every 5 minutes at a rate of 20 milligrams per minute. This should be discontinued if any of the following occur:

- Arrhythmia is suppressed
- Hypotension ensues
- QRS complex is widened by 50% of its original width
- A total of 17 mg/kg of the medication has been administered

The maintenance infusion of procainamide is 1 to 4 milligrams per minute. The duration of procainamide's effect is shorter than lidocaine, requiring a more rigorous approach.

Procainamide should be administered by slow IV bolus (20 milligrams per minute) followed by a maintenance infusion. Generally, one gram of procainamide is placed in 500 ml of D_5W. This gives a final concentration of 2 mg/ml (see Figure 7-13).

How Supplied

Procainamide is supplied in the following dosages: 10-milliliter vials containing 1,000 milligrams of the drug; 2-milliliter vials containing 1,000 milligrams of the drug (for infusion).

Bretylium Tosylate (Bretylol)

Class: Antiarrhythmic

Description

Bretylium is an antiarrhythmic that exhibits both adrenergic and direct myocardial effects.

Mechanism of Action

Bretylium tosylate causes two effects on adrenergic nerve endings. Once administered, bretylium causes release of norepinephrine from adrenergic nerve endings. This causes a slight increase in heart rate, blood pressure, and cardiac output. These sympathomimetic effects last approximately 20 minutes in the non-cardiac arrest setting. Then, norepinephrine release is inhibited, which results in an adrenergic blockade. At this time, hypotension may develop (particularly orthostatic hypotension). Adrenergic blockade usually begins 15–20 minutes after drug administration and lasts for several hours (see Figure 7-14). The antiarrhythmic effect of bretylium is poorly understood, but it appears that it elevates the ventricular fibrillation threshold much like lidocaine. Bretylium will sometimes convert ventricular fibrillation or ventricular tachycardia to a supraventricular rhythm. Because of this action, bretylium is sometimes referred to as a "chemical defibrillator."

Indications

- Ventricular fibrillation refractory to lidocaine
- Ventricular tachycardia refractory to lidocaine

At present, bretylium is not considered a first-line antiarrhythmic.

Contraindications

There are no contraindications to bretylium when used in the treatment of life-threatening ventricular arrhythmias.

Precautions

Postural hypotension occurs in approximately 50 percent of the patients receiving bretylium. This side effect should be anticipated, and the patient should be kept in a supine position.

Side Effects

Bretylium may cause dizziness, syncope, seizures, hypotension, hypertension, angina, nausea, and vomiting.

Interactions

Arrhythmias caused by digitalis toxicity may be worsened by the initial release of norepinephrine that accompanies bretylium usage. Bretylium can interact with other antiarrhythmic agents causing antagonistic or additive effects. The hypotensive effects of bretylium may be worsened if administered with Class IA antiarrhythmics such as procainamide, quinidine, or disopyramide.

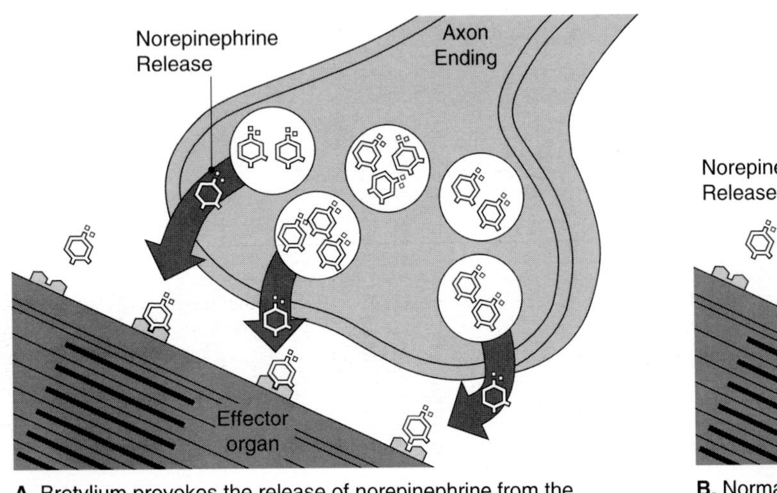

A. Bretylium provokes the release of norepinephrine from the axon ending.

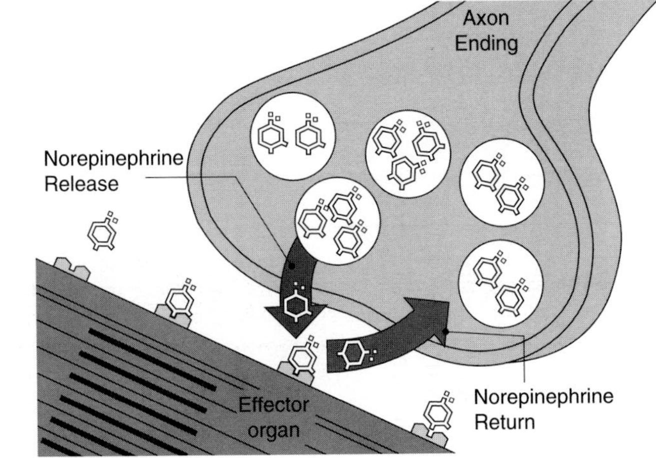

B. Normally, norepinephrine is released and then taken back up to the axon ending.

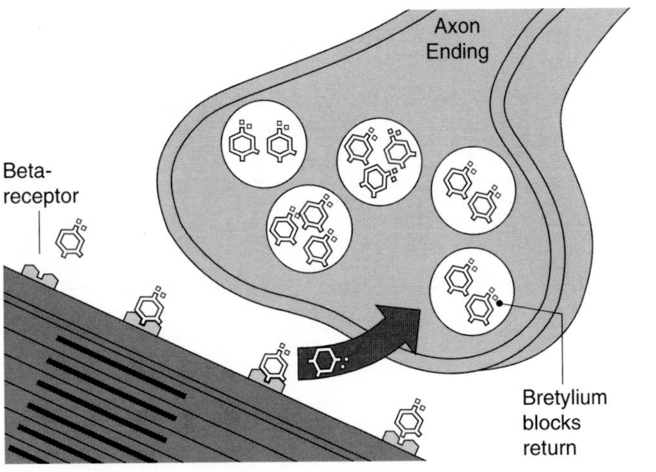

C. Bretylium blocks the return of norepinephrine to the axon ending.

Figure 7-14 The pharmacological effects of bretylium.

Dosage

Bretylium should be administered at a dose of 5 milligrams per kilogram body weight. If the arrhythmia persists, subsequent doses of 10 milligrams per kilogram can be administered at five minute intervals. The total dose should not exceed 30 milligrams per kilogram. Because bretylium is somewhat slow in its onset, it should be administered by IV bolus.

How Supplied

Bretylium is supplied in ampules containing 500 milligrams of the drug in 10 milliliters of solvent.

Adenosine (Adenocard)

Class: Antiarrhythmic

Description

Adenosine is a naturally occurring nucleoside that slows AV conduction through the AV node. It has an exceptionally short half-life and a relatively good safety profile.

Mechanism of Action

Adenosine is a naturally occurring substance (purine nucleoside) that is present in all body cells. Adenosine decreases conduction of the electrical impulse through the AV node and interrupts AV reentry pathways in paroxysmal supraventricular tachycardia (PSVT). It can effectively terminate rapid supraventricular arrhythmias such as PSVT. The half-life of adenosine is approximately 5 seconds. Because of its rapid onset of action and very short half-life, the administration of adenosine is sometimes referred to as "chemical cardioversion." A single bolus of the drug was effective in converting PSVT to a normal sinus rhythm in a significant number (90%) of patients in the initial drug studies. Adenosine does not appear to cause hypotension to the same degree as does verapamil.

Indication

- PSVT (including that associated with Wolff-Parkinson-White syndrome) refractory to common vagal maneuvers

Contraindications

Adenosine is contraindicated in patients with second- or third-degree heart block, sick sinus syndrome, or those with known hypersensitivity to the drug.

Precautions

Adenosine will typically cause arrhythmias at the time of cardioversion. These will generally last a few seconds or less and may include PVCs, premature atrial contractions, sinus bradycardia, sinus tachycardia, and various degrees of AV block. In extreme cases, transient asystole may occur. If this occurs, appropriate therapy should be initiated. Adenosine should be used cautiously in patients with asthma.

Side Effects

Adenosine can cause facial flushing, headache, shortness of breath, dizziness, and nausea, among others. Because the half-life of adenosine is so brief, side effects are generally self-limited.

Interactions

Methylxanthines (aminophylline, theophylline) may decrease the effectiveness of adenosine, thus requiring larger doses. Dipyridamole (Persantine) can potentiate the effects of adenosine. The dosage of adenosine may need to be reduced in patients receiving dipyridamole.

Dosage

The initial dose of adenosine is 6 milligrams given as a rapid intravenous bolus over a 1- to 2-second period. To be certain that the drug rapidly reaches the central circulation, it should be given directly into a vein or into a proximal medication port of a functioning IV line. It should be followed immediately by a rapid saline flush.

If the initial dose does not result in conversion of the PSVT within 1 to 2 minutes, a 12-milligram dose may be given as a rapid IV bolus. The 12-milligram dose may be repeated a second time if required. Doses greater than 12 milligrams should not be administered (see Figure 7-15).

Adenosine should only be given by rapid IV bolus, directly into the vein, or into the medication administration port closest to the patient.

How Supplied

Adenosine (Adenocard) is supplied in vials containing 6 milligrams of the drug in 2 milliliters of saline solvent.

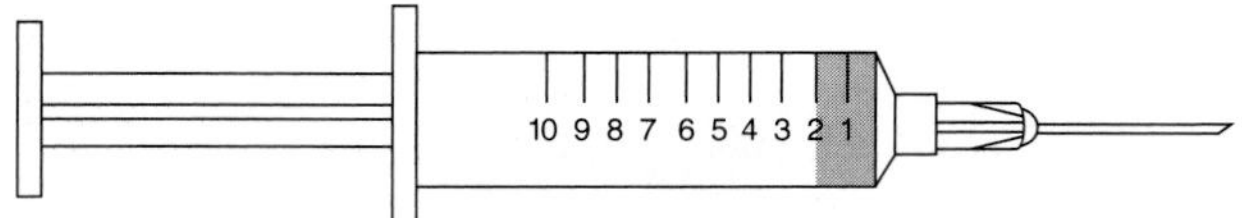

Figure 7-15 Administration of adenosine.

CASE PRESENTATION

At 2130 hours paramedics are dispatched to the library at the University for a 22-year-old female complaining of palpitations and chest pain. The patient is conscious and breathing. On arrival the paramedics are met by campus security and are directed to the library. They find the patient seated in a chair in an office in the library. The patient looks anxious, scared, and pale.

On Examination

CNS: The patient is conscious, alert, and oriented × 4; appears anxious and scared

Resp: Respirations are 26 and shallow, with difficulty breathing normally, lung sounds clear bilaterally, trachea is midline, no signs of trauma

CVS: Carotid and radial pulses are present and rapid, pulse weaker radially; skin is pale, cool

ABD: Soft and non-tender

Vitals:

Pulse: 240/min, regular, weak

Resp: 26/min, shallow, with difficulty breathing normally

BP: 132/76

SpO_2: 95%

ECG: Supraventricular tachycardia

HX:
- **P** studying
- **Q** palpitations, squeezing discomfort with choking sensation
- **R** non-radiating
- **S** 5/10
- **T** started suddenly about 20 minutes ago

Past Hx: The patient states that this has happened twice before. The first time it went away after 5 minutes. The second time she was taken to the hospital by her boyfriend. At the hospital they gave her a medication to slow down her heart. Her doctor told her to call the ambulance if it happened again. She does not take any medication except birth control pills and is not allergic to anything.

Treatment:

Oxygen was administered by non-rebreather at 12 l/min and an IV was initiated. The SVT was confirmed in MCL leads and contact was made with the base hospital. Paramedics were advised to administer 6 mg of adenosine by rapid IV push. They advised the patient about adenosine, explaining the potential side effects. The patient stated that she thought this was the drug they used in the hospital. The paramedics administered the adenosine and after a brief two-second interval of asystole, the patient's rhythm converted to a regular sinus rhythm. The patient stated that she was free of the previous symptoms. She was transported to the hospital for further assessment.

Verapamil (Isoptin) (Calan)

Class: Calcium Channel Blocker

Description

Verapamil is a calcium ion antagonist (calcium channel blocker). Calcium channel blockers cause a relaxation of vascular smooth muscle and slow conduction through the AV node. Verapamil has a greater effect on conduction and a lesser effect on vascular smooth muscle than do other agents in the same class.

Mechanism of Action

Verapamil causes vascular dilation and slows conduction through the atrioventricular (AV) node. The advantages of this are twofold. First, verapamil will inhibit arrhythmias caused by a reentry mechanism such as with paroxysmal supraventricular tachycardia. Second, it will decrease the rapid ventricular response seen with atrial tachyarrhythmias such as atrial flutter and fibrillation. Verapamil also reduces myocardial oxygen demand because of its negative inotropic effects and causes coronary and peripheral vasodilation.

Indication

- Paroxysmal supraventricular tachycardia (PSVT) refractory to adenosine

Contraindications

Verapamil should not be administered to any patient with severe hypotension or cardiogenic shock. In addition, verapamil should not be administered to patients with ventricular tachycardia in the prehospital setting.

Before attempting to treat a patient suffering atrial flutter or atrial fibrillation, it is essential that the paramedic assure that the patient does not suffer from Wolff-Parkinson-White syndrome.

Precautions

Verapamil can cause systemic hypotension. Because of this, it is essential that the blood pressure be constantly monitored following verapamil administration. Calcium chloride can be used to prevent the hypotensive effects of calcium channel blockers and in the management of calcium channel blocker overdosage.

Side Effects

Verapamil can cause nausea, vomiting, dizziness, headache, bradycardia, heart block, hypotension, and asystole.

Interactions

Verapamil should not be administered to patients receiving intravenous β blockers because of an increased risk of congestive heart failure, bradycardia, and asystole.

Dosage

In the treatment of paroxysmal supraventricular tachycardia, a 2.5- to 5-milligram IV dose should be given initially during a 2- to 3-minute interval. A repeat dose of 5 to 10 milligrams can be given in 15–30 minutes if PSVT persists and there have not been any adverse responses to the initial dose. The total dose of verapamil should not exceed 30 milligrams in 30 minutes.

How Supplied

Verapamil (Isoptin) is supplied in 2-milliliter ampules containing 5 milligrams of the drug.

Diltiazem (Cardizem)

Class: Calcium Channel Blocker

Description

Diltiazem is a calcium-ion antagonist (calcium channel blocker). Calcium channel blockers cause a relaxation of vascular smooth muscle and slow conduction through the AV node. Diltiazem has a nearly equal effect on vascular smooth muscle and AV conduction.

Mechanism of Action

Diltiazem causes vascular dilation and slows conduction through the atrioventricular (AV) node. It slows the rapid ventricular rate associated with atrial fibrillation and atrial flutter. It is also used in the treatment of angina because of its negative inotropic effect and because it dilates the coronary arteries.

Indications

- To control rapid ventricular rates associated with atrial fibrillation and atrial flutter
- Angina pectoris
- Paroxysmal supraventricular tachycardia (PSVT) refractory to adenosine

Contraindications

Diltiazem should not be administered to any patient with severe hypotension or cardiogenic shock. In addition, diltiazem should not be administered to patients with ventricular tachycardia (wide-complex tachycardia) in the prehospital setting.

Before attempting to treat a patient suffering atrial flutter or atrial fibrillation, it is essential that the paramedic assure that the patient does not suffer from Wolff-Parkinson-White syndrome.

Precautions

Diltiazem can cause systemic hypotension. Because of this, it is essential that the blood pressure be constantly monitored following diltiazem administration. Calcium chloride can be used to prevent the hypotensive effects of calcium channel blockers and in the management of calcium channel blocker overdosage. Diltiazem should be kept refrigerated. However, it can be kept at room temperature for one month, but must be discarded if unused.

Side Effects

Diltiazem can cause nausea, vomiting, dizziness, headache, bradycardia, heart block, hypotension, and asystole.

Interactions

Diltiazem should not be administered to patients receiving intravenous β blockers because of an increased risk of congestive heart failure, bradycardia, and asystole.

Dosage

In the treatment of rapid ventricular rates associated with atrial fibrillation and atrial flutter, a 20-milligram intravenous bolus (0.25 mg/kg) of diltiazem should be administered over 2 minutes. The bolus dose should be followed by a maintenance infusion of 5–15 mg/hour. For paroxysmal supraventricular tachycardia, a 0.25 mg/kg intravenous bolus should be administered over 2 minutes (see Figure 7-16).

How Supplied

Diltiazem (Cardizem) is supplied in 5-milliliter vials containing 25 milligrams of the drug and in 10-milliliter vials containing 50 milligrams of the drug.

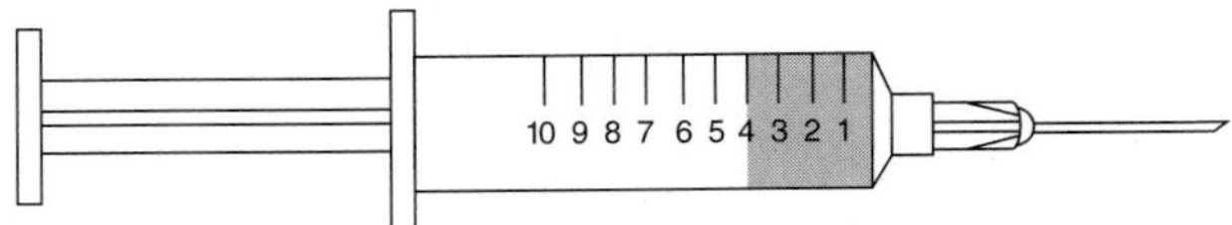

Figure 7-16 Loading dose of diltiazem.

Phenytoin (Dilantin)

Class: Antiarrhythmic/Anticonvulsant

Description

Phenytoin is an anticonvulsant and antiarrhythmic that depresses spontaneous ventricular depolarization.

Mechanism of Action

Phenytoin (Dilantin) is used frequently in the treatment of epilepsy but also has antiarrhythmic properties. It has proved effective in the management of arrhythmias caused by digitalis toxicity or tricyclic drug overdoses. It depresses spontaneous depolarization of ventricular tissues and appears to improve atrioventricular conduction. Its use in the management of status epilepticus is discussed in Chapter 10.

Indication

- Life-threatening arrhythmias resulting from digitalis toxicity or tricyclic antidepressant overdose.

Ventricular arrhythmias in the setting of acute myocardial infarction should first be treated with lidocaine.

Contraindications

Phenytoin is contraindicated in cases of bradycardia and high-grade heart block. It should not be administered to patients who take the drug chronically for seizures until the blood level has been determined.

Precautions

Intravenous administration of phenytoin should not exceed 50 milligrams per minute. Signs of central nervous system depression or hypotension may occur. Elderly patients are at increased risk of developing side effects from phenytoin administration. Avoid extravasation. Any patient receiving intravenous phenytoin should have continuous cardiac monitoring as well as frequent monitoring of vital signs.

Side Effects

Phenytoin can cause drowsiness, dizziness, headache, hypotension, arrhythmias, itching, rash, nausea, and vomiting.

Interactions

Phenytoin must never be diluted in dextrose-containing solutions such as D_5W. It should be diluted in normal saline or other non-glucose-containing crystalloids.

Dosage

The recommended dose of phenytoin is 100 milligrams over 5 minutes to a maximum loading dose of 1,000 milligrams, until the arrhythmia is suppressed, or until symptoms of central nervous system depression appear. In the emergency setting, phenytoin should be given by slow IV bolus or IV infusion with constant EKG monitoring.

How Supplied

Phenytoin (Dilantin) is supplied in 2- and 5-milliliter vials containing 50 milligrams per milliliter of the drug. Dilantin is incompatible with solutions containing dextrose. If an infusion of Dilantin is prepared, the drug should be placed in normal saline.

Edrophonium Chloride (Tensilon)

Class: Antiarrhythmic/Cholinesterase Inhibitor

Description

Edrophonium belongs to a class of drugs referred to as "anticholinesterase agents." It is used in the treatment of paroxysmal supraventricular tachycardia refractory to first-line agents.

Mechanism of Action

Edrophonium inhibits the actions of the enzyme *acetylcholinesterase*. This enzyme plays an important role in neurophysiology as it deactivates the neurotransmitter of the parasympathetic nervous system, acetylcholine. Physostigmine, an emergency drug used in the management of atropine-type poisonings and tricyclic antidepressant overdoses, is chemically similar to edrophonium. The neurophysiology of the parasympathetic nervous system is discussed in more detail in the following section on parasympatholytics. Edrophonium has proven effectiveness in the management of paroxysmal supraventricular tachycardias that do not respond to vagal maneuvers. The inhibition of acetylcholinesterase by edrophonium serves to enhance the acetylcholine secreted by the vagus nerve on the heart. This increased parasympathetic effect has been successful in slowing and eventually terminating paroxysmal supraventricular tachycardias.

With the introduction of adenosine and the calcium channel blockers (verapamil), edrophonium has fallen into relative disuse.

Indication

- PSVT refractory to vagal maneuvers and adenosine

Contraindications

Edrophonium should not be administered to patients with a history of hypersensitivity to the drug. It should not be used in patients who are hypotensive or bradycardic as it can worsen these conditions.

Precautions

The respiratory pattern should be carefully monitored during and following administration of edrophonium. Also, the patient should be constantly monitored for signs of bradycardia. Atropine sulfate should be readily available in those cases of bradycardia causing hemodynamic problems. Edrophonium should be used with caution in the elderly.

Side Effects

Edrophonium can cause dizziness, weakness, sweating, increased salivation, constricted pupils, hypotension, bradycardia, abdominal cramps, nausea, and vomiting.

Interactions

Do not administer edrophonium in dextrose solutions as it tends to crystalize in the tubing. The chances of developing a significant bradycardia are enhanced when edrophonium is administered to patients taking digitalis.

Dosage

The standard dosage is 5 milligrams initially intravenously. If unsuccessful after 10 minutes or so, a second dose of 10 milligrams may be administered. Physicians frequently order the administration of a test dose of 0.1 to 0.5 milligrams, particularly to elderly patients, before the administration of the full dose. Edrophonium should be administered intravenously only.

How Supplied

Edrophonium is supplied in ampules containing 10 milligrams of the drug in 1 milliliter of solvent.

Magnesium Sulfate

Class: Antiarrhythmic

Description

Magnesium sulfate is a salt that dissociates into the magnesium cation (Mg^{++}) and the sulfate anion when administered. Magnesium is an essential element in numerous biochemical reactions that occur within the body.

Mechanism of Action

Magnesium is an essential element in many of the biochemical processes that occur in the body. It acts as a physiological calcium channel blocker and blocks neuromuscular transmission. A decreased magnesium level (hypomagnesemia) is associated with cardiac arrhythmias, symptoms of cardiac insufficiency, and sudden death. Hypomagnesemia can cause refractory ventricular fibrillation.

Administration of magnesium sulfate in the emergency setting appears to reduce the incidence of ventricular arrhythmias that may follow an acute myocardial infarction. It also appears to decrease the complications associated with acute myocardial infarction.

Magnesium sulfate has been used for years in the management of preterm labor and the hypertensive disorders of pregnancy (pre-eclampsia and eclampsia). Its usage in obstetrics is discussed in Chapter 11.

Indications

- Severe refractory ventricular fibrillation/pulseless ventricular tachycardia
- Post-myocardial infarction for prophylaxis of arrhythmias
- Torsades de pointes (multi-axial ventricular tachycardia)

Contraindications

Magnesium sulfate should not be administered to patients who are in shock, who have persistent severe hypertension, who have a third degree AV block, who routinely undergo dialysis, or who are known to have a decreased calcium level (hypocalcemia).

Precautions

Magnesium sulfate should be administered slowly to minimize side effects. Any patient receiving intravenous magnesium sulfate should have continuous cardiac monitoring as well as frequent monitoring of vital signs. If possible, the knee and biceps deep tendon reflexes should be checked prior to magnesium therapy. It should be used with caution in patients with known renal insufficiency. Hypermagnesemia (elevated magnesium) can occur following magnesium sulfate administration. Calcium salts (calcium chloride or calcium gluconate) should be available as an antidote for magnesium sulfate should serious side effects occur.

Side Effects

Magnesium sulfate can cause flushing, sweating, bradycardia, decreased deep tendon reflexes, drowsiness, respiratory depression, arrhythmias, hypotension, hypothermia, itching, and a rash.

Interactions

Magnesium sulfate can cause cardiac conduction abnormalities if administered in conjunction with digitalis.

Dosage

- ***Ventricular Fibrillation/Ventricular Tachycardia.*** 1–2 grams of magnesium sulfate should be diluted in 10 ml of D_5W and administered by slow IV push over 1–2 minutes. Alternatively, 1–2 grams of magnesium sulfate can be diluted in 100 ml of D_5W and administered IV piggyback over 1–2 minutes.
- ***Torsades de Pointes.*** Higher doses are often required in the treatment of torsades de pointes. Typically, 5–10 grams are diluted in 100 ml of D_5W and administered at a rate of 1 gram per minute until the arrhythmia is suppressed or the maximum dose has been administered.
- ***Post-Myocardial Infarction Prophylaxis.*** 1–2 grams of magnesium sulfate can be diluted in 100 ml of D_5W and administered over 5–30 minutes as an IV piggyback.

Magnesium should be administered intravenously in the prehospital setting. However, it can be administered intramuscularly if IV access cannot be obtained. Because of the volume of the drug (5–10 ml), the dose should be divided in half and each half administered intramuscularly at a separate site (usually each gluteus.)

How Supplied

Magnesium sulfate is supplied in vials and prefilled syringes. The drug is supplied in both 10% and 50% solutions. Closely examine the solution prior to preparation to avoid dosing errors.

PARASYMPATHOLYTICS

Drugs that inhibit the actions of the parasympathetic nervous system are referred to as *parasympatholytics*. Sometimes they are referred to as *anticholinergics*. To fully understand the role and actions of the parasympatholytics, we must first review the parasympathetic nervous system.

The parasympathetic, or *cholinergic*, system plays a major role in the maintenance of homeostasis. Parasympathetic stimulation induces peristalsis and causes pupillary constriction and a decrease in the heart rate. The primary nerve of the parasympathetic nervous system is the *vagus nerve*. The vagus nerve descends from the brain along the carotid arteries. It then innervates the heart and the digestive system. Paramedics should be familiar with the manual method of vagal stimulation, carotid sinus massage. Carotid sinus massage is used to slow the heart rate in paroxysmal supraventricular tachycardia.

When the vagus nerve is stimulated, it causes acetylcholine to be released from the presynaptic nerve endings. It then activates acetylcholine receptors on the target organs. These receptors cause the heart rate to slow. Then, after only a fraction of a second, cholinesterase is released, which deactivates acetylcholine. Several drugs act on these junctions. The primary drug of this type is atropine sulfate. Atropine binds to the acetylcholine receptors, thus inhibiting activation. Besides increasing the heart rate, atropine is used frequently as a preoperative medication because it decreases digestive secretions, especially salivation. Certain chemicals, especially the organophosphate insecticides, tend to block, in an irreversible manner, the action of cholinesterase. Excessive levels of acetylcholine can cause serious problems.

Research has shown that some cases of asystole can be caused by an increase in parasympathetic tone. The reason for the increase is not clear. Based on this data, however, the American Heart Association recommends administering 1 milligram of atropine sulfate as soon as possible to any patient encountered in asystole.

It is important to remember that abdominal distension with air from CPR can increase parasympathetic tone. This can often go unrecognized and make it difficult to restore a spontaneous rhythm from asystole. It should be a routine part of advanced life support (ALS) to decompress the stomach if distended. The use of proper CPR, Sellicks' maneuver, and endotracheal intubation can help minimize abdominal distension.

Atropine Sulfate

Class: Anticholinergic

Description

Atropine is a parasympatholytic (anticholinergic) that is derived from parts of the *Atropa belladonna* plant.

Mechanism of Action

Atropine sulfate is a potent parasympatholytic and is used to increase the heart rate in hemodynamically-significant bradycardias. Hemodynamically-significant bradycardias are those slow heart rates accompanied by hypotension, shortness of breath, chest pain, altered mental status, congestive heart failure, and shock.

Atropine acts by blocking acetylcholine receptors, thus inhibiting parasympathetic stimulation. Although it has positive chronotropic properties, it has little or no inotropic effect. It plays an important role as an antidote in organophosphate poisonings.

Atropine has shown to be of some use in asystole, presumably because some cases of asystole may be caused by a sudden and tremendous increase in parasympathetic tone. The mechanism by which atropine is effective in asystole is not clear. However, despite no definite proof of its value in asystole, there is little evidence that its use is harmful in this setting.

Indications

- Hemodynamically-significant bradycardia
- Asystole

Contraindications

None in emergency situations

Precautions

Atropine may actually worsen the bradycardia associated with second-degree Mobitz II and third-degree AV blocks. In these cases, go straight to transcutaneous pacing instead of trying atropine.

A maximum dose of 0.04 milligrams per kilogram body weight of atropine should not be exceeded except in the setting of organophosphate poisoning. If the heart rate fails to increase after a total of 0.04 mg/kg has been given, then transcutaneous pacing is indicated.

Side Effects

Atropine sulfate can cause blurred vision, dilated pupils, dry mouth, tachycardia, drowsiness, and confusion.

Interactions

Few in the prehospital setting

Dosage

- ***Hemodynamically-significant bradycardia***. An initial dose of 0.5 milligram should be administered intravenously. This can be repeated every 3–5 minutes until a maximum dose of 0.04 mg/kg has been administered.
- ***Asystole***. In the treatment of asystole, the dose should be increased to 1.0 mg. When an IV cannot be placed, atropine can be administered endotracheally. However, the dose should be increased to 2–2.5 times the intravenous dose.

Atropine should be given as an IV bolus in emergency situations or endotracheally when an IV cannot be placed.

How Supplied

Atropine is supplied in prefilled syringes containing 1.0 milligrams in 10 milliliters of solution.

CASE PRESENTATION

Paramedics are called to a local shopping mall for a medical emergency. Reportedly, a patient collapsed and is unconscious and breathing. On arrival the patient is found lying on the floor in the center court with a pillow under her head. The patient appears to be in her early 60s.

On Examination

CNS: The patient is conscious, slow to respond to verbal commands, and disoriented to person, place, and time

Resp: Respirations are 12 and shallow, lung sounds clear bilaterally, trachea is midline, no signs of trauma

CVS: Weak, regular, slow carotid pulse, and radial pulses are present; skin is pale, cool, and diaphoretic; no complaint of chest pain

ABD: Soft and non-tender

Vitals:

Pulse: 36/min, regular, weak

Resp: 12/min, shallow

BP: 72/56

SpO2: 86%

ECG: Sinus bradycardia

HX: Unknown. Patient was in the mall alone. The patient is unable to give a history or answer questions.

Past Hx: Unknown; no Medic Alert

Treatment:

Oxygen was administered by non-rebreather at 12 l/min and well tolerated by the patient. An IV of normal saline was established. The patient was given 0.5 mg of atropine. Following the atropine the patient's pulse rate increased slightly to 42/min and her blood pressure was 80/62. At this point the pacing pads were placed on the patient as a precautionary measure. A second dose of atropine 0.5 mg was given and the heart rate improved to 68/min with a blood pressure of 108/82. The patient's level of consciousness improved. The patient was moved to the ambulance and transported to the hospital.

En route to the hospital the patient stated that she was shopping alone when she felt faint. She sat down to let the faintness pass. She didn't remember what happened until she saw the paramedics with her.

CARDIAC GLYCOSIDES

Digitalis, the principal drug in the cardiac glycoside class, is one of the oldest medications known to humans. For hundreds of years it has been used in the treatment of congestive heart failure. Digitalis and the related cardiac glycosides increase the force (inotropic effect) of the myocardial contraction. When given to patients in congestive heart failure, it significantly increases the cardiac output reducing left ventricular diameter, decreases venous pressure, and hastens reduction of peripheral and pulmonary edema. In recent years digitalis has also proved effective in the management of patients with atrial flutter and atrial fibrillation. In these patients rapid atrial rates produce accelerated ventricular rates, which can be reduced by digitalis therapy.

Several digitalis preparations are available. These include the following:

- *Digitoxin.* Digitoxin is the longest-acting cardiac glycoside. It must not be confused with the shorter-acting digoxin.
- *Digoxin (Lanoxin).* Digoxin is the most commonly prescribed form of digitalis.
- *Ouabain.* Ouabain has a rapid rate of onset and a relatively short duration of effect. Its use is reserved for cases in which rapid digitalization is required.
- *Deslanoside (Cedilanid-D).* Deslanoside is the most rapidly acting digitalis preparation.

Cardiac glycosides have profound effects on cardiac function and rhythm. The therapeutic index (therapeutic dose/toxic dose) is low, which means that the possibility of digitalis toxicity should always be considered in patients with this medication. Signs of digitalis toxicity include cardiac arrhythmias (PVCs, PSVT with 2:1 block, and so on), nausea, vomiting, headache, visual disturbances (yellow vision), and drowsiness. Almost any arrhythmia can be associated with digitalis toxicity.

Digitalis is a potent and potentially toxic drug. Extreme care must be used whenever it is administered. Constant monitoring of vital signs and EKG is essential. In almost all cases digitalization should be deferred until the patient is in the emergency department and under the care of the emergency department physician.

Digoxin (Lanoxin)

Class: Cardiac Glycoside

Description

Digoxin is a moderately rapid-acting cardiac glycoside used in the management of congestive heart failure and to control the heart rate in atrial fibrillation and atrial flutter.

Mechanism of Action

Digoxin is a cardiac glycoside effective in the treatment of congestive heart failure and rapid atrial arrhythmias. It increases the force of the cardiac contraction through its effects on the sodium/potassium ATPase system. Digoxin significantly increases the stroke volume, thus increasing the cardiac output. It also decreases AV nodal conduction, thus slowing the heart rate. Therapeutic effects begin in about 0.5 hour and peak at 24 hours.

Indications

- Congestive heart failure
- Supraventricular tachyarrhythmias, especially atrial flutter and atrial fibrillation

Contraindications

Digoxin should not be given to any patient showing any of the signs or symptoms of digitalis toxicity. It also should not be administered to patients in ventricular fibrillation.

Precautions

Patients receiving digoxin should be constantly monitored for signs and symptoms of digitalis toxicity. Extreme care should be used when administering digoxin to patients with myocardial infarction, as they are prone to digitalis toxicity. Digitalis toxicity is potentiated in patients with hypokalemia, hypomagnesemia, and hypercalcemia. Digitalis crosses the placenta and thus can affect the fetal heart in much the same manner as the mother's.

Side Effects

Digoxin can cause numerous side effects. Non-cardiac side effects include anorexia, nausea, vomiting, abdominal pain, diarrhea, fatigue, depression, drowsiness, yellow vision, headache, dizziness, hallucinations, sweating, itching, and rash. Cardiac side effects include arrhythmias, bradycardias, tachycardias, various degrees of heart block, hypotension, and cardiac arrest.

Interactions

Many drugs have potential interaction problems with digoxin. Quinidine and the calcium channel blockers (verapamil, nifedipine, diltiazem) can increase serum digoxin levels. The administration of digoxin concomitantly with beta blockers can cause severe bradycardia. Diuretics can cause potassium depletion, which can lead to digitalis toxicity.

Dosage

The dosage is 0.25 to 0.5 milligrams given by slow IV push. Digoxin is generally given intravenously in the treatment of supraventricular tachyarrhythmias.

How Supplied

Digoxin (Lanoxin) is supplied in 2-milliliter ampules containing 0.5 milligrams of the drug.

THROMBOLYTICS

A myocardial infarction begins with the formation of a blood clot (thrombus) in a coronary artery. This results in complete occlusion of the artery and subsequent interruption of blood flow to the area of the myocardium supplied by that artery. Usually, the coronary artery is already partially obstructed by atherosclerosis. These obstructions are often the narrowest (or "tightest") portions of the artery and the site of thrombus formation.

Following arterial occlusion, the portion of the myocardium supplied by the obstructed artery becomes ischemic. At this point the ischemia can be reversed with minimal permanent injury to the muscle if the blood supply can be restored. However, if the occlusion continues, the myocardium will become injured and will eventually die. There is a window of 6 hours after the onset of pain to restore perfusion to the injured myocardium. There are several ways perfusion can be restored, including percutaneous transluminal coronary angioplasty (PTCA), coronary artery bypass grafting (CABG), and thrombolytic therapy. PTCA requires access to a cardiac catheterization lab and subsequent coronary arteriogram to identify the occlusion. Then, a special balloon catheter is introduced into the diseased artery. The balloon is placed at the site of the occlusion and filled, resulting in dilation of the occlusion. This process is time consuming and not available at every hospital. Likewise, coronary bypass grafting requires an initial arteriogram followed by major surgery to bypass the obstruction. Thrombolytic therapy, unlike the other procedures, does not require coronary angiography and can be performed in any community hospital and, in some places, in the prehospital setting.

Thrombolytic therapy is the administration of a drug to dissolve the blood clot in the coronary artery causing an acute myocardial infarction. There are three major types of thrombolytics available in the United States. These are streptokinase (Streptase), anistreplase (Eminase), and alteplase (tPA, Activase). Aspirin, a platelet aggregation inhibitor, is included in this discussion as it has proven highly effective in reducing mortality following myocardial infarction.

Aspirin

Class: Platelet Aggregator Inhibitor/Anti-Inflammatory Agent

Description

Aspirin is an anti-inflammatory agent and an inhibitor of platelet function. This makes it a useful agent in the treatment of various thromboembolic diseases such as acute myocardial infarction.

Mechanism of Action

Aspirin blocks the formation of the substance Thromboxane A_2, which causes platelets to aggregate and arteries to constrict. This results in an overall reduction in mortality associated with myocardial infarction. It also appears to reduce the rate of nonfatal reinfarction and nonfatal stroke.

Indications

- New chest pain suggestive of acute myocardial infarction (AMI)
- Signs and symptoms suggestive of recent stroke (CVA)

Contraindications

Aspirin is contraindicated in patients with known hypersensitivity to the drug. It is relatively contraindicated in patients with active ulcer disease and asthma.

Precautions

Aspirin can cause gastrointestinal upset and bleeding. Enteric-coated aspirin, if available, should be used in patients who have a tendency for gastric irritation and bleeding with aspirin. Use aspirin with caution in patients who report allergies to the non-steroidal anti-inflammatory (NSAID) class of drugs. Doses higher than recommended can actually interfere with possible benefits.

Side Effects

Aspirin can cause heartburn, GI bleeding, nausea, vomiting, wheezing, and prolonged bleeding.

Interactions

When administered together, aspirin and other anti-inflammatory agents may cause an increased incidence of side effects and increased blood levels of both drugs. Administration of aspirin with antacids may reduce the blood levels of the drug by decreasing absorption.

Dosage

The recommended dosage for aspirin is 160–325 mg taken as soon as possible after the onset of chest pain. Baby aspirin (160 mg) is often preferred as it can be chewed and swallowed and is often a little more palatable as many MI patients are nauseated. Aspirin is often given as part of a thrombolytic therapy protocol.

How Supplied

Aspirin is supplied in tablets (chewable and standard) containing 160 mg and 325 mg of the drug. Enteric-coated aspirin (Ecotrin) is available for those with a tendency for GI upset with aspirin therapy.

Streptokinase (Streptase)

Class: Thrombolytic

Description

Streptokinase is a potent thrombolytic. It is derived from the bacteria group C, β-hemolytic streptococci.

Mechanism of Action

Streptokinase acts with plasminogen (present in the blood) to produce a so-called "activator complex." This "activator complex" converts plasminogen to the enzyme plasmin. Plasmin then digests fibrin and fibrinogen causing the dissolution of clots causing coronary occlusion.

Indication

- Acute myocardial infarction

Contraindications

Streptokinase is absolutely contraindicated in:

- persons with active internal bleeding
- suspected aortic dissection
- traumatic CPR (rib fractures, pneumothorax)
- severe persistent hypertension
- recent head trauma or known intracranial tumor
- history of stroke in the last 6 months
- pregnancy

It is relatively contraindicated (that is, the risks must be weighed against the potential benefits) in:

- history of trauma or major surgery in the last two months
- initial blood pressure greater than 180 systolic or 110 diastolic that is controlled by medical treatment
- active peptic ulcer or blood in stool
- history of stroke, tumor, brain surgery, or head injury
- known bleeding disorder or current use of warfarin (Coumadin)

- significant liver dysfunction or kidney failure
- exposure to streptokinase or anistreplase during the preceding 12 months
- known cancer or illness with possible thoracic, abdominal, or intracranial abnormalities
- prolonged CPR

Precautions

Streptokinase may be ineffective if administered within 12 months of prior streptokinase or anistreplase therapy. Anaphylaxis can occur with streptokinase therapy. Emergency resuscitative drugs and equipment should be immediately available. Reperfusion arrhythmias are common once the occluded artery opens. Antiarrhythmic medications should be immediately available.

Side Effects

Streptokinase can cause bleeding, allergic reactions, anaphylaxis, fever, nausea, and vomiting.

Interactions

Streptokinase should be used with caution in patients on anticoagulation therapy.

Dosage

1.5 million units of streptokinase should be administered over one hour. This is typically part of a "streptokinase protocol" where aspirin, an antihistamine, and a corticosteroid are administered before administering streptokinase. The antihistamine and corticosteroid are given to prevent a possible allergic reaction to the drug.

Streptokinase must be reconstituted immediately prior to administration. The manufacturer's recommendations for reconstitution, which accompany the drug, should be followed explicitly. Streptokinase should be administered intravenously, preferably through an IV pump.

How Supplied

Streptokinase is supplied in a box containing a 50-ml infusion bottle and a 6.5-ml vial containing the drug.

Anistreplase (Eminase)

Class: Thrombolytic

Description

Anistreplase is a potent thrombolytic. It a derivative of the plasminogen-streptokinase activator complex and is derived from the bacteria group C, β-hemolytic streptococci.

Mechanism of Action

Anistreplase is an inactive derivative that is activated when administered. Plasmin is produced from plasminogen (present in the blood). Plasmin then digests fibrin and fibrinogen, causing the dissolution of clots that cause coronary occlusion.

Indication

- Acute myocardial infarction

Contraindications

Anistreplase is absolutely contraindicated in:

- persons with active internal bleeding
- suspected aortic dissection
- traumatic CPR (rib fractures, pneumothorax)
- severe persistent hypertension
- recent head trauma or known intracranial tumor
- history of stroke in the last 6 months
- pregnancy

It is relatively contraindicated (that is, the risks must be weighed against the potential benefits) in:

- history of trauma or major surgery in the last two months
- initial blood pressure greater than 180 systolic or 110 diastolic that is controlled by medical treatment
- active peptic ulcer or blood in stool
- history of stroke, tumor, brain surgery, or head injury
- known bleeding disorder or current use of warfarin (Coumadin)
- significant liver dysfunction or kidney failure
- exposure to streptokinase or anistreplase during the preceding 12 months
- known cancer or illness with possible thoracic, abdominal, or intracranial abnormalities
- prolonged CPR

Precautions

Anistreplase may be ineffective if administered within 12 months of prior streptokinase or anistreplase therapy. Anaphylaxis can occur with anistreplase therapy. Emergency resuscitative drugs and equipment should be immediately available. Reperfusion arrhythmias are common once the occluded artery opens. Antiarrhythmic medications should be immediately available.

Side Effects

Anistreplase can cause bleeding, allergic reactions, anaphylaxis, fever, nausea, and vomiting.

Interactions

Anistreplase should be used with caution in patients on anticoagulation therapy.

Dosage

30 units of anistreplase should be injected slowly over 2–5 minutes in a one-time dose. This is typically part of an "Eminase protocol" where aspirin, an antihistamine, and a corticosteroid are administered before administering anistreplase. The antihistamine and corticosteroid are given to prevent a possible allergic reaction to the drug.

Anistreplase must be reconstituted immediately prior to administration and used within 30 minutes of reconstitution. The manufacturer's recommendations for reconstitution, which accompany the drug, should be followed explicitly. When mixing the drug, be careful not to shake it. Instead, it should be gently rolled in the vial to mix it.

Anistreplase should be administered by slow intravenous bolus.

How Supplied

Anistreplase is supplied in a 30-unit vial. Anistreplase is very expensive and should be handled carefully.

Alteplase, Tissue Plasminogen Activator (tPA) (Activase)

Class: Thrombolytic

Description

Alteplase (tPA) is a potent thrombolytic. It is a tissue plasminogen activator produced through recombinant DNA technology.

Mechanism of Action

Alteplase is an enzyme that converts plasminogen (present in the blood) to the enzyme plasmin. It also produces a limited amount of fibrinogen in the absence of fibrin. When administered, alteplase binds to the fibrin in a thrombus and converts the plasminogen into plasmin. Plasmin then digests fibrin and fibrinogen, causing the dissolution of clots that cause coronary occlusion.

Indication

- Acute myocardial infarction

Contraindications

Alteplase is absolutely contraindicated in:

- persons with active internal bleeding
- suspected aortic dissection
- traumatic CPR (rib fractures, pneumothorax)

- severe persistent hypertension
- recent head trauma or known intracranial tumor
- history of stroke in the last 6 months
- pregnancy

It is relatively contraindicated in:

- history of trauma or major surgery in the last two months
- initial blood pressure greater than 180 systolic or 110 diastolic that is controlled by medical treatment
- active peptic ulcer or blood in stool
- history of stroke, tumor, brain surgery, or head injury
- known bleeding disorder or current use of warfarin (Coumadin)
- significant liver dysfunction or kidney failure
- known cancer or illness with possible thoracic, abdominal, or intracranial abnormalities
- prolonged CPR

Precautions

Alteplase does not appear to have the problem associated with readministration of streptokinase or anistreplase. Anaphylaxis can occur with alteplase therapy but is very rare. Emergency resuscitative drugs and equipment should be immediately available. Reperfusion arrhythmias are common once the occluded artery opens. Antiarrhythmic medications should be immediately available.

Side Effects

Alteplase can cause bleeding, allergic reactions, anaphylaxis, fever, nausea, and vomiting.

Interactions

Alteplase should be used with caution in patients on anticoagulation therapy.

Dosage

The dosage regimen for alteplase is controversial. The manufacturer recommends a total dose of 100 milligrams. 10 milligrams is administered as an IV bolus over 1–2 minutes followed by an infusion of 50 milligrams over the first hour, 20 milligrams over the second hour, and 20 milligrams over the third hour.

A more popular dosing regimen is the "accelerated" or "front-loaded" regimen. In this case, 15 milligrams of the drug is administered as an IV bolus over 1–2 minutes. This is followed by an IV infusion of 50 milligrams over the first hour and 35 milligrams over the second hour.

Alteplase must be reconstituted immediately prior to administration. The manufacturer's recommendations for reconstitution, which accompany the drug, should be followed explicitly. Alteplase should be administered intravenously. An initial bolus should be administered over 1–2 minutes followed by an IV infusion, preferably through an IV pump.

How Supplied

Alteplase is supplied in a box containing vials with 20, 50, or 100 milligrams of the drug. Alteplase is very expensive and should be handled carefully.

ALKALINIZING AGENTS

Alkalinizing drugs, such as sodium bicarbonate, are used to buffer the acids present in the body during and after cardiac arrest and other serious conditions. Normal body pH is 7.4 (7.35 to 7.45). During hypoxia, the serum pH may fall quickly. Sodium bicarbonate will help correct metabolic (usually lactic acid) acidosis until hypoxia is corrected. The following reaction illustrates the role of sodium bicarbonate in acid-base balance.

H^+	+	HCO_3^-	$\Leftrightarrow$	H_2CO_2	$\Leftrightarrow$	H_2O	+	CO_2
Acids (Strong)		Bicarbonate		Carbonic Acid		Water		Carbon Dioxide

Bicarbonate combines with the strong acids, usually lactic acid, and forms a weak, volatile acid (carbonic acid). This acid then is broken down into carbon dioxide and water. The two end-products are then removed via the lungs and the kidneys respectively.

Excessive administration of sodium bicarbonate may cause metabolic alkalosis, which may be worse than the metabolic acidosis being treated. Primary treatment of metabolic acidosis in the setting of hypoxia or cardiac arrest is adequate oxygenation and blood pressure support.

Sodium Bicarbonate

Class: Alkalinizing Agent

Description

Sodium bicarbonate is a salt that provides bicarbonate to buffer metabolic acidosis, which can accompany several disease processes.

Mechanism of Action

For many years sodium bicarbonate was the cornerstone of advanced cardiac life support care. Controlled studies have shown that sodium bicarbonate was ineffective in the treatment of cardiac arrest. In many instances it has actually been associated with many adverse reactions.

Sodium bicarbonate is occasionally used in the treatment of certain types of drug overdose. The most common example is drugs in the tricyclic class of antidepressants. Overdosage of these drugs has serious effects including life-threatening cardiac arrhythmias. Tricyclic antidepressant excretion from the body is enhanced by making the urine more alkaline (raising the pH). Sodium bicarbonate is sometimes administered to increase the pH of the urine to speed excretion of the drug from the body.

Indications

- Late in the management of cardiac arrest, if at all. Hyperventilation, prompt defibrillation, and the administration of epinephrine and lidocaine should always precede use of sodium bicarbonate. Because these therapies take at least 10 minutes to carry out, sodium bicarbonate should rarely be administered in the first 10 minutes of a resuscitation.
- Tricyclic antidepressant overdose
- Phenobarbital overdose
- Severe acidosis refractory to hyperventilation
- Known hyperkalemia

Contraindications

When used in the management of the situations described earlier, there are no absolute contraindications.

Precautions

Sodium bicarbonate can cause metabolic alkalosis when administered in large quantities. It is important to calculate the dosage based on patient weight and size.

Side Effects

Few when used in the emergency setting

Interactions

Most catecholamines and vasopressors (i.e., dopamine and epinephrine) can be deactivated by alkaline solutions like sodium bicarbonate. Sodium bicarbonate should not be administered in conjunction with calcium chloride. A precipitate can form, which may clog the IV line.

Dosage

The usual dose of sodium bicarbonate is 1 milliequivalent per kilogram of body weight initially followed by 0.5 milliequivalent per kilogram of body weight every 10 minutes. When possible, the dosage of sodium bicarbonate should be based on the results of arterial blood gas studies. Sodium bicarbonate should be administered only as an IV bolus.

How Supplied

Sodium bicarbonate comes in prefilled syringes containing 50 milliequivalents of the drug in 50 milliliters of solvent.

CARDIAC PAIN MANAGEMENT (ANALGESICS)

Drugs that have proved to be effective in alleviating pain are referred to as "analgesics." Although they may be administered in many different types of emergencies, they are used most often for the treatment of emergencies involving the cardiovascular system, especially myocardial infarction.

Analgesics are covered in detail in chapter 15. This section will cover morphine and nitrous oxide.

Morphine is derived from the opium plant. It has impressive analgesic and hemodynamic effects. Nitronox, a 50% mixture of oxygen and nitrous oxide that can be easily inhaled by the patient, is entirely different from the other analgesic agents discussed. Its analgesic effects are also very potent yet disappear within a few minutes after the cessation of administration. Thus, Nitronox can be given for many types of pain in the field without fear of impairing subsequent physical examination in the emergency department. In addition to its analgesic effects, Nitronox delivers oxygen to the patient, which makes it useful in cardiac emergencies.

Morphine Sulfate

Class: Narcotic Analgesic

Description

Morphine is a central nervous system depressant and a potent analgesic. Although morphine sulfate is one of the most potent analgesics known to humans, it also has hemodynamic properties that make it extremely useful in emergency medicine.

Mechanism of Action

Morphine sulfate is a central nervous system depressant that acts on opiate receptors in the brain providing both analgesia and sedation. It increases peripheral venous capacitance and decreases venous return. This effect is sometimes called a "chemical phlebotomy." Morphine also decreases myocardial oxygen demand. This action is due to both the decreased systemic vascular resistance and the sedative effects of the drug. Patient apprehension and fear can significantly increase myocardial oxygen demand, and in some cases can conceivably increase the size of myocardial infarction. The hemodynamic properties of morphine make it one of the most important drugs used in the treatment of pulmonary edema. Morphine is frequently administered to patients with signs and symptoms of pulmonary edema who are not having chest pain.

Indications

- Severe pain associated with myocardial infarction, kidney stones, etc.
- Pulmonary edema either with or without associated pain

Contraindications

Morphine should not be used in patients who are volume depleted or severely hypotensive because of the hemodynamic effects described earlier. Morphine should not be administered to any patient with a history of hypersensitivity to the drug, or to patients with undiagnosed head injury or abdominal pain.

Precautions

Morphine is a narcotic derivative of opium. It has a high tendency for addiction and abuse and is thus covered under the Controlled Substances Act of 1970. It is classified as a Schedule II drug. Because of this, there are special considerations involved in the handling of the drug. Many emergency medical services (EMS) have opted to use the synthetic analgesics, like nalbuphine and pentazocine, instead of morphine and meperidine because of these problems.

Morphine causes severe respiratory depression in higher doses. This is especially true in patients who already have some form of respiratory impairment. The narcotic antagonist naloxone (Narcan) should be readily available whenever the drug is administered.

Side Effects

Morphine can cause nausea, vomiting, abdominal cramps, blurred vision, constricted pupils, altered mental status, headache, and respiratory depression.

Interactions

The CNS depression associated with morphine can be enhanced when administered with antihistamines, antiemetics, sedatives, hypnotics, barbiturates, and alcohol.

Dosage

There are many different approaches to the administration of morphine. An initial dose in the range of 2 to 10 milligrams intravenously is standard. This can be augmented with additional doses of 2 milligrams every few minutes and can be continued until the pain is relieved or until signs of respiratory depression occur.

To attain desired effects, intramuscular injection usually requires 5 to 15 milligrams based on the patient's weight. However, morphine is routinely given intravenously in emergency medicine and is often administered with an antiemetic agent such as promethazine (Phenergan). This helps prevent nausea and vomiting, which often accompany morphine administration. The antiemetics also tend to potentiate morphine's effects. Morphine can also be given intramuscularly and subcutaneously.

How Supplied

Morphine comes in tamper-proof ampules and Tubex prefilled cartridges. To ease administration, the 10 milligrams in 1-milliliter dilution is preferred.

CASE PRESENTATION

At 1300 hours an ALS unit is dispatched to a mobile home park for a 61-year-old male complaining of chest pain. The patient is conscious and breathing.

On arrival paramedics are met at the door by the patient's wife. She states that she and her husband had attended church. During the service he began to feel short of breath. She noticed that he was sweating heavily and appeared pale. She drove him home. The patient took two nitro sprays (0.4 mg) with no relief. Initially, he would not let her call the ambulance. Finally, he agreed that she could call the ambulance.

As paramedics approach the patient, they see a 61-year-old male sitting in a reclining chair. The patient looks anxious and scared.

On Examination

CNS: The patient is conscious, alert, and oriented × 4; appears in obvious distress

Resp: Respirations are 24 and shallow, lung sounds clear bilaterally, trachea is midline, no signs of trauma

CVS: Carotid and radial pulses are present and weak; skin is pale, cool, and diaphoretic

ABD: Soft and non-tender

Vitals:

Pulse: 96/min, regular, weak

Resp: 24/min, shallow

BP: 144/94

SpO_2: 88%

ECG: Regular sinus rhythm with ST elevation

HX:

P no provoking factors

Q squeezing pain

R radiating to left shoulder and jaw

S 8/10, worst pain ever

T started suddenly about 2 hours ago

Past Hx: The patient's wife states that her husband has had several episodes of chest pain in the last month but has not seen his doctor during that time. He was diagnosed with angina 2 years ago. He has nitro spray, which he has used more often this month than ever in the past. Nitro is the patient's only prescription home medication. The patient has no recent history of operations, ulcers, or hypertension.

Treatment:

Oxygen was administered by non-rebreather at 12 l/min and tolerated by the patient. The patient was hooked up to the ECG monitor, and a regular sinus rhythm with ST elevation was noted. The ST elevation was confirmed in MCL leads 1 and 6. An intravenous line with an 18 gauge catheter was established and run TKO. Paramedics administered nitro spray (0.4 mg) from their drug kit. The patient stated that the pain was not relieved by the oxygen or the nitro. The base hospital ordered 2.5 mg of morphine IV. The morphine was given and transport to the hospital was started. En route the patient stated that the chest pain was

6/10 and a second dose of 2.5 mg of morphine was given with moderate relief. A second 18 gauge IV was started and run TKO. ASA 325 mg was given P.O. The patient stated the pain was now 2/10. He was pale, cool, and diaphoretic but appeared less anxious. The base hospital was contacted and advised of the patient findings. The base hospital physician agreed with the findings of the paramedics and prepared to follow through with the thrombolytic protocol on the patient's arrival at the hospital pending evaluation of a 12 lead ECG.

Nitrous Oxide (Nitronox)

Class: Analgesic/Anesthetic Gas

Description

Nitronox is a blended mixture of 50% nitrous oxide and 50% oxygen that has potent analgesic effects.

Mechanism of Action

Nitrous oxide is a CNS depressant with analgesic properties. In the prehospital setting it is delivered in a fixed mixture of 50% nitrous oxide and 50% oxygen. When inhaled, it has potent analgesic effects. These quickly dissipate, however, within 2 to 5 minutes after cessation of administration.

The Nitronox unit consists of one oxygen and one nitrous oxide cylinder. The gases are fed into a blender that combines them at the appropriate concentration. The mixture is then delivered to a modified demand valve for administration to the patient.

Nitronox must be self-administered. It is effective in treating many varieties of pain encountered in the prehospital setting including pain from many types of trauma. The high concentration of oxygen delivered along with the nitrous oxide will increase the oxygen tension in the blood, thus reducing hypoxia.

Indications

- Pain of musculoskeletal origin, particularly fractures
- Burns
- Suspected ischemic chest pain
- States of severe anxiety including hyperventilation

Contraindications

Nitronox should not be used with any patient who cannot comprehend verbal instructions or who is intoxicated with alcohol or other drugs. It should not be administered to any patient with a head injury who exhibits an altered mental status. Nitronox should not be administered to any patient with COPD where the high concentration of oxygen (50%) might result in respiratory depression. Nitrous oxide tends to diffuse into closed spaces more readily than either carbon dioxide or oxygen. Many COPD patients have air-containing blebs in their lungs, and nitrous oxide can concentrate in these blebs causing them to swell. Swollen blebs may rupture causing a pneumothorax.

Nitronox should not be administered to patients with a thoracic injury suspicious of pneumothorax, as the gas may accumulate in the pneumothorax increasing its size. Also, patients with severe abdominal pain and distention, suggestive of bowel obstruction, should not receive Nitronox. Nitrous oxide can concentrate in pockets of an obstructed bowel possibly leading to rupture.

Precautions

Nitronox should only be used in areas that are well ventilated. When the gas is used in the patient compartment of an ambulance, it is recommended that a scavenging system be in place.

Nitrous oxide exists in a liquid state inside the gas cylinder. Heat present in the air, the cylinder wall, or the various regulators and lines causes the liquid to vaporize. This vaporization process makes the cylinder tank and lines cool to touch. Following prolonged use, frost may develop on the cylinder, regulator, or lines. In very cold environments, generally less than 21°F (6°C), the liquid may be slow to vaporize, and administration may be impossible.

Side Effects

Nitrous oxide/oxygen mixture can cause dizziness, light-headedness, altered mental status, hallucinations, nausea, and vomiting.

Interactions

Nitrous oxide can potentiate the effects of other CNS depressants such as narcotics, sedatives, hypnotics, and alcohol.

Dosage

Nitronox should only be self-administered. Continuous administration may take place until the pain is significantly relieved or the patient drops the mask. The patient care record should document the duration of drug administration.

How Supplied

Nitrous oxide/oxygen mixture is supplied in a cylinder system where both gases are fed into a blender that delivers a fixed 50%/50% mixture to the patient. The blender is designed to shut off if the oxygen cylinder becomes depleted. It will allow continued administration of oxygen if the nitrous oxide cylinder becomes depleted.

In several countries (England, Canada, Australia) the nitrous oxide/oxygen mixture (Entonox, Dolonox) is premixed and supplied in a single cylinder. This setup is much lighter than the system used in the United States.

DIURETICS

One of the most common cardiovascular emergencies that emergency personnel are called on to treat is congestive heart failure. Congestive heart failure occurs when the heart loses its ability to pump blood effectively. When this occurs, the venous vessels leading to the heart become engorged. Failure of the left side of the heart causes a buildup of blood in the pulmonary circulation. Failure of the right side of the heart results in congestion of the peripheral circulation, which usually manifests as peripheral edema. Common signs of right heart failure include jugular venous distention, ascites, and pedal (ankle or pretibial) edema.

In the treatment of congestive heart failure, the primary objectives are to increase the cardiac output and to reduce pulmonary and peripheral edema. Although the inotropic effects of digitalis preparations will increase cardiac output, the rate of onset is relatively slow, making this drug less than ideal in acute pulmonary edema. In acute heart failure the most effective therapy is to reduce venous filling pressure. This can be done mechanically by applying rotating tourniquets, which are placed on three of the extremities to decrease venous return. Phlebotomy (drawing blood out of the circulatory system) can also be employed. The preferred method, however, is the administration of potent diuretics.

Furosemide (Lasix)

Class: Diuretic

Description

Furosemide is a potent diuretic that inhibits sodium and chloride reabsorption in the kidneys and that causes venous dilatation.

Mechanism of Action

Furosemide is a loop diuretic that inhibits the reabsorption of both sodium and chloride in the kidneys. It is extremely useful in the treatment of congestive heart failure and pulmonary edema. The effects of furosemide are two-fold. First, following administration furosemide causes venous dilation. This effect usually occurs within five minutes and causes a reduction in preload, thus decreasing cardiac work. The second effect of furosemide is the diuretic effect, which begins 5 to 15 minutes following administration.

Indications

- Congestive heart failure
- Pulmonary edema

Contraindications

Usage in pregnancy should be limited to life-threatening situations in which the benefits of furosemide outweigh the risks. Furosemide has been known to cause fetal abnormalities. It should not be administered to patients with a known allergy to the sulfa class of medications.

Precautions

Dehydration, electrolyte depletion, and hypotension can result from excessive doses of potent diuretics. Thus, the blood pressure should be frequently monitored when furosemide is administered. Furosemide should be protected from light.

Side Effects

Furosemide can cause headache, dizziness, hypotension, volume depletion, potassium depletion, arrhythmias, diarrhea, nausea, and vomiting.

Interactions

Furosemide should not be administered in the same line as amrinone (Inocor) because a chemical reaction can occur between the two, causing the formation of a precipitate in the intravenous line.

Administration of furosemide with other diuretics can lead to severe volume depletion and electrolyte imbalance.

Dosage

The standard dosage of furosemide is 40 milligrams given by slow IV push in patients already on chronic oral furosemide therapy, and 20 milligrams intravenously in patients who are not taking the drug orally on a regular basis. Dosages as high as 80–120 milligrams intravenously may be indicated in severe cases. Furosemide should be given intravenously in emergency situations.

How Supplied

Furosemide is supplied in ampules and prefilled syringes. These containers contain 10 milligrams per milliliter.

CASE PRESENTATION

ALS is called at 0900 hours for a woman having difficulty breathing. Dispatch states that the woman is conscious and breathing. The response time is 2 minutes.

Upon arrival paramedics find a 51-year-old female lying in a semi-Fowler's position, in bed, and in severe respiratory distress. Paramedics immediately place the patient in a sitting position propped up by pillows and supported by her husband.

On Examination

CNS: The patient is conscious, alert, and oriented × 4; appears in obvious distress and is very restless

Resp: Respirations are 32 and shallow, lung sounds are diminished bilaterally with loud rales (crackles) audible, 1–2 word dyspnea, trachea is midline, no signs of trauma

CVS: Carotid and radial pulses are weak and regular; skin is ashen, lips are blue, and the patient is cool and diaphoretic

ABD: Soft and non-tender

Vitals:

Pulse: 130/min, regular, weak

Resp: 32/min, shallow, bilateral loud rales

BP: 244/112

SpO_2: 74%

ECG: Sinus tachycardia

HX: The patient's husband states that his wife had a very restless night and when she awoke at 0800 she complained of shortness of breath. By 0845 she could hardly talk. He wasn't sure what to do and finally called the ambulance.

Past Hx: The patient has a history of congestive heart disease and is currently taking Lasix 40 mg, Slo-K (potassium), Digoxin, and a bronchodilator. This is the worst episode ever.

Treatment:

Oxygen was administered by non-rebreather at 12 l/min and not well tolerated by the patient. An IV of normal saline was initiated and run TKO. Nitro spray was administered with no relief. The base hospital was contacted and the paramedics received the order to administer two more sprays of nitroglycerin. Following the nitro spray, they administered 2.5 mg of morphine followed by 80 mg of Lasix (the patient was already taking Lasix).

The patient did not experience any improvement from the nitro spray but did seem more relaxed following the morphine. En route the patient began to experience some relief after the Lasix was given. Upon arrival at the hospital, the patient was given another 80 mg of Lasix with significant improvement.

Bumetanide (Bumex)

Class: Diuretic

Description

Bumetanide is a potent diuretic with a rapid rate of onset and a short duration of action.

Mechanism of Action

Like furosemide, bumetanide is a loop diuretic that inhibits the reabsorption of sodium chloride in the kidneys. This causes a net diuresis. One milligram of bumetanide has the diuretic potency of 40 milligrams of furosemide.

Indications

- Congestive heart failure
- Pulmonary edema

Contraindications

Usage in pregnancy should be limited to life-threatening situations in which the benefits of using bumetanide outweigh the risks.

Precautions

Dehydration and electrolyte depletion can result from excessive doses of potent diuretics. Patients who have experienced allergic reactions to furosemide have not experienced those same reactions when administered bumetanide, which suggests that this drug may be used in patients with furosemide allergy who are in need of rapid diuresis.

Side Effects

Bumetanide can cause muscle cramps, dizziness, hypotension, headache, nausea, and vomiting.

Interactions

Bumetanide can potentiate the effect of the various antihypertensive agents and should be used with caution in patients taking these.

Dosage

The usual initial dose of bumetanide is 0.5 to 1.0 milligram given during a period of 1 to 2 minutes. A second or third dose can be administered at 2- to 3-hour intervals if required. The total daily dosage should not exceed 10 milligrams. Bumetanide injection can be given by either the IV or intramuscular routes. In the emergency setting, the IV route is preferred.

How Supplied

Bumetanide (Bumex) is supplied in ampules containing 0.5 milligrams in 2 milliliters of solvent (0.25 milligrams per milliliter). It is also supplied in 2-, 4-, and 10-milliliter vials containing 0.25 milligrams per milliliter.

ANTIANGINAL AGENTS

A common manifestation of advanced cardiovascular disease is angina pectoris, which results from a narrowing of the coronary arteries due to the buildup of atherosclerotic plaques, or coronary artery vasospasm. In exercise and other stressful situations, the amount of blood that can be carried by the coronary arteries may not be sufficient to meet the oxygen demands of the myocardium. This results in myocardial hypoxia, causing the classic pain syndrome called angina pectoris. Sublingual nitroglycerin usually gives immediate relief by dilating the coronary arteries and decreasing cardiac work. In recent years there have been trials in which nitroglycerin has been administered to patients suffering myocardial infarction in the hope of decreasing the extent of myocardial damage. Nitroglycerin is often administered to patients complaining of chest pain to rule out angina as the cause. When cardiac pain is not relieved by nitroglycerin, morphine and other potent analgesics are administered.

Nitroglycerin is usually administered sublingually. Recently, however, it can be given intravenously in certain cases of unstable angina and acute myocardial infarction.

Calcium-ion antagonists, such as nifedipine (Procardia), have proved effective in the management of angina, especially when there is coronary artery vasospasm.

Nitroglycerin (Nitrostat)

Class: Nitrate

Description

Nitroglycerin is a potent smooth-muscle relaxant used in the treatment of angina pectoris.

Mechanism of Action

Nitroglycerin is a rapid smooth-muscle relaxant that reduces cardiac work and, to a lesser degree, dilates the coronary arteries. This results in increased coronary blood flow and improved perfusion of the ischemic myocardium. Relief of ischemia causes reduction and alleviation of chest pain. Pain relief following nitroglycerin administration usually occurs within 1 to 2 minutes, and therapeutic effects can be observed up to 30 minutes later. Nitroglycerin also causes vasodilation, which decreases preload. Decreased preload leads to decreased cardiac work. This feature, in conjunction with coronary vasodilation, reverses the effects of angina pectoris.

Indications

- Chest pain associated with angina pectoris
- Chest pain associated with acute myocardial infarction
- Acute pulmonary edema (unless accompanied by hypotension)

Contraindications

Nitroglycerin is contraindicated in patients who are hypotensive or who may have increased intracranial pressure. It should not be administered to patients in shock.

Precautions

Patients taking nitroglycerin may develop a tolerance for the drug, which necessitates increasing the dose. Headache is a common side effect of nitro-

POTENTIALLY FATAL TO PT'S TAKING VIAGRA

glycerin administration and results from vasodilation of cerebral vessels. Nitroglycerin deteriorates quite rapidly once the bottle is opened. When a bottle of nitroglycerin is opened, it should be dated. Nitroglycerin should also be protected from light.

Always monitor the blood pressure and the other vital signs during nitroglycerin administration.

Side Effects

Nitroglycerin can cause headache, dizziness, weakness, tachycardia, hypotension, orthostasis, skin rash, dry mouth, nausea, and vomiting.

Interactions

Nitroglycerin can cause severe hypotension when administered to patients who have recently ingested alcohol. It can cause orthostatic hypotension when used in conjunction with beta blockers.

Dosage

One tablet (0.4-milligram) sublingually for routine angina pectoris. This can be repeated in 3–5 minutes as required. Usually, more than three tablets should not be administered in the prehospital setting. Nitroglycerin should be administered sublingually. Care should be taken to assure that it is not swallowed. IV nitroglycerin is used in the emergency department and intensive care units, but the sublingual route is adequate for most prehospital situations. Nitroglycerin is also available in patches and in ointment form for transdermal administration.

How Supplied

Nitroglycerin is supplied in bottles containing 0.4-milligram tablets (1/150 grain). The tablets must be protected from light and air to prevent deterioration.

Nitroglycerin Paste (Nitro-Bid Ointment)

Class: Nitrate

Description

Nitroglycerin paste contains a 2% solution of nitroglycerin in a special absorbent paste. When placed on the skin, nitroglycerin is absorbed into the systemic circulation. In many cases it may be preferred over nitroglycerin tablets because of its longer duration of action.

Mechanism of Action

Nitroglycerin is a rapid smooth-muscle relaxant that reduces cardiac work and, to a lesser degree, dilates the coronary arteries. This results in increased coronary blood flow and improved perfusion of the ischemic myocardium. Relief of ischemia causes reduction and alleviation of chest pain. Pain relief following transcutaneous nitroglycerin administration usually occurs within 5 to 10 minutes, and therapeutic effects can be observed up to 30 minutes later. Nitroglycerin also causes vasodilation, which decreases preload. Decreased preload leads to decreased cardiac work. This feature, in conjunction with coronary vasodilation, reverses the effects of angina pectoris.

Indications

- Chest pain associated with angina pectoris
- Chest pain associated with acute myocardial infarction

Contraindications

Nitroglycerin paste is contraindicated in patients with increased intracranial pressure. It should not be administered to patients who are hypotensive or in shock.

Precautions

Patients taking the drug routinely may develop a tolerance and require an increased dose. Headache is a common side effect of nitroglycerin administration and occurs as a result of vasodilatation of the cerebral vessels.

Postural syncope sometimes occurs following the administration of nitroglycerin. This should be anticipated and the patient kept supine when possible. It is important to monitor the blood pressure constantly.

Side Effects

Nitroglycerin can cause headache, dizziness, weakness, tachycardia, hypotension, orthostasis, skin rash, dry mouth, nausea, and vomiting.

Interactions

Nitroglycerin can cause severe hypotension when administered to patients who have recently ingested alcohol. It can cause orthostatic hypotension when used in conjunction with beta blockers.

Dosage

Generally 1/2 to 1 inch (1.25 to 2.50 centimeters) of the Nitro-Bid Ointment is applied. Measuring applicators are supplied.

How Supplied

Nitro-Bid Ointment is supplied in 20-gram and 60-gram tubes. Several dose-measuring applicators are also included.

Nitroglycerin Spray (Nitrolingual Spray)

Class: Nitrate

Description

Nitroglycerin spray is a special preparation of nitroglycerin in an aerosol form that delivers precisely 0.4 milligram of nitroglycerin per spray.

Mechanism of Action

Nitroglycerin is a rapid smooth-muscle relaxant that reduces cardiac work and, to a lesser degree, dilates the coronary arteries. This results in increased coronary blood flow and improved perfusion of the ischemic myocardium. Relief of ischemia causes reduction and alleviation of chest pain. Pain relief following nitroglycerin administration usually occurs within 1 to 2 minutes and peak effects occur within 4 minutes. Therapeutic effects can be observed up to 30 minutes later. Nitroglycerin also causes vasodilation, which decreases preload. Decreased preload leads to decreased cardiac work. This feature, in conjunction with coronary vasodilation, reverses the effects of angina pectoris.

Indications

- Chest pain associated with angina pectoris
- Chest pain associated with acute myocardial infarction

Contraindications

Nitroglycerin is contraindicated in patients who are hypotensive, in shock, or who may have increased intracranial pressure.

Precautions

Patients taking nitroglycerin routinely may develop a tolerance for the drug. Headache is a common side effect of nitroglycerin administration and results from dilation of cerebral blood vessels. This should be anticipated. The blood pressure should be monitored during nitroglycerin therapy.

Side Effects

Nitroglycerin can cause headache, dizziness, weakness, tachycardia, hypotension, orthostasis, skin rash, dry mouth, nausea, and vomiting.

Interactions

Nitroglycerin can cause severe hypotension when administered to patients who have recently ingested alcohol. It can cause orthostatic hypotension when used in conjunction with beta blockers.

Dosage

One spray (0.4 milligram) should be sprayed under the tongue at the onset of an attack of angina. No more than three sprays are recommended in a 25-minute period. (The spray should not be inhaled.) Nitroglycerin spray should be applied to the sublingual mucous membranes in the manner described earlier.

How Supplied

Nitroglycerin spray is supplied in an aerosol container containing 200 doses of nitroglycerin.

ANTIHYPERTENSIVES

A dangerously elevated blood pressure is a hypertensive emergency. A "hypertensive crisis" is defined as a sudden increase in the systolic and diastolic blood pressure, causing a functional disturbance of the central nervous system, the heart, or the kidneys. Hypertensive emergencies call for prompt and efficient care by prehospital providers.

Hypertensive emergencies are often divided into two categories: hypertensive emergencies and hypertensive urgencies. A "hypertensive emergency" is a situation in which the blood pressure must be lowered within 1 hour. A "hypertensive urgency" is a situation in which the blood pressure should be lowered within 24 hours. Hypertensive emergencies develop when the blood pressure exceeds 130 millimeters of mercury diastolic pressure (with or without symptoms) or any elevated blood pressure associated with end-organ symptoms. End-organ symptoms include chest pain, dyspnea, altered mental status, seizures, stroke, nose bleed, or hypertensive encephalopathy. In many cases the emergency develops not from the absolute blood pressure value, but often from how rapid the value is achieved. Rapid elevations in blood pressure are poorly tolerated by the body and more apt to cause end-organ symptoms.

Hypertensive encephalopathy is the most devastating complication of hypertension. Signs and symptoms include severe headache, nausea and vomiting, and an altered mental state. This can range from lethargy or confusion to coma. Neurological symptoms may be present as well. These can include blindness, inability to speak, muscle twitches, weakness, or paralysis. The treatment is to lower blood pressure as rapidly and as safely as possible.

There are several agents available to lower blood pressure acutely. The most popular of these is nifedipine (Procardia). Procardia can be administered sublingually with an onset of action in less than 10 minutes. In hypertension refractory to nifedipine, sodium nitroprusside is often used. Labetalol (previously discussed) is a β blocker used in the management of hypertensive emergencies. Sodium nitroprusside is administered as a controlled infusion that can be titrated to obtain the desired pressure. Hydralazine is often used to lower the blood pressure in pregnancy to prevent eclampsia. Diazoxide (Hyperstat), once used commonly in emergency care, has fallen into relative disuse with nifedipine being the preferred agent.

Nifedipine (Procardia) (Adalat)

Class: Calcium Channel Blocker

Description

Nifedipine is a calcium channel blocker that is widely used in emergency medicine in the treatment of hypertension.

Mechanism of Action

Nifedipine causes relaxation of the smooth muscles that encircle the peripheral blood vessels, principally the arterioles. This relaxation results in peripheral vasodilation, decreased peripheral vascular resistance, and a decrease in both the systolic and diastolic blood pressure. Nifedipine is also effective in reducing coronary artery spasm in angina. Nifedipine can be used in hypertension associated with pregnancy if hydralazine is not available.

Indications

- Severe hypertension
- Angina pectoris

Contraindications

Nifedipine is contraindicated in patients with known hypersensitivity to the drug. It should not be administered to patients who are hypotensive.

Precautions

Nifedipine can cause a significant drop in blood pressure. Thus, the blood pressure should be frequently monitored. Nifedipine should be used with caution in patients with heart failure. Nifedipine should not be administered to patients receiving IV β blockers.

Side Effects

Nifedepine can cause nausea, vomiting, dizziness, headache, bradycardia, heart block, hypotension, and asystole.

Interactions

Nifedepine should not be administered to patients receiving intravenous β blockers because of an increased risk of congestive heart failure, bradycardia, and asystole.

Dosage

Several small puncture holes should be placed in one 10-milligram capsule before placing it under the tongue where it can be absorbed. Alternatively, the capsule can be bitten by the patient and swallowed with approximately the same rate of onset. In severe hypertension the medical control physician may order an initial dose of 20 milligrams. Nifedipine should only be administered orally or sublingually as described earlier.

How Supplied

Nifedipine is supplied in 10- and 20-milligram tablets.

Sodium Nitroprusside (Nitropress, Nipride)

Class: Antihypertensive/Vasodilator

Description

Sodium nitroprusside is a potent vasodilating agent used in the management of hypertensive crisis when a prompt reduction in blood pressure is required.

Mechanism of Action

Sodium nitroprusside acts by dilating both peripheral arteries and peripheral veins. This reduction in peripheral vascular resistance results in an immediate reduction in blood pressure, which is generally proportional to the rate of drug administration. Sodium nitroprusside administration is usually accompanied by an increase in heart rate.

Although not approved, sodium nitroprusside is occasionally used in the management of severe congestive heart failure. The dilation of the peripheral veins results in decreased blood return to the heart (preload). In addition, the dilation of the peripheral arteries reduces the pressure against which the heart has to pump (afterload). This results in a net increase in cardiac output in patients with severe congestive heart failure (see Figure 7-17).

Because sodium nitroprusside is such a potent agent, the blood pressure, pulse rate, respiratory status, and EKG should be constantly monitored during drug administration.

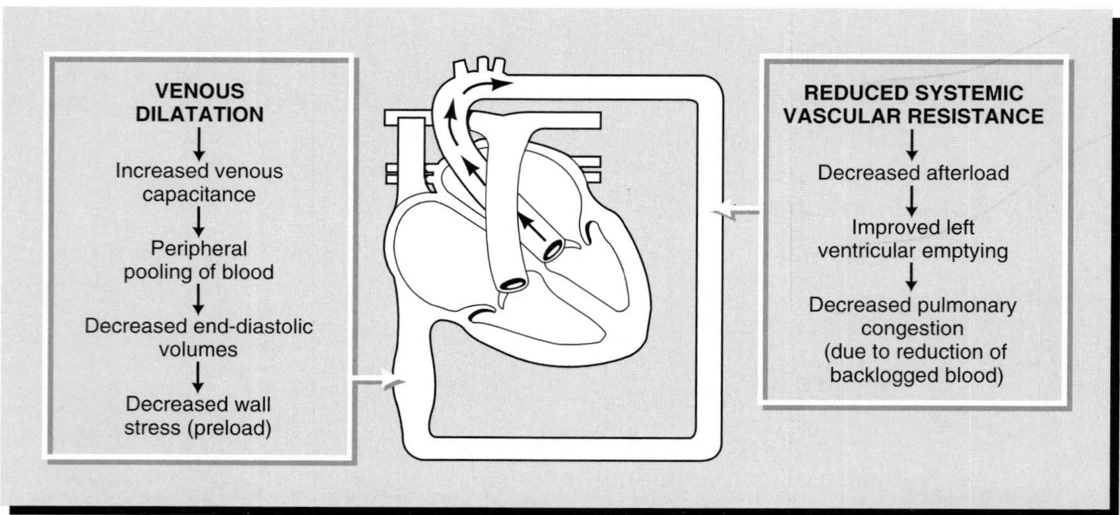

Figure 7-17 Actions of sodium nitroprusside.

Indication

- Hypertensive crisis in which a prompt reduction in blood pressure is essential

Contraindications

None when used in the management of life-threatening hypertensive crisis

Precautions

Once the sodium nitroprusside infusion is prepared, it should be immediately wrapped in an opaque material, usually aluminum foil, to protect it from light. Once exposed to light the drug is quickly inactivated.

Sodium nitroprusside should not be used in children or pregnant women in the prehospital setting. The dosage should be reduced somewhat in elderly patients. The constant monitoring of blood pressure and pulse is essential throughout sodium nitroprusside administration.

Side Effects

Sodium nitroprusside can cause dizziness, headache, hypotension, chest pain, dyspnea, palpitations, nausea, and vomiting.

Interactions

The effects of sodium nitroprusside can be potentiated when administered with other antihypertensive agents.

Dosage

Fifty milligrams of sodium nitroprusside should be diluted in 500 milliliters of D_5W. This will give a concentration of 100 micrograms per milliliter. The initial dose should be 0.5 micrograms per kilogram per minute (see Figure 7-18). The typical dosage range is from 0.5–8.0 micrograms/kilogram/minute. Sodium nitroprusside should only be diluted in D_5W or normal saline and administered by slow IV infusion using a minidrip administration set (preferably through an IV pump). *This medication should never be given by IV bolus.*

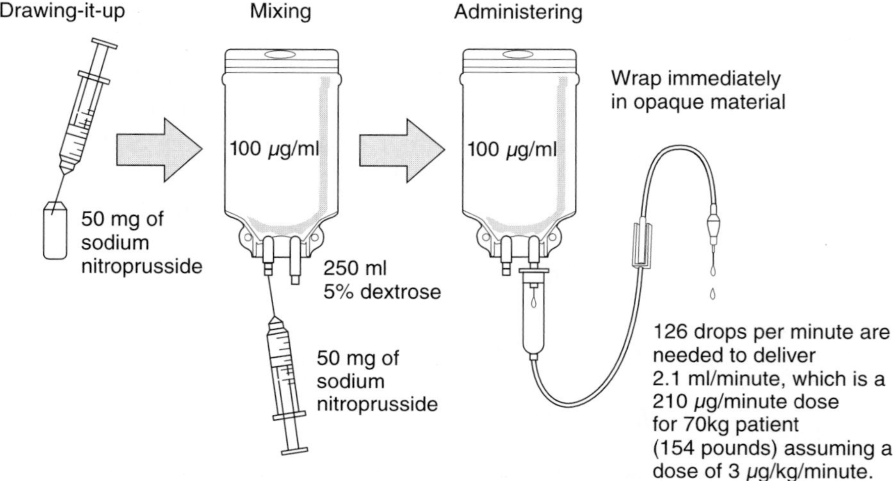

Figure 7-18 Preparation of sodium nitroprusside infusion.

How Supplied

Sodium nitroprusside is supplied in 5-milliliter vials containing 50 milligrams of the drug.

Hydralazine (Apresoline)

Class: Antihypertensive/Vasodilator

Description

Hydralazine is a potent vasodilating agent used to lower blood pressure in cases of hypertensive crisis.

Mechanism of Action

Hydralazine, like sodium nitroprusside, relaxes vascular smooth muscle, primarily in the arterial system, thus causing decreased arterial pressure (diastolic greater than systolic), decreased peripheral resistance, and increased cardiac output. Hydralazine causes postural hypotension to a lesser degree than sodium nitroprusside. The effects of hydralazine are usually seen within 5 to 10 minutes after the initiation of therapy.

Indications

- Hypertensive crisis in which a prompt reduction in blood pressure is required
- Hypertension complicating pregnancy (preeclampsia)

Contraindications

Hydralazine should not be administered to patients with a known history of hypersensitivity to the drug, coronary artery disease, or rheumatic heart disease involving the mitral valve.

Precautions

The administration of hydralazine may cause angina pectoris or EKG changes because of the increased cardiac output. This drug should not be used in the prehospital phase of emergency medical care to children because of limited experience with the drug in these cases. The blood pressure, pulse rate, respiratory status, and EKG should be monitored at all times during hydralazine therapy. Headache, nausea, and vomiting have been known to occur following hydralazine therapy and should be expected.

Side Effects

Hydralazine can cause headache, dizziness, altered mental status, tachycardia, arrhythmias, orthostasis, chest pain, nausea, and vomiting.

Interactions

The effects of hydralazine can be potentiated when administered with other antihypertensive agents.

Dosage

The usual dosage of hydralazine in the management of hypertensive crisis is 20 to 40 milligrams given by slow IV bolus. This can be repeated in 4–6 hours if required. If an IV line cannot be established, then the same dosage of the drug can be given by intramuscular injection. The blood pressure and EKG should be continuously monitored. Parenteral hydralazine should be administered by slow IV bolus. When necessary, however, the drug can be administered by intramuscular injection.

How Supplied

Hydralazine is supplied in 1-milliliter ampules containing 20 milligrams of the drug.

Diazoxide (Hyperstat)

Class: Antihypertensive/Vasodilator

Description

Diazoxide relaxes vascular smooth muscle and is effective in the treatment of hypertensive crisis.

Mechanism of Action

Diazoxide causes a decrease in both systolic and diastolic pressure by causing vasodilatation of the peripheral arterioles. This results in decreased peripheral vascular resistance and a subsequently lowered systolic and diastolic blood pressure.

Indication

- Severe hypertension in which a prompt decrease in diastolic blood pressure is indicated

Contraindications

Diazoxide should not be administered to patients with a known hypersensitivity to the drug or to the thiazide class of diuretics. Although there are some additional medical conditions for which diazoxide is contraindicated, the paramedic will most likely be unaware of these in the field.

Precautions

Hypotension may occur and, if severe, should be treated with sympathomimetics. Because of the rapid onset of action of diazoxide, frequent blood pressure monitoring (every minute) to detect possible hypotension is mandatory.

Side Effects

Diazoxide can cause headache, dizziness, altered mental status, tachycardia, arrhythmias, chest pain, congestive heart failure, edema, hyperglycemia, nausea, and vomiting.

Interactions

The effects of diazoxide can be potentiated when administered with other antihypertensive agents. It can also decrease the blood levels of phenytoin and precipitate a seizure.

Dosage

The standard dose of diazoxide is 1 to 3 milligrams per kilogram of body weight given intravenously over 30 seconds up to 150 milligrams per kilogram. The dose may be repeated at 5- to 15-minute intervals as required. Diazoxide is administered intravenously.

How Supplied

Diazoxide is supplied in ampules containing 300 milligrams of the drug in 20 milliliters of solvent.

OTHER CARDIOVASCULAR DRUGS

The following agent does not readily fit into the classes of drugs discussed thus far.

Calcium Chloride

Class: Calcium Supplement

Description

Calcium chloride provides elemental calcium in the form of the cation (Ca^{++}). Calcium is required for many physiological activities.

Mechanism of Action

Calcium chloride replaces calcium in cases of hypocalcemia. Calcium chloride causes a significant increase in the myocardial contractile force and appears to increase ventricular automaticity. Although frequently used for many years in the management of cardiac arrest, especially that resulting from asystole and electromechanical dissociation, recent studies have presented data that seriously question the role of calcium chloride, even in these situations. Calcium chloride is an antidote for magnesium sulfate and can minimize some of the side effects of calcium channel blocker usage.

Indications

- Acute hyperkalemia (elevated potassium)
- Acute hypocalcemia (decreased calcium)
- Calcium-channel-blocker toxicity (nifedipine, verapamil, diltiazem)

Contraindications

Caution is warranted when calcium chloride is administered to patients receiving digitalis, as it may precipitate digitalis toxicity.

Precautions

It is extremely important to flush the IV line between administrations of calcium chloride and sodium bicarbonate to avoid precipitation. Calcium chloride can cause tissue necrosis at the injection site. It should always be administered through an IV that is patent and running well.

Side Effects

Calcium chloride can cause bradycardia, arrhythmias, syncope, nausea, vomiting, and cardiac arrest.

Interactions

Calcium chloride will interact with sodium bicarbonate and form a precipitate. In addition, calcium chloride can cause elevated digoxin levels, and possibly digitalis toxicity, when administered to patients receiving digitalis preparations.

Dosage

The standard dose for calcium chloride is 2 to 4 milligrams per kilogram intravenously. This may be repeated every 10 minutes as required. Calcium chloride should only be given intravenously in the emergency setting.

How Supplied

Calcium chloride comes in prefilled syringes containing 1 gram of the drug in 10 milliliters of solvent (10 milliliters of a 10% solution).

SUMMARY

All of the medications discussed in this chapter are only of value when used in conjunction with other treatment modalities. Without appropriate cardiopulmonary resuscitation, the medications used in the management of cardiac arrest are not effective.

As mentioned, the dosages presented in this chapter are based on nationally accepted regimens. You should become familiar with the routine dosages and protocols used in your area.

KEY WORDS AND PHRASES

adrenergic receptors. Receptors specific to norepinephrine and epinephrine-like substances.

adrenergic system. The part of the nervous system that prepares the body to deal with various stresses, whether real or imagined. Also referred to as the sympathetic nervous system.

aerobic metabolism. The process of generating energy with the aid of oxygen.

agonist. A drug or other substance that causes a physiological response.

anaerobic metabolism. The process of generating energy without the aid of oxygen.

antagonist. A drug or other substance that blocks a physiological response or that blocks the action of another drug or substance.

automaticity. The capacity of self-depolarization. Refers to the pacemaker cells of the heart.

catecholamine. A class of hormones that act upon the autonomic nervous system. They include epinephrine, norepinephrine, and similar compounds.

cholinergic system. A division of the autonomic nervous system that is responsible for controlling vegetative functions. Also called the parasympathetic nervous system.

chronotrope. A drug or substance that affects the heart rate.

concomitant. Occurring at the same time.

dopaminergic receptor. Receptor in the renal and splanchnic vessels that maintains vasodilation.

dromotrope. A drug or substance that affects the conduction velocity of the heart.

endogenous. Coming from inside the body.

homeostasis. The natural tendency of the body to maintain the internal environment relatively constant.

hypoxic drive. Respiratory control system commonly present in patients with chronic obstructive pulmonary disease whereby respirations are dependent upon changes in the concentration of oxygen concentration as opposed to changes in the concentration of carbon dioxide.

inotrope. A drug or substance that affects the contractile force of the heart.

lactic acid. An organic acid normally present in tissue. One form of lactic acid in muscle and blood is a product of the change of the carbohydrates, glucose and glycogen, to energy during physical exercise.

neurotransmitter. A substance that is released from the axon terminal of a presynaptic neuron upon excitation and that travels across the synaptic cleft to either excite or inhibit the target cell. Examples include acetylcholine, norepinephrine, and dopamine.

pheochromocytoma. A tumor of the adrenal gland that causes too much release of two hormones (epinephrine and norepinephrine). Signs include high blood pressure, headache, sweating, excess blood sugar, nausea, vomiting, and fainting spells.

pulse oximetry. An assessment modality that measures the oxygen saturation level of the blood through a noninvasive sensor placed on a finger or earlobe.

retrolental fibroplasia. A disorder caused by giving excess amounts of oxygen to premature infants. A fiberlike tissue forms behind the lens of the eye.

stroke volume. The amount of blood ejected by the heart in one cardiac contraction.

sympathomimetic. A drug or substance that causes effects like those of the sympathetic nervous system (also called adrenergic).

Torsades de pointes. A form of ventricular tachycardia where the morphology of the QRS appears to change (the axis rotates). It is often drug-induced, but may be the result of low potassium levels in the blood (hypokalemia) or profound slow heart beat (bradycardia).

Wolff-Parkinson-White syndrome. A disorder of the heart characterized by early contraction of the heart muscle.

chapter 8

Drugs Used in the Treatment of Respiratory Emergencies

OBJECTIVES

1. Discuss the devices commonly used to administer oxygen in the field.
2. Discuss pulse oximetry and end-tidal carbon dioxide detection, and describe the prehospital use of both.
3. Discuss the pathophysiology and prehospital management of asthma and status asthmaticus.
4. Describe and list the indications, contraindications, and dosages for the following beta-agonists used in respiratory emergencies: epinephrine 1:1,000, albuterol, racemic epinephrine, terbutaline, isoetharine, metaproterenol, and aminophylline.
5. Describe and list the indications, contraindications, and dosages for the following anticholinergics: atropine and ipratropium.
6. Describe and list the indications, contraindications, and dosages for the following corticosteroids: methylprednisolone and hydrocortisone.
7. Discuss the indications and considerations in the use of neuromuscular blockers.
8. List the steps in performing rapid sequence intubation.
9. Describe and list the indications, contraindications, and dosages for the following medications used as neuromuscular blocking agents: succinylcholine, pancuronium, and vecuronium.

INTRODUCTION

Oxygen is the most important drug for use in the management of respiratory emergencies. In addition to oxygen, however, several pharmacologic agents have proved quite effective in relieving respiratory distress. In this chapter medications commonly used in the prehospital treatment of respiratory emergencies are discussed. These include:

Gases

- Oxygen

Beta Agonists

- Epinephrine 1:1,000
- Albuterol
- Racemic Epinephrine
- Terbutaline
- Isoetharine
- Metaproterenol

Xanthines

- Aminophylline

Anticholinergics

- Atropine
- Ipratropium

Corticosteroids

- Methylprednisolone
- Hydrocortisone

Neuromuscular Blockers

- Succinylcholine
- Vecuronium
- Pancuronium

Sympathomimetics are among the most frequently used agents in the treatment of respiratory emergencies. The principal sympathomimetics include epinephrine, isoetharine, terbutaline, metaproterenol, and albuterol. In treating cardiovascular emergencies it is highly desirable to activate β_1 adrenergic receptors. When treating patients in respiratory distress, however, it is desirable to activate β_2 receptors. Unfortunately, most of the agents that activate β_2 receptors also have some effect on β_1 receptors. When activated, β_1 receptors cause an increase in heart rate and myocardial contractile force while β_2 receptors cause peripheral vasodilation and, most important, bronchodilation. Common side effects of these medications include palpitations, anxiety, and dizziness. Considerable effort has been devoted to isolation of pharmacological agents that act principally on β_2 receptors. Currently, metaproterenol and albuterol are the sympathomimetic agents most frequently used in the prehospital phase of emergency medical care. They are chemically related to epinephrine but tend to be more selective for β_2 receptors than epinephrine.

Another agent used in the management of respiratory emergencies is aminophylline. Aminophylline, chemically unrelated to the catecholamines, belongs to a class of drugs called *xanthines*. A commonly encountered drug within the xanthines class is caffeine. Aminophylline causes relaxation of the bronchiole smooth musculature and bronchodilation.

Although not discussed here, corticosteroids play a major role in the treatment of respiratory diseases. Asthma, and many cases of COPD, have inflammation as the underlying cause. While the β-agonists will help reverse bronchospasm, they do little for the underlying inflammation. Corticosteroids have a very long rate of onset (1– 4 hours) and thus their effects are not usually seen in the prehospital setting.

Some systems have added neuromuscular blocking agents to their paramedic drug lists. These medications are very effective in providing muscle relaxation for endotracheal intubation. However, as they remove a patient's protective reflexes and cause apnea, they should only be used by personnel with experience in their use.

OXYGEN

Oxygen administration is an important aspect of patient care. It is essential in cases that involve suspected hypoxia of any cause, chest pain due to myocardial ischemia, asthma, and cardiorespiratory arrest.

Oxygen Administration

Administering oxygen to a hypoxic patient raises his or her oxygen level by:

- Increasing the inspired percentage of oxygen
- Increasing oxygen concentration at the alveolar level
- Increasing arterial oxygen levels
- Increasing the amount of oxygen delivered to the patient's cells

Oxygen administration decreases hypoxia and reduces the volume of respiration necessary to oxygenate the blood. It also reduces the myocardial work demanded to maintain given arterial oxygen tension.

There are no absolute contraindications to oxygen administration. However, it should be used with caution in premature infants and patients who are prone to carbon dioxide retention (hypoxic drive). It should be administered at lower flow rates with COPD patients: 1–3 liters delivered via nasal cannula. If your patient develops respiratory depression, breathing should be assisted with a bag-valve-mask device. When ventilating via a bag-valve-mask device, use 100 percent oxygen. When providing oxygen to a premature infant, hold the mask over the face, not directly on it.

Oxygen Devices

Devices commonly used to administer oxygen in the field include the nasal cannula, the simple face mask, the nonrebreather mask, and to a lesser extent, the Venturi mask.

Nasal Cannula The *nasal cannula* is a frequently used device that is comfortable and is easily tolerated by the patient. It can deliver oxygen concentrations ranging from 24–44 percent. The oxygen flow rates for the nasal cannula vary from 1–6 liters per minute.

Simple Face Mask The *simple face mask* will deliver an oxygen concentration of 40–60 percent. Flow rates administered through the simple face mask range from 8–12 liters per minute. No fewer than 6 liters per minute should be administered through this device, as expired carbon dioxide can otherwise accumulate in the mask. Flow rates in excess of 8 liters per minute are needed to "wash out" any expired carbon dioxide.

The simple face mask provides oxygen to patients who are suffering from moderate hypoxia. Disadvantages include: it may feel confining to the patient, it muffles the patient's speech, and it requires a tight face seal. Because the mask covers the patient's face, it should be used with caution in cases that involve nausea or vomiting. With the pediatric patient, a flow rate of 6–8 liters per minute is generally considered acceptable.

Nonrebreather Mask When the patient inhales, the 100 percent oxygen contained in the reservoir is drawn into the mask and the patient's respiratory passages. Ambient air is prevented from entering the mask by the rubber flap that closes over the inlet/outlet ports during inspiration. When the patient exhales, the flapper valve is open to allow the expired air an exit. A one-way valve situated between the mask and the reservoir prevents the expired air from entering the reservoir bag.

The *nonrebreather mask* delivers the highest concentration of oxygen. When supplied at a flow rate of 10–15 liters per minute, it can deliver an 80–100 percent oxygen concentration. No fewer than 8 liters of oxygen per minute should be administered through this device. Because the nonrebreather mask is a relatively closed system, it restricts the inspiration of ambient air. Therefore, its reservoir bag should not be allowed to deflate totally or be allowed to kink. Otherwise, the patient might suffocate.

The nonrebreather mask is similar to the simple face mask in that it requires a tight seal. This may be difficult to obtain with some patients because they find the mask confining. This device should be employed with caution in nauseated patients. Its main application lies in the treatment of severely hypoxic patients—those suffering respiratory compromise, shock, acute myocardial infarction, trauma, or carbon monoxide poisoning.

Venturi Mask With the *Venturi mask*, relatively precise concentrations of oxygen can be provided. This device is not commonly used in prehospital care and is used in the treatment of COPD patients. To control the amount of ambient air taken in by a patient, some venturi masks are supplied with dial selection, while others come with interchangeable caps. These devices deliver oxygen concentrations of 24 percent, 28 percent, 35 percent, or 40 percent. The liter flow depends on the oxygen concentration desired.

VENTILATION

In the field you will be called upon in many cases to provide ventilatory support. Situations will range from those that involve apneic patients to less obvious cases in which patients are experiencing depressed respiratory function.

Remember that when a patient is unconscious, his or her respiratory center may not function at a satisfactory level. A significant decrease in the patient's rate or depth of breathing will lead to decreased respiratory minute volume, hypercarbia, hypoxia, and a lowered pH. If not corrected, respiratory or cardiac arrest may occur. To achieve effective ventilatory support, an adequate rate and volume of oxygen must be delivered—at least 800 mL of oxygen at a rate of 12–20 breaths per minute.

PULSE OXIMETRY

Pulse oximetry is now widely used in emergency care. The pulse oximeter is a quick and accurate tool that can objectively determine the oxygenation status of the patient. The pulse oximeter provides immediate and continuous evaluation of oxygen delivery to body tissues. It quantifies the effects of interventions including oxygen therapy, medication, suctioning, and ventilatory assistance. As well, oximetry often detects problems with oxygenation before blood pressure, pulse, and respirations would reveal such a problem. Use pulse oximetry, when available, in virtually any patient care situation. In fact, it has been referred to as the "fifth vital sign." It should be used during the patient assessment process to determine the patient's baseline value. It should also be used to guide patient care and to monitor the patient's response to your interventions. Normal SpO_2 varies between 95 percent and 100 percent. Readings between 91 percent and 94 percent indicate mild hypoxia and warrant further evaluation and supplemental oxygen administration. Readings between 86 percent and 91 percent indicate moderate hypoxia. These patients should receive 100 percent supplemental oxygen. Readings of 85 percent or lower indicate severe hypoxia and warrant immediate intervention, including the administration of 100 percent oxygen, ventilatory assistance, or both. The goal of therapy is to maintain the SpO_2 in the normal (95–99 percent) range.

The incidence of false readings with pulse oximetry is small. When it does occur, the oximeter generates an error signal or a blank screen. Causes of false readings include carbon-monoxide poisoning, high-intensity lighting, and certain hemoglobin abnormalities. The absence of a pulse in an extremity will give a false reading. In hypovolemia, and in severely anemic patients, the pulse oximetry reading may be misleading. While the SpO_2 reading may be normal, the total amount of hemoglobin available to carry oxygen may be so markedly decreased that the patient will remain hypoxic at the cellular level.

Pulse oximetry is now an important part of emergency care, including prehospital care. Like the ECG monitor, it provides important information related to the patient. It is important to remember that it is only an additional tool. It does not replace other assessment or monitoring skills. Do not depend solely on pulse oximetry reading to guide care. Always consider and treat the whole patient. The reliability and validity of the pulse oximeter is well-documented.

CAPNOGRAPHY

Devices that measure the concentration of exhaled carbon dioxide are increasingly used in prehospital care. These devices, called *end-tidal carbon dioxide ($ETCO_2$) detectors*, are most commonly used to assess proper placement of an endotracheal tube. A lack of carbon dioxide in the exhaled air strongly indicates that the tube is placed in the esophagus, while the presence of carbon dioxide probably indicates proper tube placement.

End-tidal carbon dioxide detectors are available either as a disposable colormetric device or an electronic monitor. The device is attached in-line between the endotracheal tube and the ventilation device. Proper tube placement is confirmed by a color change in the colormetric device or by a light on the electronic monitor.

As with pulse oximetry, you should use an $ETCO_2$ detector only as an adjunct to assessment of endotracheal placement. Use the device in conjunction with other methods of assessment. It is not a replacement for actually visualizing the endotracheal tube passing through the vocal cords.

ASTHMA

Asthma is a common respiratory illness that affects many persons. During a time when deaths from other respiratory diseases are steadily declining, deaths from asthma have significantly increased during the last decade. Most of the increased asthma deaths have occurred in patients who are 45 years of age or older. Approximately 50 percent of patients who die from asthma do so before reaching the hospital. Thus, EMS personnel are frequently called upon to treat patients suffering an asthma attack. Prompt recognition, followed by appropriate treatment, can significantly improve the patient's condition and enhance chances of survival.

Pathophysiology

Asthma is a chronic inflammatory disorder of the airways. In susceptible individuals, this inflammation causes symptoms usually associated with widespread but variable airflow obstruction. The major characteristic of asthma is reversible lower airway obstruction. This obstruction is caused by edema, mucus, and smooth muscle spasm; typically, all three factors are involved. Obstruction narrows the diameter of the smaller, smooth muscle-walled bronchioles. The natural dilation of the airways during inhalation allows air to enter these narrowed airways. However, contraction of the airways on exhalation and the obstruction caused by asthma combine to prevent air from escaping.

Air becomes trapped behind the obstruction. This prevents continued ventilation of the alveoli, and oxygen/carbon dioxide exchange may be severely impaired. Hypoxemia and hypercarbia result, with the degree of respiratory distress increasing with the severity of obstruction and number of airways involved.

Asthma may be triggered by one of many different factors. These items, commonly referred to as "triggers" or "inducers," vary from one individual to the next. In allergic individuals, environmental allergens are a major cause of inflammation. These may occur both indoors and outdoors. In addition to allergens, asthma may be triggered by cold air, exercise, foods, irritants, and certain medications. Often a specific trigger cannot be identified.

Within minutes of exposure to the offending trigger, a two-phase reaction occurs. The first phase of the reaction is characterized by the release of chemical mediators such as histamine. These mediators cause contraction of the bronchial smooth muscle and leakage of fluid from peribronchial capillaries. This results in both bronchoconstriction and bronchial edema. These two factors can significantly decrease expiratory airflow causing the typical "asthma attack." Often, the asthma attack will resolve spontaneously in 1–2 hours or may be aborted by the use of inhaled bronchodilator medications such as albuterol. However, within 6–8 hours after exposure to the trigger, a second reaction occurs. This late phase is characterized by inflammation of the bronchioles as cells of the immune system (eosinophils, neutrophils, and lymphocytes) invade the mucosa of the respiratory tract. This leads to additional edema and swelling of the bronchioles and a further decrease of expiratory airflow.

The second phase of the reaction will not typically respond to inhaled beta-agonist drugs such as epinephrine or albuterol. Instead, anti-inflammatory agents such as corticosteroids are often required. It is important to point out that the severe inflammatory changes seen in an acute asthma attack do not develop over a few hours or even a few days. The inflammation will often begin several days or several weeks before the onset of the actual asthma attack.

Status Asthmaticus: Status Asthmaticus is defined as a severe, prolonged asthma attack that cannot be broken by repeated doses of epinephrine or albuterol. It is a serious medical emergency that requires prompt recognition, treatment, and transport. The patient suffering from status asthmaticus frequently will have a greatly distended chest from continual air trapping. Breath sounds, and often wheezing, may be absent. The patient is usually exhausted, severely acidotic, and dehydrated. You should recognize that respiratory arrest is imminent and be prepared for endotracheal intubation. Transport should be immediate, with aggressive treatment continued en route.

Management of Asthma

Treatment of asthma is designed to correct hypoxia, reverse any bronchospasm, and treat inflammatory changes associated with the disease. Oxygen should be administered at a high concentration (100 percent). Intravenous access should be established and the patient placed on an ECG monitor. Initial treatment should be directed at reversing any bronchospasm present. The most commonly used drugs are inhaled beta-agonist preparations such as albuterol (Ventolin, Proventil). These can be easily administered with a small volume, oxygen-powered nebulizer. The patient's response to these medications should be monitored and documented.

In addition to beta-agonists, early administration of corticosteroids should be considered. While the inhaled beta-agonists will help with bronchoconstriction, they will do little for the underlying inflammation, which is the principle problem. If you anticipate a long transport time, medical control may request the administration of methylprednisolone or similar corticosteroid. It is important to point out that the beneficial effects of corticosteroid administration will probably not be detected until 6–8 hours following administration.

If symptoms are severe and do not improve with administration of the inhaled beta-agonists, the intravenous administration of aminophylline may be indicated. If the patient is not currently taking a theophylline preparation, administer a loading dose of 5–6 mg/kg of aminophylline over 20–30 minutes. This should be followed by a maintenance infusion of 0.8–1.0 mg/kg/hr. Remember that both the inhaled beta-agonists and aminophylline may increase heart rates and/or cause tremors, nausea, and vomiting.

Epinephrine 1:1,000

Class: Sympathetic Agonist

Description

Epinephrine is a naturally occurring catecholamine. It is a potent α and β adrenergic stimulant; however, its effect on β receptors is more profound.

Mechanism of Action

Epinephrine acts directly on α and β adrenergic receptors. Its effect on β receptors is much more profound than its effect on α receptors. The effects of epinephrine include increased heart rate, cardiac contractile force, systemic vascular resistance, and blood pressure. It also causes bronchodilation due to its effects on β_2 adrenergic receptors. It is occasionally used to treat the bronchoconstriction accompanying asthma, COPD, and is also effective in treating bronchoconstriction associated with anaphylaxis.

Epinephrine's effects usually appear within 90 seconds of administration, and they are usually of short duration. Occasionally it must be readministered in 15–30 minutes if needed. Epinephrine 1:1,000 is given subcutaneously to ensure a steady and prolonged action. Inhaled β agonists are preferred over epinephrine in the treatment of bronchospasm as they have fewer undesirable side effects.

Indications (Respiratory)

- Bronchial asthma
- Exacerbation of some forms of COPD
- Anaphylaxis

Contraindications

Because of the cardiac effects seen with the administration of epinephrine, it should not be administered to patients with underlying cardiovascular disease or hypertension. Patients with profound anaphylactic reactions, characterized by hypotension and shock, are usually peripherally vasoconstricted, which will delay absorption of the drug from the subcutaneous site of injection. In these cases, epinephrine 1:10,000 should be administered intravenously.

Precautions

Epinephrine should be protected from light. Also, as with the other catecholamines, it tends to be deactivated by alkaline solutions. Any patient receiving epinephrine 1:1,000 should be carefully monitored for changes in blood pressure, pulse, and EKG. Palpitations, anxiety, nausea, and headache are fairly common side effects.

Side Effects

Epinephrine can cause palpitations, anxiety, tremulousness, headache, dizziness, nausea, and vomiting. Because of its strong inotropic and chronotropic properties, epinephrine increases myocardial oxygen demand. Even in low doses it can cause myocardial ischemia. These effects should be kept in mind when administering epinephrine in the emergency setting.

Interactions

The effects of epinephrine can be intensified in patients who are taking antidepressants.

Dosage

The standard dose of epinephrine 1:1,000 ranges from 0.3 to 0.5 milligram subcutaneously depending on the patient's weight and overall medical condition. Typically, 0.3 milligram is the usual starting dose for adults. The dose for pediatric patients is 0.01 mg/kg subcutaneously. In the prehospital phase of emergency medical care, epinephrine 1:1,000 should only be administered subcutaneously (except in the case of pediatric cardiac arrest).

How Supplied

Epinephrine is supplied in ampules and prefilled syringes containing 1 milligram of the drug in 1 milliliter of solvent.

Albuterol (Proventil, Ventolin)

Class: Sympathetic Agonist

Description

Albuterol is a sympathomimetic that is selective for β_2-adrenergic receptors.

Mechanism of Action

Albuterol is a selective β_2 agonist with a minimal amount of side effects. It causes prompt bronchodilation and has a duration of action of approximately 5 hours.

Indications

- Bronchial asthma
- Reversible bronchospasm associated with chronic bronchitis and emphysema

Contraindications

Albuterol should not be administered to any patient with a known history of hypersensitivity to the drug.

Precautions

As with any sympathomimetic, the patient's vital signs must be monitored. Caution should be used when administering albuterol to elderly patients and those with cardiovascular disease or hypertension. Lung sounds should be auscultated before and after each treatment. Ideally, the patient's peak flow rate should be measured both before and after drug administration.

Side Effects

Albuterol can cause palpitations, anxiety, dizziness, headache, nervousness, tremor, hypertension, arrhythmias, chest pain, nausea, and vomiting.

Interactions

The possibility of developing unpleasant side effects increases when albuterol is administered with other sympathetic agonists. β blockers may blunt the pharmacological effects of albuterol.

Dosage

Albuterol can be administered by metered-dose inhaler or small-volume nebulizer. A common initial dose is two sprays when using a metered-dose inhaler. Each spray delivers 90 micrograms of albuterol.

When using a small-volume nebulizer, the standard adult dose is 2.5 milligrams (0.5 milliliter of a 0.5% solution diluted in 2.5 milliliters of normal saline). This amount is typically delivered during 5 to 15 minutes.

Albuterol (Ventolin) is also available in the Rotohaler form. A special 200-microgram Rotocap is placed in the device and inhaled by the patient. Albuterol should only be administered by inhalation.

How Supplied

Albuterol is supplied in metered-dose inhalers that contain approximately three hundred 90-microgram sprays. The solution for inhalation is supplied in single-patient vials containing 0.5 milliliter of the drug in 2.5 milliliters of normal saline. Rotocaps for inhalation are supplied in special 200-microgram capsules.

CASE PRESENTATION

EMS is called to a high school for a male patient complaining of shortness of breath. The patient is conscious and breathing. Enroute Dispatch informs the paramedics that the patient is an asthmatic and takes Ventolin by inhaler, but left it at home today.

On arrival paramedics are met by a teacher who takes them to the first aid room. The patient, a 17-year-old male, is sitting on an examining table hunched forward and struggling to breathe.

On Examination

CNS: The patient is conscious, alert, and oriented × 4; he is able to answer questions with a "yes" or "no" only; patient is clearly frightened

Resp: Respirations are 30 and shallow; patient is wheezing; wheezes are heard throughout all lung fields on expiration; trachea is midline; no signs of trauma

CVS: Carotid and radial pulses are present and weak, skin is warm and dry

ABD: Soft and non-tender

Vitals:

Pulse: 120/min, regular, weak

Resp: 30/min, shallow

BP: 114/54

SpO_2: 86%

ECG: Regular sinus rhythm

HX: Patient has been an asthmatic for 12 years. He had a cold for the previous two weeks. He was playing basketball and couldn't catch his breath. He stopped playing basketball to use his Ventolin and realized he forgot it at home. He became more anxious and short of breath.

Treatment:

Paramedics realized that this patient required medications to relieve the bronchospasm. Oxygen was administered by nasal cannula at 6 l/min and albuterol, 2.5 mg, was administered by an oxygen-powered nebulizer. With coaching, the patient relaxed and his breathing improved. On arrival at the hospital, the patient was able to speak in short sentences and his wheezing had diminished significantly. The SpO_2 had increased to 96%.

Racemic Epinephrine (microNEFRIN, Vaponefrin)

Class: Sympathetic Agonist

Description

Racemic epinephrine is slightly different chemically from the epinephrine compounds that have been discussed previously. Compounds that differ only in their chemical arrangement are called *isomers*. This particular form is frequently used in children to treat croup.

Mechanism of Action

Racemic epinephrine stimulates both α and β adrenergic receptors. However, racemic epinephrine has a slight preference for β_2 adrenergic receptors and causes bronchodilation. It also has some effect in relieving the subglottic edema associated with croup. Racemic epinephrine should only be administered by inhalation.

Indication

- Croup (laryngotracheobronchitis)

Contraindications

Racemic epinephrine should not be used in the management of epiglottitis.

Precautions

Racemic epinephrine can result in tachycardia and possibly arrhythmias. Vital signs should be monitored. Many patients will develop "rebound worsening" 30–60 minutes after the initial treatment and the effects of racemic epinephrine have worn off. Because of this, all children who receive racemic epinephrine should be transported to the hospital. Most hospitals have an institutional policy that requires all children who have received racemic epinephrine to be admitted for at least 24 hours in case rebound worsening occurs.

Dosage

A standard dose is 0.25–0.75 ml racemic epinephrine diluted with 2 ml normal saline (2.25%) and administered via a standard aerosol nebulizer. It should only be used initially and not repeated. Racemic epinephrine should be given only by inhalation, generally by small-volume nebulizer, diluted with 2 to 3 milliliters of normal saline.

How Supplied

Racemic epinephrine is supplied in inhaler or nebulizer bottles containing either 7.5, 15, or 30 milliliters.

Terbutaline (Brethine, Bricanyl)

Class: Sympathetic Agonist

Description

Terbutaline is a synthetic sympathomimetic that is selective for β_2-adrenergic receptors.

Mechanism of Action

Terbutaline, because of its effects on β_2-adrenergic receptors, causes immediate bronchodilation with minimal cardiac effects. Its onset of action is similar to that of epinephrine. Terbutaline is also used to suppress preterm labor.

Indications

- Bronchial asthma
- Reversible bronchospasm associated with chronic bronchitis and emphysema

Contraindications

Terbutaline should not be administered to any patient with a history of hypersensitivity to the drug.

Precautions

As with any sympathomimetic, the patient's vital signs must be monitored. Caution should be used when administering terbutaline to elderly patients and those with cardiovascular disease or hypertension. Lung sounds should be auscultated before and after each treatment. Ideally, the patient's peak flow rate should be measured both before and after drug administration.

Side Effects

Terbutaline can cause palpitations, anxiety, dizziness, headache, nervousness, tremor, hypertension, arrhythmias, chest pain, nausea, and vomiting.

Interactions

The possibility of developing unpleasant side effects increases when terbutaline is used with other sympathetic agonists. β blockers may blunt the pharmacological effects of terbutaline.

Dosage

The standard dose is two inhalations, 1 minute apart, from a metered-dose inhaler.

Terbutaline can also be administered by subcutaneous injection. The usual dose is 0.25 milligram. This can be repeated in 15 to 30 minutes if needed. Terbutaline should only be administered by inhalation or by subcutaneous injection as described herein.

How Supplied

Terbutaline is supplied in aerosol canisters. Each spray delivers approximately 0.20 mg of the drug. Terbutaline for subcutaneous injection is supplied in vials containing 1 milligram of the drug in 1 milliliter of solvent.

Isoetharine (Bronkosol)

Class: Sympathetic Agonist

Description

Isoetharine is a sympathomimetic similar in chemical structure to epinephrine. It exhibits a slight specificity for β_2-adrenergic receptors, thus reducing the potential for cardiac toxicity.

Mechanism of Action

Isoetharine is a β-agonist with slight selectivity for β_2-adrenergic receptors causing pulmonary bronchodilation. Its onset of action is similar to that of epinephrine. However, it has a longer duration of effect.

Indications

- Bronchial asthma
- Reversible bronchospasm associated with chronic bronchitis and emphysema

Contraindications

Isoetharine should not be administered to any patient with a history of hypersensitivity to any of the ingredients.

Precautions

As with any sympathomimetic, the patient's vital signs must be monitored. Caution should be used when administering isoetharine to elderly patients and those with cardiovascular disease or hypertension. Lung sounds should be auscultated before and after each treatment. Ideally, the patient's peak flow rate should be measured both before and after drug administration.

Side Effects

Isoetharine can cause palpitations, anxiety, dizziness, headache, nervousness, tremor, hypertension, arrhythmias, chest pain, nausea, and vomiting.

Interactions

The possibility of developing unpleasant side effects increases when isoetharine is administered with other sympathetic agonists. β blockers may blunt the pharmacological effects of isoetharine.

Dosage

There are three major ways to administer isoetharine, each with different dosages. They are as follows:

Method of Administration	Usual Dose	Dilution
Metered-Dose Inhaler	2 inhalations	Undiluted
Oxygen Aerosolization	0.5 milliliter	1:3 with saline
Intermittent positive-pressure breathing	0.5 milliliter	1:3 with saline

Isoetharine should be administered only by one of the methods listed above.

How Supplied

Isoetharine is supplied in a 2-milliliter unit dose containing a 1% solution.

Metaproterenol (Alupent)

Class: Sympathetic Agonist

Description

Metaproterenol is a sympathomimetic that is selective for β_2-adrenergic receptors.

Mechanism of Action

Metaproterenol is a selective β_2 agonist and is an effective bronchodilator. Its duration of effect is up to 4 hours.

Indications

- Bronchial asthma
- Reversible bronchospasm associated with chronic bronchitis and emphysema

Contraindications

Metaproterenol should not be used in patients with cardiac arrhythmias or significant tachycardia.

Precautions

As with any sympathomimetic, the patient's vital signs must be monitored. Caution should be used when administering metaproterenol to elderly patients and those with cardiovascular disease or hypertension. Lung sounds should be auscultated before and after each treatment. Ideally, the patient's peak flow rate should be measured both before and after drug administration.

Side Effects

Metaproterenol can cause palpitations, anxiety, dizziness, headache, nervousness, tremor, hypertension, arrhythmias, chest pain, nausea, and vomiting.

Interactions

The possibility of developing unpleasant side effects increases when metaproterenol is administered with other sympathetic agonists. β blockers may blunt the pharmacological effects of metaproterenol.

Dosage

Metaproterenol may be administered by metered-dose inhaler. Each spray contains 0.65 milligram of metaproterenol. The usual single dose is two to three inhalations, a minute apart, as needed.

Metaproterenol may also be administered by small-volume nebulizer. The typical adult dose is 0.2 to 0.3 milliliter of metaproterenol diluted in 2.5 milliliters of normal saline. This is usually administered during 5 to 15 minutes. Metaproterenol should be administered by inhalation only in the emergency setting.

How Supplied

Metaproterenol is supplied in metered-dose inhalers with each spray delivering 0.65 milligram of the drug. The solution for nebulization is supplied in single-dose units of 0.4% (0.2 milliliter of Alupent in 2.5 milliliters of saline) and 0.6% (0.3 milliliter of Alupent in 2.5 milliliters of saline).

Aminophylline (Somophyllin)

Class: Xanthine

Description

Aminophylline is a xanthine bronchodilator that sometimes proves effective in cases in which sympathomimetics have not been effective.

Mechanism of Action

Aminophylline achieves its bronchodilation effects via a different mechanism than the sympathomimetics. It relaxes bronchial smooth muscle, but does not act on adrenergic receptors. Aminophylline also stimulates the respiratory center in the brain. This effect is particularly useful in the treatment of infants with apnea. In addition to bronchodilation, aminophylline has mild diuretic properties, increases the heart rate and cardiac output, and may precipitate arrhythmias. Owing to its mild diuretic and inotropic effects, aminophylline is also used in the management of congestive heart failure and pulmonary edema. In prehospital emergency care, aminophylline is usually given by slow IV infusion. Some systems also carry aminophylline suppositories for use in special situations.

Indications

- Bronchial asthma
- Reversible bronchospasm associated with chronic bronchitis and emphysema

- Congestive heart failure
- Pulmonary edema

Contraindications

Aminophylline should not be administered to any patient with a history of hypersensitivity to the drug. It should not be used in patients who have uncontrolled cardiac dysrhythmias.

Precautions

Extreme caution should be used when administering aminophylline to any patient with a history of cardiovascular disease or hypertension. Any patient receiving aminophylline should have a cardiac monitor. One should be alert for any signs of cardiac irritability, especially PVCs and tachycardia. Hypotension can occur following rapid administration.

Side Effects

Aminophylline can cause tachycardia, arrhythmias, palpitations, chest pain, nervousness, headache, seizures, nausea, and vomiting.

Interactions

Aminophylline should not be administered to patients who are on chronic theophylline therapy (Slo-Bid, Theo-Dur, and so on) until the amount of drug in the blood has been obtained (theophylline level). Concomitant use with β blockers and drugs of the erythromycin class of antibiotics may lead to theophylline toxicity.

Dosage

Two major regimens are used in administering aminophylline. The first is for use in patients in whom fluid overload or edema does not appear to be present (that is, acute bronchial asthma):

> Place 250 or 500 milligrams in 90 or 80 milliliters of 5% dextrose, respectively. This can be done with a 100-milliliter IV bag or with a Buretrol or Volutrol-type administration set. This is then infused during 20 to 30 minutes. This mechanism of slow infusion tends to reduce the chances of arrhythmias.

In patients with congestive heart failure, or for whom any additional fluid might be dangerous, a more concentrated infusion is prepared:

> Place 250 or 500 milligrams (2 to 5 milligrams per kilogram) in 20 milliliters of 5% dextrose in water. This is then infused during 20 to 30 minutes using a Buretrol or Volutrol-type administration set.

Parenteral aminophylline should only be given by slow IV infusion by one of the regimens discussed above.

How Supplied

Aminophylline is supplied in ampules containing 250 milligrams in 10 milliliters of solvent or containing 500 milligrams in 20 milliliters of solvent.

Atropine Sulfate

Class: Anticholinergic

Description

Atropine is a parasympatholytic (anticholinergic) that is derived from parts of the *Atropa belladonna* plant.

Mechanism of Action

Atropine sulfate is a potent parasympatholytic. It is used in the treatment of respiratory emergencies, as it causes bronchodilation and drying of respiratory tract secretions. Atropine acts by blocking acetylcholine receptors thus inhibiting parasympathetic stimulation. With the release of ipratropium, atropine has fallen into relative disuse in the treatment of reactive airway disease.

Indications

- Bronchial asthma
- Reversible bronchospasm associated with chronic bronchitis and emphysema

Contraindications

Atropine sulfate should not be used in patients hypersensitive to the drug. It is not indicated for the acute treatment of bronchospasm where rapid response is required.

Precautions

The patient's vital signs must be monitored during therapy with atropine. Caution should be used when administering atropine to elderly patients and those with cardiovascular disease or hypertension. Lung sounds should be auscultated before and after each treatment. Ideally, the patient's peak flow rate should be measured both before and after drug administration.

Side Effects

Atropine can cause palpitations, anxiety, dizziness, headache, nervousness, rash, nausea, and vomiting.

Interactions

Few in the prehospital setting

Dosage

Atropine is usually administered with a β agonist. Typically, 0.5–1.0 milligram of atropine is placed in 2–3 ml of normal saline. This is administered by small-volume nebulizer with or without a β agonist.

How Supplied

Atropine is supplied in ampules and vials containing 1.0 milligram in 1 milliliter of solution.

Ipratropium (Atrovent)

Class: Anticholinergic

Description

Ipratropium is an anticholinergic (parasympatholytic) bronchodilator that is chemically related to atropine.

Mechanism of Action

Ipratropium is a parasympatholytic used in the treatment of respiratory emergencies. It causes bronchodilation and dries respiratory tract secretions. Ipratropium acts by blocking acetylcholine receptors thus inhibiting parasympathetic stimulation.

Indications

- Bronchial asthma
- Reversible bronchospasm associated with chronic bronchitis and emphysema

Contraindications

Ipratropium should not be used in patients hypersensitive to the drug. It is not indicated for the acute treatment of bronchospasm where rapid response is required.

Precautions

The patient's vital signs must be monitored during therapy with ipratropium. Caution should be used when administering it to elderly patients and those with cardiovascular disease or hypertension. Lung sounds should be auscultated before and after each treatment. Ideally, the patient's peak flow rate should be measured both before and after drug administration.

Side Effects

Ipratropium can cause palpitations, anxiety, dizziness, headache, nervousness, rash, nausea, and vomiting.

Interactions

Few in the prehospital setting

Dosage

Ipratropium is usually administered with a β agonist. Typically, 500 micrograms of Atrovent is placed in a small-volume nebulizer. A β agonist can be added if desired. This solution is then administered by small-volume nebulizer with or without a β agonist. Atrovent is also available in a metered-dose inhaler.

How Supplied

Atrovent is supplied in unit dose vials containing 500 micrograms (0.02% inhalation solution) of the drug already diluted in 2.5 ml saline.

CASE PRESENTATION

At 1830 hours paramedics are called to a rural residence 45 minutes from the hospital for a woman complaining of shortness of breath. She is conscious and breathing. On arrival paramedics are met by the patient's husband who leads them to the living room. There paramedics find a patient sitting forward on a chair. The patient is using home oxygen by nasal cannula and is using an oxygen-powered nebulizer. The patient appears very anxious and in respiratory distress.

On Examination

CNS: The patient is conscious, alert, and oriented × 4; in extreme respiratory distress

Resp: Respirations are 32 and shallow; wheezes are heard unaided by stethoscope; there are tight, barely audible wheezes in the apices bilaterally, no sounds heard in the bases; trachea is midline; no signs of trauma

CVS: Carotid and radial pulses are present and weak, skin is pale and cool

ABD: Soft and non-tender

Vitals:

Pulse: 140/min, regular, weak

Resp: 32/min, shallow

BP: 144/94

SpO_2: 87%

ECG: Sinus tachycardia

Hx: Patient has a 20 year history of asthma and was taking Ventolin by inhaler twice a day, Beclofort twice a day, and home oxygen by nasal cannula at 4 l/min PRN and during sleep. The patient was talking to her granddaughter on the phone. She became very upset during the telephone call and then became short of breath. The patient put on her oxygen with no relief and also took one dose (2.5 mg) of albuterol with an oxygen-powered nebulizer with no relief.

Treatment:

The patient's home oxygen was continued, a second dose of albuterol was administered, and the patient was coached to take a breath and hold it. The patient was very agitated and the coaching had little effect. An IV was initiated and run TKO. The base hospital was contacted and the paramedics were directed to administer 125 mg of Solu-Medrol IV push and to administer Atrovent through the oxygen-powered nebulizer along with the albuterol. The patient's condition improved slightly with the combination of medications. The patient was admitted to ICU upon arrival at the hospital.

Methylprednisolone (Solu-Medrol)

Class: Corticosteroid/Anti-Inflammatory

Description

Methylprednisolone is a synthetic steroid with potent anti-inflammatory properties.

Mechanism of Action

The pharmacological actions of the steroids are vast and complex. In general medical practice, steroids have a wide range of uses. Effective as anti-inflammatory agents, they are used in the management of allergic reactions, asthma, and anaphylaxis. Methylprednisolone is considered an intermediate-acting steroid with a plasma half-life of about 3 to 4 hours.

Indications

- Severe anaphylaxis
- Asthma/COPD
- Urticaria

Contraindications

There are no major contraindications to the use of methylprednisolone in the acute management of severe anaphylaxis.

Precautions

A single dose of methylprednisolone is all that should be given in the prehospital phase of care. Long-term steroid therapy can cause gastrointestinal bleeding, prolonged wound healing, and suppression of adrenocortical steroids.

Side Effects

Methylprednisolone can cause fluid retention, congestive heart failure, hypertension, abdominal distention, vertigo, headache, nausea, malaise, and hiccups.

Interactions

Few in the prehospital setting

Dosage

The standard dosage of methylprednisolone in the management of severe anaphylaxis is 125 to 250 milligrams intravenously. Methylprednisolone may be administered intravenously or intramuscularly. The intravenous route is preferred in emergency medicine.

How Supplied

Methylprednisolone is supplied in Mix-O-Vials containing 125 milligrams of the drug. Methylprednisolone is supplied in powder form that must be reconstituted in the supplied Mix-O-Vial system. Once reconstituted, it should be used within 48 hours.

Hydrocortisone (Solu-Cortef)

Class: Corticosteroid/Anti-Inflammatory

Description

Hydrocortisone is a potent corticosteroid with anti-inflammatory properties.

Mechanism of Action

The pharmacological actions of the steroids are vast and complex. Hydrocortisone is considered a short-acting steroid with a plasma half-life of 90 minutes. Like the other adrenocorticosteroids, it is effective as an adjunct in the management of severe anaphylaxis.

Indications

- Severe anaphylaxis
- Asthma/COPD
- Urticaria (hives)

Contraindications

There are no major contraindications to the use of hydrocortisone in the acute management of anaphylaxis.

Precautions

A single dose of hydrocortisone is all that should be given in the prehospital phase of care. Long-term steroid therapy can cause gastrointestinal bleeding, prolonged wound healing, and suppression of adrenocortical steroids.

Side Effects

Hydrocortisone can cause fluid retention, congestive heart failure, hypertension, abdominal distention, vertigo, headache, nausea, malaise, and hiccups.

Interactions

Few in the prehospital setting

Dosage

The standard dosage of hydrocortisone in the management of severe anaphylaxis is 40 to 250 milligrams intravenously.

Route

The IV route is preferred in emergency medicine. However, hydrocortisone can be administered intramuscularly when an IV cannot be started.

How Supplied

Hydrocortisone is supplied in Mix-O-Vials containing 100 and 250 milligrams of the drug.

NEUROMUSCULAR BLOCKERS

Establishment and protection of the airway has the highest priority in emergency care. On certain occasions patients who are still responsive may have trouble maintaining their airway and may require endotracheal intubation. This situation most commonly occurs in drug overdoses, status epilepticus, and in trauma patients with closed head injuries. Often, however, intubation is difficult because of the presence of gag reflexes, clenched teeth, or general combativeness. In these cases endotracheal intubation can be carried out following administration of a neuromuscular blocking agent.

Neuromuscular blocking agents are drugs that cause muscle relaxation, thus facilitating endotracheal intubation. All skeletal muscles, including the muscles of respiration, respond to these drugs. Following administration, the patient will become apneic and require mechanical ventilation. Neuromuscular blocking agents have no effect on the patient's level of consciousness or pain sensation. Neuromuscular blocking drugs are classified as *depolarizing* and *non-depolarizing* based on their mechanism of action. The most commonly used depolarizing drug is succinylcholine, while vecuronium and pancuronium are the most frequently used non-depolarizing agents.

- *Succinylcholine (Anectine).* Succinylcholine is a depolarizing neuromuscular blocker commonly used in emergency medicine. It acts in approximately 60 to 90 seconds and lasts approximately 3 to 5 minutes. Following administration, succinylcholine causes muscle fasciculations. This progresses to total paralysis, including the diaphragm.

- *Pancuronium (Pavulon)*. Pancuronium is a long-acting, non-depolarizing neuromuscular blocking agent. It acts in 2 to 5 minutes and lasts 40 to 60 minutes.
- *Vecuronium (Norcuron)*. Vecuronium is a non-depolarizing neuromuscular blocking agent with a rapid onset and short duration of action. It has fewer cardiovascular side effects than succinylcholine and does not cause fasciculations.

Before administering a neuromuscular blocking agent, it is essential that you have equipment ready for airway management as soon as the patient becomes apneic. In addition, because a neuromuscular blocking agent has no effect on pain sensation and mental status, it should not be administered to alert patients without first administering a sedative or analgesic.

Most emergency patients have eaten or drunk something in the hours prior to the onset of the emergency. Thus, virtually every emergency patient is considered to have a full stomach. Neuromuscular blockade and endotracheal intubation may cause vomiting, which increases the risk of aspiration. Because of this, special precautions must be taken to gain rapid control of the airway as soon as the drug is administered. As a result, this procedure is often referred to as *rapid sequence intubation*. The following steps will help you perform a rapid sequence intubation correctly.

1. Assemble the required equipment.
2. Assure that the IV line is functioning and secure.
3. Place the patient on a cardiac monitor and pulse oximeter.
4. Preoxygenate the patient with 100% oxygen using a bag-valve-mask unit.
5. Premedicate the patient if appropriate:
   - diazepam (Valium)—5–10 milligrams intravenously
   - morphine sulfate—5–10 milligrams intravenously
   - atropine—0.01 mg/kg IV push for children and adolescents (blocks vagal effects and helps prevent muscle fasciculations)
6. Have another rescuer apply Sellick's maneuver to occlude the esophagus and maintain it until the ET tube is in place and the cuff inflated.
7. Administer 1.5 mg/kg succinylcholine or 0.08 mg/kg vecuronium IV push and continue ventilation.
8. Apnea and jaw relaxation are indications that the patient is sufficiently relaxed to proceed with endotracheal intubation.
9. Perform endotracheal intubation. If you are unable to place the tube in 20 seconds, stop, and ventilate the patient with 100% oxygen for 30–60 seconds before attempting the procedure again.
10. Once the tube is in place, inflate the cuff and confirm tube placement by auscultating bilateral breath sounds and, if available, by use of an end-tidal CO_2 detector.
11. Release cricoid pressure and properly seal the endotracheal tube. The effects of succinylcholine will wear off in 3 to 5 minutes. A bite block should be placed to prevent the patient from

biting the endotracheal tube. Medical control may request the administration of pancuronium or vecuronium if continued paralysis is warranted.

Succinylcholine (Anectine)

Class: Depolarizing Neuromuscular Blocker

Description

Succinylcholine is a short-acting, depolarizing skeletal muscle relaxant used to facilitate endotracheal intubation.

Mechanism of Action

Succinylcholine is a short-acting, depolarizing skeletal muscle relaxant. Like acetylcholine, it combines with cholinergic receptors in the motor nerves to cause depolarization. Neuromuscular transmission is thus inhibited, which renders the muscles unable to be stimulated by acetylcholine. Following IV injection, complete paralysis is obtained within 1 minute and persists for approximately 2 minutes. Effects then start to fade, and a return to normal is seen within 6 minutes.

Muscle relaxation begins in the eyelids and jaw. It then progresses to the limbs, the abdomen, and finally the diaphragm and intercostals. It has no effect on the consciousness whatsoever.

Indication

- To achieve temporary paralysis where endotracheal intubation is indicated and where muscle tone or seizure activity prevents it

Contraindications

Succinylcholine is contraindicated in patients with a history of hypersensitivity to the drug. It should not be used with penetrating eye injuries or in patients with a history of narrow-angle glaucoma. *Succinylcholine should not be administered by persons inexperienced with its use.*

Precautions

Succinylcholine should not be administered unless personnel skilled in endotracheal intubation are present and ready to perform the procedure. Oxygen therapy equipment should be readily available as should all emergency resuscitative drugs and equipment. Fractures have been reported in children following the use of depolarizing neuromuscular blockers due to strong and sustained muscle fasciculations. Cardiac arrest and ventricular arrhythmias have been reported when succinylcholine was administered to patients with severe burns and severe crush injuries.

Side Effects

Succinylcholine can cause wheezing, respiratory depression, apnea, aspiration, arrhythmias, bradycardia, sinus arrest, hypertension, hypotension, increased intraocular pressure, and increased intracranial pressure.

Interactions

Certain drugs can enhance the neuromuscular blocking action of succinylcholine. These include: lidocaine, procainamide, β blockers, magnesium sulfate, and other neuromuscular blockers.

Dosage

The dosage for succinylcholine is 1–1.5 milligram per kilogram intravenously. The preferred route for succinylcholine administration is intravenously. It can be administered intramuscularly if required, however.

How Supplied

Succinylcholine is supplied in vials containing 10 milliliters of a 20 milligrams per milliliter concentration (200 total milligrams).

Pancuronium Bromide (Pavulon)

Class: Non-depolarizing Neuromuscular Blocker

Description

Pancuronium bromide is a derivative of curare and is used to provide muscle relaxation in order to facilitate endotracheal intubation.

Mechanism of Action

Pancuronium competes with acetylcholine for cholinergic receptor sites on the post-junctional membrane. This results in paralysis of muscle fibers served by the occupied neuromuscular junction. It does not cause an initial depolarization wave as does succinylcholine. The onset of action of pancuronium is 3–5 minutes and the effect may persist for up to 60 minutes.

Indication

- To achieve temporary paralysis where endotracheal intubation is indicated and where muscle tone, seizures, or laryngospasm prevents it

Contraindications

Pancuronium is contraindicated in patients with a history of hypersensitivity to the drug. *Pancuronium should not be administered by persons inexperienced with its use.*

Precautions

Pancuronium should not be administered unless personnel skilled in endotracheal intubation are present and ready to perform the procedure. Oxygen therapy equipment should be readily available as should all emergency resuscitative drugs and equipment. Hypotension can occur. Thus, the vital signs must be constantly monitored. Pancuronium can increase intracranial pressure. In patients with head injuries, vecuronium is often preferred.

Side Effects

Pancuronium can cause wheezing, respiratory depression, apnea, aspiration, arrhythmias, bradycardia, sinus arrest, hypertension, hypotension, increased intraocular pressure, and increased intracranial pressure.

Interactions

Certain drugs can enhance the neuromuscular blocking action of pancuronium. These include: lidocaine, procainamide, β blockers, magnesium sulfate, certain antibiotics (aminoglycosides) and other neuromuscular blockers.

Dosage

The adult and pediatric dosage for pancuronium is 0.04–0.1 mg/kg intravenously. Repeat doses of 0.01–0.02 mg/kg intravenously may be required every 20–40 minutes.

How Supplied

Pancuronium is supplied in 2 and 5 milliliter vials containing 2 milligrams/milliliter of the drug.

Vecuronium (Norcuron)

Class: Non-depolarizing Neuromuscular Blocker

Description

Vecuronium is a derivative of pancuronium and is used to provide muscle relaxation in order to facilitate endotracheal intubation.

Mechanism of Action

Vecuronium has a similar mechanism of action as pancuronium. However, it is approximately 1/3 more potent with a shorter duration of effect.

Vecuronium competes with acetylcholine for cholinergic receptor sites on the post-junctional membrane. This results in paralysis of muscle fibers served by the occupied neuromuscular junction. It does not cause an initial depolarization wave as does succinylcholine. The onset of action of vecuronium is 1 minute with good to excellent intubation conditions within 2.5–3 minutes.

Indication

- To achieve temporary paralysis where endotracheal intubation is indicated and where muscle tone or seizure activity prevents it

Contraindications

Vecuronium is contraindicated in patients with a history of hypersensitivity to the drug.

Precautions

Vecuronium should not be administered unless personnel skilled in endotracheal intubation are present and ready to perform the procedure. Oxygen therapy equipment should be readily available as should all emergency resuscitative drugs and equipment.

Side Effects

Vecuronium can cause wheezing, respiratory depression, apnea, aspiration, arrhythmias, bradycardia, sinus arrest, hypertension, hypotension, increased intraocular pressure, and increased intracranial pressure.

Interactions

Certain drugs can enhance the neuromuscular blocking action of vecuronium. These include: lidocaine, procainamide, β blockers, magnesium sulfate, and other neuromuscular blockers.

Dosage

The adult dosage for vecuronium is 0.08–0.10 milligram per kilogram intravenously. Neuromuscular blockade should last 25–30 minutes.

How Supplied

Vecuronium is supplied in 10-milliliter vials containing 10 milligrams of the drug. It must be reconstituted with the diluent provided.

SUMMARY

Respiratory emergencies are a serious and potentially fatal condition if not treated immediately. Prompt recognition of the signs and symptoms of respiratory distress is essential. Oxygen is the primary drug for treating any respiratory problem. Many types of medical problems, especially asthma and anaphylaxis, respond only to the medications discussed in this chapter.

KEY WORDS

allergens. A foreign substance that can cause an allergic response in the body, but is only harmful to some people.

bronchospasm. An abnormal contraction of the bronchi, resulting in narrowing and blockage of the airway. A cough with wheezing is the usual symptom. Bronchospasm is the main feature of asthma and bronchitis.

capnography. A system for measuring the concentration of exhaled carbon dioxide.

COPD. (Chronic Obstructive Pulmonary Disease) A pulmonary disease characterized by a decreased ability of the lungs to perform the function of ventilation.

edema. An abnormal pooling of fluid in the tissues.

hypercapnia. An increased level of carbon dioxide in the body.

hypoxia. A state in which insufficient oxygen is available to meet the oxygen requirements of the cells.

pH. A scientific method of expressing the acidity or alkalinity of a solution. It is the logarithm of the hydrogen ion concentration divided by one. The higher the pH, the more alkaline the solution. The lower the pH, the more acidic the solution.

pulse oximetry. An assessment modality that measures the oxygen saturation level of the blood through a non-invasive sensor placed on a finger or earlobe.

chapter 9

Drugs Used in the Treatment of Metabolic-Endocrine Emergencies

OBJECTIVES

1. Define the term *hormone.*
2. Discuss the function and location of the pancreas.
3. List two functions of the islets of Langerhans.
4. Discuss the function of glucagon.
5. Define *diabetes mellitus.*
6. Discuss the function of insulin and its relation to glucose metabolism.
7. Compare and contrast Type I (insulin-dependent) and Type II (non-insulin dependent) diabetes mellitus.
8. Compare and contrast diabetic ketoacidosis and hypoglycemia.
9. Describe and list the indications, contraindications, and dosages for insulin, glucagon, $D_{50}W$, and thiamine.

INTRODUCTION

Glands that secrete hormones directly into the blood, without the aid of ducts, are called *endocrine glands*. With the exception of the pancreas, they rarely cause emergency disorders. Occasionally the thyroid, the endocrine gland that controls metabolic rate, will begin secreting excess thyroid hormones. This disorder, called hyperthyroidism, is characterized by increased heart rate, loss of body weight, insomnia, dry skin, hair loss, and nervousness. A rare, but severe form of thyroid dysfunction is "thyroid storm." Thyroid storm causes fever, tachycardia, dehydration, and a change in mental status. Although this chapter is devoted to metabolic-endocrine emergencies, we will primarily discuss the pancreatic disorder diabetes mellitus.

DIABETES MELLITUS

The pancreas is located in the retroperitoneal space within the folds of the small intestine. Within the pancreas is an area called the *islets of Langerhans*. The islets of Langerhans have three types of cells that secrete three different hormones. The α cells secrete the hormone *glucagon*. The β cells secrete *insulin*. A third hormone, called *somatostatin*, is secreted from the ∂ (delta) cells. Insulin is required for the passage of glucose into the cells. Without insulin the blood glucose level rises. Glucagon causes stored carbohydrates, especially glycogen, to be broken down to glucose. When the blood sugar level falls, glucagon is released, which then causes a release of stored carbohydrates. Somatostatin inhibits the secretion of both insulin and glucagon. Functionally, it is similar to growth hormone.

Diabetes mellitus is caused when β cells of the pancreas reduce the amount of insulin secreted. In addition, the relative number of insulin receptors decrease. These two factors contribute to an increasing level of glucose in the blood. This will result in increased thirst, increased hunger, and increased urination. The hunger is due to the fact that the various body cells are glucose depleted. The thirst is due to a relative dehydration that occurs when glucose spills over into the urine. Glucose spillage into the urine takes water with it. This results in the polyuria and polydipsia characteristic of hyperglycemia. If allowed to progress untreated, the patient will eventually lapse into diabetic coma. Patients in diabetic coma have warm, dry skin. Clinically they are dehydrated. They may exhibit rapid, deep respirations (Kussmaul Respirations), which are part of the body's attempt to rid itself of accumulated acids. Because the signs and symptoms occur early, most patients seek medical care before coma ensues. Once diagnosed, the patient will most likely be placed on hypoglycemic agents. If an excessive amount of insulin is taken, or if the patient fails to eat properly, then *hypoglycemia* can develop (see Table 9-1).

TYPES OF DIABETES

Generally, diabetes mellitus can be divided into two different categories. Type I diabetes, or insulin-dependent diabetes, usually begins in the early years. Patients who have Type I diabetes must take insulin. Type II, or non-insulin-dependent diabetes, usually begins later in life and tends to be associated with obesity. Type II diabetes can often be controlled without using insulin. It is important for you to understand the difference between these two forms of diabetes.

TABLE 9-1

Diabetic Emergencies

Diabetic Ketoacidosis	*Hypoglycemia*
Causes	**Causes**
Patient has not taken insulin.	Patient has taken too much insulin.
Patient has overeaten, flooding the body with carbohydrates.	Patient has overexerted, thus reducing glucose levels.
Patient has infection that disrupts glucose/insulin balance.	
Signs and Symptoms	**Signs and Symptoms**
Polyuria, polydypsia, polyphagia	Weak, rapid pulse
Nausea/vomiting	Cold, clammy skin
Tachycardia	Weakness/uncoordination
Deep, rapid respirations	Headache
Warm, dry skin	Irritable, nervous behavior
Fruity odor on breath	May appear intoxicated
Abdominal pain	Coma (severe cases)
Falling blood pressure	
Fever (occasionally)	
Decreased LOC	
Management	**Management**
Fluids, insulin	Dextrose

Type I Diabetes Mellitus

Type I diabetes mellitus is a serious disease characterized by inadequate production of insulin by the endocrine pancreas. The cause of Type I diabetes is not well understood. One theory is that a viral infection attacks the pancreatic beta cells, thus slowing or stopping insulin production. Another theory proposes that the body's immune system mistakenly targets the pancreatic beta cells as foreign and attacks them. In either case, heredity appears to be a factor in increasing a person's chance in contracting the disease.

With Type I diabetes mellitus, the patient must take daily doses of insulin. In the normal state, the intake of glucose, such as in a meal, results in the release of insulin. Insulin promotes the uptake of glucose by the cells. Type I diabetes generally begins with decreased insulin secretion, subsequently leading to elevated blood glucose levels. However, since insulin is required for glucose to enter into the various body cells, they become glucose-depleted despite increased blood glucose levels.

In diabetes, a drop in insulin levels is accompanied by a steady accumulation of glucose in the blood. As the cells become glucose-depleted, they begin to use other sources of energy. Therefore, various harmful byproducts, such as *ketones* and *organic acids*, are produced. When these start to accumulate, several of the classic findings of diabetic ketoacidosis appear. If the various acids and ketones continue to collect in the blood, severe metabolic acidosis occurs and coma ensues. Severe acidosis can result in serious brain damage or death.

As the concentration of glucose in the blood continues to rise, the kidneys will begin excreting glucose in the urine. When glucose is spilled into the urine, it takes water with it, resulting in osmotic diuresis, which dehydrates the patient.

Type II Diabetes Mellitus

Type II diabetes mellitus occurs more commonly than Type I does. Like Type I, it is characterized by decreased insulin production by the endocrine pancreas. As mentioned previously, Type II diabetes usually begins later in life. It is often associated with obesity, but can occur in non-obese patients. Increased body weight causes a relative decrease in the number of available insulin receptors. In addition, the insulin receptors become defective and less responsive to insulin. The pancreas also becomes less responsive to stimulation from increased blood glucose levels. Thus, insulin is not secreted as needed, increasing blood glucose levels even further.

The first approach in treating Type II diabetes is to encourage the patient to lose weight by reducing the intake of carbohydrates. Physicians may also prescribe oral hypoglycemic agents. These medications tend to stimulate increased insulin secretion from the pancreas and to promote an increase in the number of insulin receptors on the cells. Both actions tend to lower blood glucose levels. If diet and oral agents fail, insulin may be required.

Type II diabetes does not usually result in diabetic ketoacidosis. In type II diabetes, the patient makes enough insulin to maintain pH homeostasis, but not enough to supply all of the body's needs. It can, however, develop into a life-threatening emergency termed *nonketotic hyperosmolar coma*. In Type II diabetes, when blood glucose levels exceed 600 mg/dL, the high osmolality of the blood causes an osmotic diuresis and dehydration of body cells. This prevents the manufacture of ketones and the complications of metabolic acidosis. However, it is difficult to distinguish diabetic ketoacidosis from nonketotic hyperosmolar coma in the field. Therefore, the prehospital treatment of both emergencies is identical.

Diabetic Ketoacidosis (Diabetic Coma)

Diabetic ketoacidosis is a serious complication of diabetes mellitus. It occurs when insulin levels become inadequate to meet the metabolic demands of the body.

Pathophysiology. Diabetic ketoacidosis develops as blood glucose levels increase and individual cells become glucose depleted. The body begins spilling sugar into the urine. This causes a significant osmotic diuresis and serious dehydration, evidenced by dry, warm skin and mucous membranes. As cellular glucose-depletion continues, ketone and acid production occur. Subsequently, the blood becomes acidotic. Deep respiration begins as the body tries to compensate for the metabolic acidosis. If ketoacidosis is uncorrected, coma will follow.

Clinical Presentation. The onset of diabetic ketoacidosis is slow, lasting from 12 to 24 hours. In its early stages, the signs and symptoms include increased thirst, excessive hunger, urination, and malaise. Increased urination results from osmotic diuresis accompanying glucose spillage into the urine. Intensified thirst is caused by the body's attempt to replace fluids lost by increased urination. Diabetic ketoacidosis is characterized by nausea, vomiting, marked dehydration, tachycardia, and weakness. The skin is usually warm and dry. Coma is not uncommon. The breath may have a sweet or acetone-like character due to the increased ketones in the blood. Very deep, rapid respirations, called *Kussmaul's respirations*, also occur. Kussmaul's respirations represent the body's attempt to compensate for the metabolic acidosis produced by ketones and organic acids present in the blood.

Diabetic ketoacidosis is often associated with infection or decreased insulin intake. It may be complicated by several electrolyte imbalances. The most significant is decreased potassium. Decreased potassium (hypokalemia) can lead to serious dysrhythmias or even death.

Ketoacidosis can occur in patients who fail to take their insulin or who take an inadequate amount over an extended period. Persons not previously diagnosed as diabetic will occasionally present in ketoacidosis.

Hypoglycemia (Insulin Shock)

Hypoglycemia occurs when insulin levels are excessive. Hypoglycemia is an urgent medical emergency as a prolonged hypoglycemic episode can result in serious brain injury.

Pathophysiology. Hypoglycemia, sometimes called insulin shock, lies at the other end of the spectrum from diabetic ketoacidosis. Hypoglycemia can occur if a patient accidentally or intentionally takes too much insulin or eats an inadequate amount of food after taking insulin. If the patient is untreated, the insulin will cause the blood glucose level to drop to a very low level. THIS IS A TRUE MEDICAL EMERGENCY. If the patient is not treated quickly, he or she can sustain serious injury to the brain since it receives most of its energy from glucose metabolism.

Clinical Presentation. The clinical signs and symptoms of hypoglycemia are many and varied. An abnormal mental status is the most important. In the earliest stages of hypoglycemia, the patient may appear restless or impatient or complain of hunger. As the blood sugar falls lower, he or she may display inappropriate anger (even rage) or display a variety of bizarre behaviors. Sometimes the patient may be placed in police custody for such behaviors or be involved in an automobile accident.

Physical signs may include diaphoresis and tachycardia. If the blood sugar falls to a critically low level, the patient may sustain a *hypoglycemic seizure* or become comatose.

In contrast to diabetic ketoacidosis, hypoglycemia can develop quickly. A change in mental status can occur without warning. When encountering a patient behaving bizarrely, you should always consider hypoglycemia.

CASE PRESENTATION

At 1630 hours on a Thursday afternoon you are called to respond to a suburban residence for a patient who is unresponsive. The emergency medical dispatcher informs you that the caller is a nine-year-old girl who just came home from school and cannot wake up her mother.

You and your partner are met by the young girl as you arrive at the small frame residence. Tearfully she tells you that her mother is a diabetic and that the ambulance has been called several times before. As you enter the residence you notice that someone had been preparing a meal. You find the mother lying on the floor in the living room. The girl tells you that her mother's name is Tanya. You call to Tanya and gently shake her shoulder, but there is no response. There is no evidence of trauma or of a fall. Your partner turns off the stove as you continue your assessment.

The patient is a thirty-year-old female who is unconscious and unresponsive. She is breathing adequately and has both a radial and a carotid pulse. Both, however, are weak. The following is a summary of your examination findings:

Examination

CNS: The patient is unconscious and unresponsive.

Resp: Respirations are 30 per minute and shallow. Her lungs are clear bilaterally with equal air entry. The trachea is midline and there are no signs of trauma.

CVS: The radial and carotid pulses are present, but weak. Her skin is pale and quite diaphoretic.

ABD: The abdomen is soft and non-tender in all 4 quadrants. There is no sign of vomiting.

Musc/Skel: No apparent injuries. No pitting edema.

Vital Signs:

Pulse: 112/minute

Resp: 30/minute, shallow

B/P: 118/78 mmHg

SpO_2: 92%

ECG: Sinus Tachycardia

Past Hx: Her daughter states that the patient has been a diabetic for as long as she can remember. She also shows you insulin vials in the refrigerator (Humulin N and Humulin R). The daughter does not know when her mother last ate. However, they usually eat at 5 P.M.

Treatment:

Based on your physical findings, the patient history obtained from the daughter, and the presence of insulin in the refrigerator, you suspect that the patient is hypoglycemic. To confirm this, you decide to determine the blood glucose level. While you prepare to do this, your partner administers oxygen by nonrebreather mask at 12 L/min. By medical control protocol, you are able to begin definitive advanced life support procedures. You perform venipuncture with an 18 gauge catheter and, prior to connecting the IV tubing, you draw a "red top" blood tube for analysis. You also use the hub of the needle to obtain a blood sample for glucose testing. An IV of D_5W (normal saline is also acceptable) is initiated and run at a TKO rate. The blood glucose reading is 40 mg/dl (2.2 mmol/L). At this time you administer 50 milliliters (25 grams) of $D_{50}W$. Following administration of the $D_{50}W$, a fluid bolus of 25 ml of D_5W is administered to flush the IV line.

Almost immediately following the $D_{50}W$ administration, the patient begins to make sounds and move about. The patient awakens and is surprised to see you there. She is very apologetic and somewhat embarrassed. She insists that she is fine now and refuses transport to the hospital. After you have assured yourself that the patient is conscious, alert, and in no further danger, you inform her of the risks of refusing transports. She acknowledges the risks and signs the release form. You aseptically discontinue the IV, apply an adhesive strip, and leave the scene.

INSULIN

In this chapter we will discuss *insulin, glucagon, 50% dextrose in water ($D_{50}W$)*, and *thiamine*. All of these agents, except thiamine, are primarily used in the management of the diabetic patient. Thiamine should be administered before $D_{50}W$ to patients with coma of an unknown origin and alcoholism is suspected.

There are three major classifications of injectable insulin. *Regular insulin* is classified as fast acting. *Lente* or *NPH insulin* is classified as intermediate acting. Long-lasting insulin is called *ultralente*. Table 9-2 helps illustrate the relationship among the three classes.

TABLE 9-2

Comparison of Insulin Types

Type	*Time of Onset (Hours)*	*Duration of Action (Hours)*
Regular Insulin	1	6
NPH or Lente	2	24
Ultralente	6	36

Insulin (Humulin, Novolin, Iletin)

Class: Hormone/Antihyperglycemic

Description

Insulin is a protein secreted by the β cells of the islets of Langerhans. It is responsible for promoting the uptake of glucose by the cells. In diabetics, where insulin secretion has diminished, supplemental insulin must be obtained by injection. Older forms of insulin are derived from animals (bovine and porcine). However, animal insulin is not identical to human insulin. Because of this, many patients will develop antibodies to animal insulin rendering it less effective. Human insulin can be manufactured through genetic engineering (recombinant DNA technology). Genetically engineered insulin (Humulin, Novolin) is chemically identical to the insulin hormone secreted by the pancreas. Patients do not develop antibodies to human insulin as they do to animal insulin.

Mechanism of Action

Insulin, when administered, is distributed throughout the body. It combines with insulin receptors present on the cell membranes. This promotes glucose entry into the cell and lowers the blood glucose level.

Indications

- Diabetic ketoacidosis
- Hyperglycemia

Contraindications

Insulin should be administered only when hyperglycemia or ketoacidosis has been confirmed. A blood glucose approximation should be obtained in all diabetic emergencies. Every EMS unit carrying insulin and 50% dextrose should also carry Dextrostix reagent strips or an electronic glucose determination device for approximating blood glucose levels. Based on the results of the blood glucose test, and in conjunction with the physical examination, the differential diagnosis between hypoglycemia and ketoacidosis can usually be made. If there is any doubt about the etiology of diabetic coma, glucose should be administered. Insulin is almost always administered in the emergency department and not during the prehospital phase of emergency medical care.

Precautions

Repeated measurements of the blood glucose, including possible administration of glucose, are necessary.

Side Effects

Insulin may cause hypoglycemia. Itching, swelling, redness, and frank allergic reactions may occur following administration of animal-derived insulins.

Interactions

Certain drugs, such as the corticosteroids, can increase the blood glucose level. Patients receiving these drugs may require a higher dose of insulin. The signs and symptoms of hypoglycemia may be masked in patients receiving β blockers. Always determine the blood glucose.

Dosage

A standard dose for diabetic coma is 5–10 units of regular insulin IV followed by an infusion at 0.1 unit per kilogram per hour. 5–20 units of regular insulin can be administered subcutaneously or intramuscularly if there is not an immediate need for intravenous insulin. In an emergency setting insulin should be given intravenously, intramuscularly, or subcutaneously.

How Supplied

Insulin injection is supplied in 10-milliliter vials containing 100 units per milliliter.

Glucagon

Class: Hormone/Antihypoglycemic

Description

Glucagon is a protein secreted by the α cells of the pancreas. Glucagon for parenteral administration is extracted from beef and pork pancreas. It is used to increase the blood glucose level in cases of hypoglycemia where an IV cannot be immediately placed.

Mechanism of Action

Glucagon is a hormone secreted by the pancreas. When released it causes a breakdown of stored glycogen to glucose. It also inhibits the synthesis of glycogen from glucose. Both actions tend to cause an increase in circulating blood glucose. In hypoglycemia the administration of glucagon increases blood glucose levels. The drug of choice in the management of insulin-induced hypoglycemia is still $D_{50}W$. A return to consciousness is seen almost immediately following the administration of glucose. A return to consciousness following the administration of glucagon usually takes from 5 to 20 minutes. Glucagon is only effective if there are sufficient stores of glycogen in the liver.

Glucagon exerts a positive inotropic action on the heart and decreases renal vascular resistance.

Indications

- Hypoglycemia
- Beta blocker overdose

Contraindications

Because glucagon is a protein, hypersensitivity may occur. Do not administer glucagon to patients with a known hypersensitivity to the drug.

Precautions

Glucagon is only effective if there are sufficient stores of glycogen within the liver. In an emergency situation intravenous glucose is the agent of choice. Glucagon should be administered with caution to patients with a history of cardiovascular or renal disease.

Side Effects

Although side effects are rare, glucagon can cause hypotension, dizziness, headache, nausea, and vomiting.

Interactions

Few interactions with glucagon are reported in the emergency setting.

Dosage

A standard initial dose is 0.25 to 0.5 units intravenously. If an IV cannot be obtained, 1 milligram of glucagon can be administered intramuscularly.

Route

Glucagon can be administered intravenously, intramuscularly, or subcutaneously.

How Supplied

Glucagon must be reconstituted before administration. It is supplied in rubber-stoppered vials containing 1 unit of powder and 1 milliliter of diluting solution. It must be used or refrigerated after reconstitution.

50% Dextrose in Water ($D_{50}W$)

Class: Carbohydrate

Description

Dextrose is used to describe the six-carbon sugar *d-glucose*, which is the principal form of carbohydrate used by the body.

Mechanism of Action

50% dextrose in water supplies supplemental glucose in cases of hypoglycemia. Serious brain injury can occur if hypoglycemia is prolonged. Thus, in hypoglycemia the rapid administration of glucose is essential. When the hypoglycemic patient is comatose, glucose cannot be given by mouth and should be given as IV $D_{50}W$ solution.

Indications

- Hypoglycemia
- Coma of unknown origin

Contraindications

There are no major contraindications to the IV administration of $D_{50}W$ to a patient with suspected hypoglycemia. Even if a patient were suffering from ketoacidosis, the amount of glucose present in 50 milliliters of 50% dextrose would not adversely affect the clinical outcome. 50% dextrose should be used with caution in patients with increased intracranial pressure as the dextrose load may worsen cerebral edema.

Precautions

It is important to perform a Dextrostix or obtain a Glucometer reading and draw a sample of blood before initiating an IV infusion and giving 50% dextrose. Localized venous irritation may occur when smaller veins are used. Infiltration of 50% dextrose may result in tissue necrosis.

Side Effects

50% dextrose can cause tissue necrosis and phlebitis at the injection site.

Interactions

None in the emergency setting

Dosage

The standard dosage of 50% dextrose in hypoglycemia is 25 grams (50 milliliters of a 50% solution) intravenously. If an initial dose is ineffective, a second dose of 25 grams may also be given. 50% dextrose should be diluted 1:1 with sterile water for pediatric administration (thus forming $D_{25}W$). The pediatric dose is 0.5–1.0 gram per kilogram of body weight by slow, intravenous bolus.

Route

50% dextrose is only given intravenously. Concentrated glucose solutions can cause venous irritation if administered for an extended period.

How Supplied

50% dextrose is supplied in prefilled syringes containing 25 grams of *d-glucose* in 50 milliliters of water.

CASE PRESENTATION

Late in the afternoon on a warm September day you are dispatched to a residence for a patient "not feeling well." The emergency medical dispatcher tells you that the patient is a 60-year-old male who is reportedly conscious and alert. On arrival you are directed into the patient's bedroom by his wife. The patient is lying in bed propped up by two pillows. The patient tells you that he has been feeling ill for over 48 hours. He also reports that he has had rather severe abdominal pain accompanied by nausea and vomiting. However, he has been able to tolerate some clear liquids. He has not been unable to keep down any food. He denies any diarrhea or any other problems and is sure that this is the "flu."

Examination

CNS: The patient is conscious, alert, and oriented × 4.

Resp: Respirations are 32/minute, deep and labored. His lungs are clear bilaterally with equal air entry. His trachea is midline and there are no signs of trauma.

CVS: Both radial and carotid pulses are present, but weak. His skin is slightly pale and dry.

ABD: Soft and non-tender in all 4 quadrants.

Musc/Skel: No apparent injuries. No pitting edema.

Vital Signs:

Pulse: 140/minute

Resp: 32/minute, shallow, labored

B/P: 92/54 mmHg

SpO_2: 94%

ECG: Sinus Tachycardia

Past Hx: Past medical history includes insulin-dependent diabetes mellitus (Type I). His wife states that the patient has not taken insulin since he has been sick.

Treatment:

Oxygen is administered by nonrebreather mask at 12 liters per minute. The rapid, deep respirations are consistent with Kussmaul-type respirations. Your partner prepares an IV of normal saline while you perform venipuncture with a 16 gauge catheter. Blood is drawn for a "red top" tube and the hub of the needle is used to obtain a blood sample for glucose testing. The IV of normal saline is connected to the catheter and run at 150 ml/hour. The blood glucose reading exceeds 400 mg/dl (approx 20 mmol/l). You suspect the patient is in early diabetic ketoacidosis. Care provided during transport to the hospital is primarily supportive and includes monitoring of vital signs and fluid replacement.

At the emergency department his blood glucose is 880 mg/dl. His serum ketones are positive at 1:16 dilution. An arterial blood gas reveals a pH of 7.16, pCO_2 of 30 Torr, and pO_2 of 190 Torr (on 40% mask), which is generally consistent with a partially compensated metabolic acidosis. He is started on an insulin drip and admitted to the hospital. A chest X-ray reveals a right lower lobe pneumonia, which the ED physician feels contributed to the development of diabetic ketoacidosis. Following a three day course of antibiotics and aggressive fluid therapy, the patient is discharged home.

Thiamine

Class: Vitamin

Description

Thiamine is an important vitamin commonly referred to as vitamin B_1. It is required for the conversion of pyruvic acid to acetyl-coenzyme-A.

Mechanism of Action

A vitamin is a substance that the body cannot manufacture but that is required for metabolism. Most of the vitamins required by the body are obtained through the diet. Thiamine is required for the conversion of pyruvic acid to acetyl-coenzyme-A. Without this step a significant amount of the energy available in glucose cannot be obtained. The brain is extremely sensitive to thiamine deficiency.

Chronic alcohol intake interferes with the absorption, intake, and use of thiamine. A significant percentage of alcoholics have thiamine deficiency. During extended periods of fasting, neurological symptoms owing to thiamine deficiency may occur. These include Wernicke's syndrome and Korsakoff's psychosis. Wernicke's syndrome is an acute and reversible encephalopathy characterized by an unsteady gait, eye muscle weakness, and mental derangement. Korsakoff's psychosis is a significant memory disorder and may be irreversible. Any comatose patients, especially those who are suspected to be alcoholic, should receive IV thiamine in addition to the administration of 50% dextrose or naloxone.

Indications

- Coma of unknown origin, especially if alcohol may be involved
- Delirium tremens

Contraindications

There are no contraindications to the administration of thiamine in the emergency setting.

Precautions

A few cases of hypersensitivity to thiamine have been reported.

Side Effects

Few side effects are reported with thiamine usage. However, hypotension, dyspnea, and respiratory failure have been reported with its use.

Interactions

None in the emergency setting

Dosage

The emergency dose of thiamine is 100 milligrams intravenously or intramuscularly.

Route

Thiamine can be given either intravenously or intramuscularly. The intravenous route is preferred in emergency medicine.

How Supplied

Thiamine is supplied in 1-milliliter ampules containing 100 milligrams of the vitamin.

SUMMARY

Diabetes mellitus is probably the most common metabolic-endocrine emergency seen in the prehospital phase of emergency medical care. Hypoglycemia, if not immediately treated, can result in serious and permanent brain damage. It is important to remember that acute metabolic-endocrine disorders can cause a wide range of signs and symptoms from bizarre behavior to coma.

Prehospital drug administration should be guided by available data. Always determine the blood glucose level. If it is low, administer 50% dextrose. If alcoholism is suspected, consider the administration of thiamine. If narcotic abuse is possible, consider the administration of naloxone. The "coma cocktail" is a thing of the past. Prehospital care should be based on physical exam findings and the patient's past medical history.

KEY WORDS

diabetes mellitus. An endocrine disorder characterized by inadequate insulin production by the beta cells of the islets of Langerhans in the pancreas.

endocrine glands. Glands that secrete hormones directly into the blood.

hormones Chemical substances released by a gland that control or affect other glands or body systems.

hyperglycemia. A complication of diabetes characterized by excessive levels of blood glucose.

hypoglycemia. A complication of diabetes characterized by low levels of blood glucose. This often occurs from too high a dose of insulin or from inadequate food intake following a normal insulin dose. Sometimes called *insulin shock*, hypoglycemia is a true medical emergency.

ketoacidosis. A complication of diabetes due to decreased insulin secretion or intake. It is characterized by high levels of glucose in the blood, metabolic acidosis, and, in advanced stages, coma. Ketoacidosis is often called *diabetic coma*.

Kussmaul's respirations. A very deep gasping respiratory pattern found in diabetic coma.

chapter 10

Drugs Used in the Treatment of Neurological Emergencies

OBJECTIVES

1. Describe the treatment for a patient with a blunt or penetrating head injury.
2. Describe and list the indications, contraindications, and dosages for:
   - Dexamethasone
   - Mannitol
   - Methylprednisolone
3. List three acute, nontraumatic neurological disorders.
4. Describe and list the indications, contraindications, and dosages for the following drugs used in the treatment of seizures:
   - Diazepam
   - Lorazepam
   - Midazolam
   - Phenytoin
   - Phenobarbital

INTRODUCTION

Emergencies involving the nervous system can be devastating. In addition, they are also notoriously difficult to manage. Signs and symptoms of neurological disorders can range from slight headache to coma. They may be temporary or permanent. Prompt recognition and treatment is essential.

NEUROLOGICAL TRAUMA

Head injuries are an all too common result of automobile and motorcycle accidents. Although encased within the protective skull, the brain is quite susceptible to injury. Following craniocerebral trauma, cerebral edema occurs within 24 hours.

The primary treatment of patients with blunt or penetrating head injury is supportive. Airway management is of paramount importance, and continuous monitoring of blood pressure to detect occult blood loss in major trauma is mandatory. Pharmacological agents that have proved effective in the management of neurological emergencies include *dexamethasone*, which is thought to be of use in reducing brain edema, and *mannitol*, an osmotic diuretic that is also useful in reducing brain edema and is faster-acting than dexamethasone.

The management of spinal cord injuries is principally supportive. Recently, a protocol has been established whereby methylprednisolone (Solu-Medrol) is promptly administered to patients with spinal cord injuries. The initial results are favorable with many patients regaining spinal cord function. The severity of the injury will depend on the anatomical location of the spinal cord damage. Sometimes, following injury to the spinal cord, shock will occur (neurogenic shock). In these cases the body loses control over peripheral vascular tone. Vasopressor agents, such as norepinephrine, are indicated to assure maintenance of blood pressure.

The drugs on the following pages are frequently used in the prehospital phase of emergency medical care in the management of traumatic neurological emergencies.

Dexamethasone (Decadron, Hexadrol)

Class: Corticosteroid

Description

Dexamethasone is a synthetic steroid chemically related to the natural hormones secreted by the adrenal cortex.

Mechanism of Action

Dexamethasone is a long-acting steroid with a plasma half-life of about 5 hours. In general medical practice, steroids have a wide range of uses. Effective as anti-inflammatory agents, they are used in the management of allergic reactions and occasionally as an adjunctive agent in the management of shock. The role of steroids in the management of cerebral edema remains controversial. The mechanism and extent to which dexamethasone decreases cerebral edema, if indeed it does, is unclear.

It is generally agreed that a large single dose of steroids has little harmful effect. Consequently, it is used frequently in patients with cerebral edema, both in the emergency department and in the prehospital setting.

Indications

- Cerebral edema
- Anaphylaxis
- Asthma
- Exacerbation of COPD

Contraindications

There are no major contraindications to the use of dexamethasone in the emergency setting.

Precautions

A single dose of dexamethasone is all that should be given in the prehospital phase of care. Long-term steroid therapy can cause gastrointestinal bleeding, prolonged wound healing, and suppression of adrenocortical steroids.

Side Effects

Dexamethasone can cause fluid retention, congestive heart failure, hypertension, abdominal distention, vertigo, headache, nausea, malaise, and hiccups.

Interactions

Few in the prehospital setting

Dosage

The dose of dexamethasone varies considerably from physician to physician. The usual range is 4 to 24 milligrams with 12 milligrams intravenously being a commonly used dose. High-dose dexamethasone therapy, however, with up to 100 milligrams of the drug, is sometimes given.

Route

Dexamethasone is administered intravenously or intramuscularly with the intravenous route preferred in the emergency setting.

How Supplied

Decadron is supplied in two concentrations. The most common is the 4 milligrams per milliliter. It is supplied in prefilled syringes containing 1 milliliter of the drug and in vials containing 5 milligrams.

A second concentration, containing 24 milligrams per milliliter, is also available. It is supplied in 5- and 10-milliliter ampules. This concentration should only be used intravenously.

Mannitol (Osmotrol)

Class: Osmotic Diuretic

Description

Mannitol is a six-carbon sugar compound that has osmotic diuretic properties.

Mechanism of Action

Mannitol is an osmotic diuretic that inhibits sodium and water absorption in the kidneys. It promotes movement of fluid from the intracellular into the extracellular space. Because it dehydrates brain tissue, mannitol has proven effective in the management of cerebral edema and reduces intracranial pressure.

Indications

- Acute cerebral edema
- Blood transfusion reactions

Contraindications

Mannitol should not be used in any patient with acute pulmonary edema or severe pulmonary congestion. It should not be used in any patient who is profoundly hypovolemic.

Precautions

Rapid administration of mannitol can cause a transitory increase in intravascular volume and can result in congestive heart failure. The diuresis that accompanies mannitol therapy can cause sodium depletion.

One problem in the use of mannitol in the prehospital phase of emergency medical care is crystallization of the drug. The more concentrated the solution, the more tendency it has to crystallize at low temperatures. Crystallization begins as temperatures approach 45°F. Anytime a concentrated solution of mannitol is used, usually 15% or greater, an in-line filter should be present. It is important to remember that microscopic crystals appear long before those that can be seen to the naked eye.

If mannitol solution does crystallize, it should be warmed slowly in boiling water until the crystals disappear. It should be removed from EMS vehicles that are not parked in heated areas during colder weather.

Side Effects

Mannitol can cause chills, headache, dizziness, lethargy, mental status change, chest pain, nausea, and vomiting.

Interactions

Mannitol should not be administered with whole blood or packed red blood cells as it can damage the red blood cells.

Dosage

The typical adult dose of mannitol is 1.5–2.0 grams per kilogram of body weight intravenously. This can be given as a slow IV bolus or IV infusion. The slower rate of infusion helps eliminate the chances of inducing circulatory overload and congestive heart failure.

Route

Mannitol should be given intravenously.

How Supplied

Mannitol is supplied in 250 and 500 milliliters of a 20% solution for IV infusion. A 25% solution in 50 milliliters is available for slow IV bolus.

CASE PRESENTATION

At 2:30 P.M. you are called with fire department first responders to a motorcycle collision. On arrival you find an 18-year-old male, unhelmeted rider. Bystanders state that he lost control of the motorcycle on a corner and slid head-first into the cement retaining wall.

The patient is unconscious and unresponsive to deep pain. He is lying on his left side. His head is being supported by a bystander who states that the patient has been unconscious and unresponsive since he arrived.

Examination

CNS: The patient is unconscious and unresponsive. The pupils are bilaterally constricted. There is abnormal flexion (decorticate posture) bilaterally.

Resp: Respirations are 30 per minute and deep. His lungs are clear bilaterally with equal air entry. His trachea is midline and there are no signs of trauma to the neck or chest.

CVS: Both radial and carotid pulses are present and weak. His skin is pale and diaphoretic.

ABD: Soft and non-tender in all 4 quadrants

Musc/Skel: No other injuries noted

Vital Signs:

Pulse: 50 per minute

Resp: 30 per minute, deep

B/P: 160 by palpation

SpO_2: 87%

ECG: Sinus Bradycardia

Past Hx: Unknown

Treatment:

Fire department first responders assist with spinal immobilization while you insert an oropharyngeal airway and begin to hyperventilate the patient with a bag-valve-mask device and 100% oxygen. The patient is moved to your ALS ambulance following rapid immobilization and stabilization on a long spine board. During transport the patient's condition remains largely unchanged with the following exceptions:

Vital Signs:

Pulse: 50 per minute
Resp: 36 per minute, deep
B/P: 210/120 mmHg
SpO_2: 91%
CNS: Uneven pupils (right > left)

Because of the critical nature of this patient's injuries, the following procedures were completed:

Endotracheal intubation, IV line × 2, 14 gauge catheter, (per trauma protocol) normal saline TKO, and Mannitol 1.5 g/kg.

Total scene time was 10 minutes, and transport time to the hospital was 8 minutes. There were no changes in patient condition en route. On arrival at the hospital the patient was immediately taken to CT where an epidural hematoma was visualized. The patient was taken emergently to surgery where the epidural hematoma was decompressed. The patient was transferred to the neuro ICU where he remains.

Methylprednisolone (Solu-Medrol)

Class: Corticosteroid/Anti-Inflammatory

Description

Methylprednisolone is an intermediate-acting corticosteroid related to the natural hormones secreted by the adrenal cortex.

Mechanism of Action

Methylprednisolone is an intermediate-acting steroid. In general medical practice, steroids have a wide range of uses. Effective as anti-inflammatory agents, they are used in the management of allergic reactions and occasionally as an adjunctive agent in the management of shock. The role of steroids in the management of neurological emergencies remains controversial.

It is generally agreed that a large single dose of steroids has little harmful effect. Consequently, it is used in patients with spinal cord injury both in the emergency department and in the prehospital setting.

Indications

- Spinal cord injury
- Anaphylaxis
- Asthma
- Exacerbation of COPD

Contraindications

There are no major contraindications to the use of methylprednisolone in the emergency setting.

Precautions

A single dose of methylprednisolone is all that should be given in the prehospital phase of care. Long-term steroid therapy can cause gastrointestinal bleeding, prolonged wound healing, and suppression of adrenocortical steroids.

Side Effects

Methylprednisolone can cause fluid retention, congestive heart failure, hypertension, abdominal distention, vertigo, headache, nausea, malaise, and hiccups.

Interactions

Few in the prehospital setting

Dosage

- ***Spinal Cord Injury.*** High-dose methylprednisolone is used in treating spinal cord injuries. An initial bolus of 30 mg/kg is administered intravenously over a fifteen-minute period. This is followed 45 minutes later by a maintenance infusion of 5.4 milligrams/kilogram/hour.
- ***Asthma/COPD/Allergic Reactions.*** For other emergencies, 80–125 milligrams is usually administered intravenously or intramuscularly.

How Supplied

Methylprednisolone is supplied in vials containing 125 and 250 milligrams of the drug. The drug must be reconstituted prior to administration.

NONTRAUMATIC NEUROLOGICAL EMERGENCIES

There are many acute nontraumatic neurological disorders. Drugs, poisonings, and metabolic derangements can precipitate neurological emergencies. There is little that can be done for stroke and brain tumors in the prehospital phase of emergency medical care. Seizures attributable to epilepsy and other disorders can be managed in the field, however.

Seizures are one of the most frequently encountered neurological emergencies. One seizure followed by another seizure, without an intervening period of consciousness, is called *status epilepticus* and constitutes a serious threat to life. Status epilepticus should be terminated as quickly as possible.

The most common drug used to terminate seizure activity is IV diazepam (Valium). Phenytoin (Dilantin) and phenobarbital are also effective, however. In the following section of this chapter, these three drugs and their roles in prehospital care are discussed.

Diazepam (Valium))

Class: Anticonvulsant/Sedative

Description

Diazepam is a benzodiazepine that is frequently used as an anticonvulsant, sedative, and hypnotic.

Mechanism of Action

In emergency medicine, diazepam is principally used for its anticonvulsant properties. It suppresses the spread of seizure activity through the motor cortex of the brain. It does not appear to abolish the abnormal discharge focus, however.

Diazepam, one of the most frequently prescribed medications in the United States, is used in the management of anxiety and stress. It is effective in treating the tremors and anxiety associated with alcohol withdrawal. It is also an effective skeletal muscle relaxant, which makes it an effective adjunct in orthopedic injuries. It is a good premedication for minor operative procedures and cardioversion because it induces amnesia, which diminishes the patient's recall of such procedures.

Indications

- Major motor seizures
- Status epilepticus
- Premedication before cardioversion
- Skeletal muscle relaxant
- Acute anxiety states

Contraindications

Diazepam should not be administered to any patient with a history of hypersensitivity to the drug.

Precautions

Because diazepam is a relatively short-acting drug, seizure activity may recur. In such cases, an additional dose may be required. Flumazenil (Romazicon), a benzodiazepine antagonist, should be available to use as antidote if required.

Injectable diazepam can cause local venous irritation. To minimize this, it should only be injected into relatively large veins and should not be given faster than 1 milliliter per minute.

Side Effects

Diazepam can cause hypotension, drowsiness, headache, amnesia, respiratory depression, blurred vision, nausea, and vomiting.

Interactions

Diazepam is incompatible with many medications. Any time diazepam is given intravenously in conjunction with other drugs, the IV line should be adequately flushed. The effects of diazepam can be additive when used in conjunction with other CNS depressants and alcohol.

Dosage

In the management of seizures, the usual dose of diazepam is 5 to 10 milligrams IV. In many instances it may be necessary to give diazepam directly into the vein, as the seizure activity will prevent the insertion of an indwelling catheter. When given directly into a vein, it is essential that a large vein, preferably in the antecubital fossa, is used.

In acute anxiety reactions, the standard dosage is 2 to 5 milligrams intramuscularly.

To induce amnesia prior to cardioversion, a dosage of 5 to 15 milligrams of diazepam is given intravenously. Peak effects are seen in 5 to 10 minutes.

Diazepam should be given intravenously by slow IV push. It can be injected intramuscularly, but absorption via this route is variable. When an IV line cannot be started, parenteral diazepam can be administered rectally with a similar onset of action.

How Supplied

Valium is supplied in ampules and prefilled syringes containing 10 milligrams in 2 milliliters of solvent.

Lorazepam (Ativan)

Class: Anticonvulsant/Sedative

Description

Lorazepam is a benzodiazepine that is used as an anti-convulsant, sedative, and hypnotic.

Mechanism of Action

Lorazepam is a benzodiazepine with a shorter half-life than diazepam. Its onset of action is approximately the same. It is used in the management of anxiety and stress. It is a good premedication for minor operative procedures and cardioversion because it induces amnesia, which diminishes the patient's recall of such procedures. Lorazepam is often used in pediatrics as an anticonvulsant because of its shorter half-life. Like diazepam, lorazepam suppresses the spread of seizure activity through the motor cortex of the brain. It does not appear to abolish the abnormal discharge focus.

Indications

- Major motor seizures
- Status epilepticus
- Premedication before cardioversion
- Acute anxiety states

Contraindications

Lorazepam should not be administered to any patient with a history of hypersensitivity to the drug.

Precautions

Lorazepam should be diluted with normal saline or D_5W prior to intravenous administration. Because lorazepam is a relatively short-acting drug, seizure activity may recur. In such cases, an additional dose may be required. Flumazenil (Romazicon), a benzodiazepine antagonist, should be available to use as antidote if required.

Side Effects

Lorazepam can cause hypotension, drowsiness, headache, amnesia, respiratory depression, blurred vision, nausea, and vomiting.

Interactions

The effects of lorazepam can be additive when used in conjunction with other CNS depressants and alcohol.

Dosage

The usual dose of lorazepam is 0.5–2.0 milligrams when given intravenously. The dose can be increased to 1.0–4.0 milligrams when given intramuscularly. It can be given rectally when an IV cannot be placed. The medication should be drawn up into a syringe. A small red rubber pediatric feeding tube can be attached to the syringe. The feeding tube should be inserted 2–4 centimeters into the rectum and the drug administered. Often it is necessary to hold the buttocks together to help the patient retain the drug.

How Supplied

Lorazepam is supplied in ampules and Tubex syringes containing 1, 2, and 4 milligrams in 2 milliliters of solvent.

Midazolam (Versed)

Class: Sedative/Hypnotic

Description

Midazolam is a benzodiazepine with strong hypnotic and amnestic properties.

Mechanism of Action

Midazolam is a potent, but short-acting benzodiazepine used widely in medicine as a sedative and hypnotic. It is 3–4 times more potent than diazepam. Its onset of action is approximately 1.5 minutes when administered intravenously and 15 minutes when administered intramuscularly. Midazolam has impressive amnestic properties. Like the other benzodiazepines, it has no effect on pain.

Indication

- Premedication before cardioversion and other painful procedures

Contraindications

Midazolam should not be administered to any patient with a history of hypersensitivity to the drug. It should not be used in patients who have narrow-angle glaucoma. Midazolam should not be administered to patients in shock, with depressed vital signs, or who are in alcoholic coma.

Precautions

Emergency resuscitative equipment must be available prior to the administration of midazolam. Vital signs must be continuously monitored during and after drug administration. Midazolam has more potential than the other benzodiazepines to cause respiratory depression and respiratory arrest. Flumazenil (Romazicon), a benzodiazepine antagonist, should be available to use as antidote if required.

Side Effects

Midazolam can cause laryngospasm, bronchospasm, dyspnea, respiratory depression and arrest, drowsiness, amnesia, altered mental status, bradycardia, tachycardia, PVCs, and retching.

Interactions

The effects of midazolam can be accentuated by CNS depressants such as narcotics and alcohol.

Dosage

When used for sedation, midazolam must be administered cautiously, as the amount of medication required to achieve sedation varies from individual to individual. Typically, 1–2.5 milligrams are administered by slow IV injection. Usually, it is best to dilute midazolam with normal saline or D_5W prior to IV administration. Midazolam can be administered intramuscularly at a dose of 0.07–0.08 mg/kg (average adult dose of 5 mg). Recently, many centers are administering midazolam intranasaly or by mouth to sedate children prior to suturing of lacerations.

How Supplied

Midazolam is supplied in ampules and vials containing 5 milligrams per milliliter of the drug.

Phenytoin (Dilantin)

Class: Anticonvulsant/Anti-Arrhythmic

Description

Phenytoin is a long-acting anticonvulsant. It is also used as an antiarrhythmic where it depresses spontaneous ventricular depolarization.

Mechanism of Action

Phenytoin is an effective anticonvulsant. Its onset of action, however, is considerably longer than for diazepam. In most emergency situations the seizure should first be controlled with Valium. If seizure activity recurs, phenytoin can be administered. Phenytoin also is used to treat arrhythmias caused by digitalis toxicity. This use of the drug is discussed in Chapter 7.

Indications

- Major motor seizures
- Status epilepticus
- Arrhythmias owing to digitalis toxicity

Contraindications

Phenytoin should not be given to any patient with a history of hypersensitivity to the drug. It is contraindicated in cases of bradycardia and high-grade heart block. It should not be administered to patients who take the drug chronically for seizures until the blood level has been determined.

Precautions

Intravenous administration of phenytoin should not exceed 50 milligrams per minute. Signs of central nervous system depression or hypotension may occur. Elderly patients are at increased risk of developing side effects from phenytoin administration. Avoid extravasation. Any patient receiving intravenous phenytoin should have continuous cardiac monitoring as well as frequent monitoring of vital signs.

Side Effects

Phenytoin can cause drowsiness, dizziness, headache, hypotension, arrhythmias, itching, rash, nausea, and vomiting.

Interactions

Phenytoin must never be diluted in dextrose-containing solutions such as D_5W. It should be diluted in normal saline or other non-glucose containing crystalloids.

Dosage

The loading dose of phenytoin is typically 10 to 15 milligrams per kilogram. This should be administered no faster than 50 milligrams per minute. Phenytoin should be diluted with normal saline, as dilution with 5% dextrose may result in precipitation of the drug. In emergency medicine phenytoin should be administered intravenously only.

How Supplied

Phenytoin is supplied in 2- and 5-milliliter ampules containing 50 milligrams per milliliter. A 2-milliliter prefilled syringe is also available. Dilantin is incompatible with solutions containing dextrose. If an infusion of Dilantin is prepared, the drug should be placed in normal saline.

Phenobarbital (Luminal)

Class: Anticonvulsant/Barbiturate

Description

Phenobarbital belongs to a class of drugs called *barbiturates*. It is used as a sedative and an anti-convulsant.

Mechanism of Action

Barbiturates have many uses in medicine. They are central nervous system depressants and are used as anticonvulsants and in the management of insomnia and anxiety. Phenobarbital is an effective anticonvulsant of relatively low toxicity. It depresses the sensory cortex, decreases motor activity, alters cerebellar function, and causes drowsiness, sedation, and hypnosis.

Indications

- Major motor seizures
- Status epilepticus
- Acute anxiety states

Contraindications

Phenobarbital should not be administered to any patient with a history of hypersensitivity to the barbiturates.

Precautions

Respiratory depression and hypotension can occur following IV administration of phenobarbital. Constant monitoring of respiratory pattern and blood pressure is essential. Administration of phenobarbital to children may result in hyperactive behavior.

Side Effects

Phenobarbital can cause drowsiness, altered mental status, agitation, hypoventilation, apnea, bradycardia, hypotension, syncope, headache, nausea, and vomiting.

Interactions

Phenobarbital may enhance the sedative effects of other sedatives including alcohol, narcotics, antihistamines, and antidepressants.

Dosage

The standard dosage of phenobarbital in the management of status epilepticus is 100 to 250 milligrams intravenously given slowly.

How Supplied

Phenobarbital is supplied in 1-milliliter ampules containing either 15, 30, 60, or 100 milligrams of the drug.

CASE PRESENTATION

At 8:30 P.M. you are called to an apartment for a 12-year-old boy with reported seizures. Dispatch informs you that the boy has had two seizures since 2:00 P.M. and is now into his third seizure. The boy has a history of epilepsy and is on medication. He is unresponsive.

Four minutes later you arrive at the apartment and are met by a very frantic mother. She leads you to the boy's bedroom. There you find the patient lying in bed with his father attempting to restrain him. The patient is in the tonic phase of a grand mal seizure.

Examination

CNS: The patient is unresponsive and in the tonic phase of a grand mal seizure.

Resp: Respirations are 30 per minute (after tonic phase) and shallow. His trachea is midline and there are no external signs of trauma.

CVS: Both the radial and carotid pulses are present, but are rapid and weak. His skin is pale and diaphoretic.

ABD: Soft and non-tender in all 4 quadrants. There are no signs of vomiting. The patient has been incontinent of urine.

Musc/Skel: The patient has lacerated his tongue several times. No other injuries are detected.

Vital Signs:

Pulse: 150 per minute

Resp: 30 per minute, shallow

B/P: Unobtainable

SpO_2: Unobtainable

ECG: Unobtainable

Past Hx: Mother states patient has been an epileptic since he was two years old. She shows you a prescription for Dilantin. The patient had first seizure at school at 2:30 P.M. His mother brought him home, and he had another seizure at 5:45 P.M. She denies recent fever or recent trauma.

Treatment:

Attempts to obtain a complete set of vital signs are unsuccessful due to seizure activity. Your partner attempts to ventilate the patient with a bag-valve-mask unit with 100% oxygen, but is unsuccessful. A nonrebreather mask is placed on the patient and held there by your partner. Following contact with the base hospital, you are preparing to give Valium IV push. With the assistance of the father, you are able to hold the patient's arm in place long enough to initiate an 18 gauge IV catheter in the right antecubital fossa and secure it with tape and kling. You then administer Valium, 2.0 mg IV push. If that doesn't terminate the seizure, a repeat of 2.0 mg may be given. You administer the first dose of Valium, and the seizure subsides in two minutes. Your partner is now able to assist respirations with the BVM. Within five minutes the patient is in the postictal stage. He is transported to the hospital without incident and without further seizure.

At the hospital a CT scan is obtained, which is reported as normal. A spinal tap is also carried out to exclude infection or bleeding as the cause. This too is negative although culture results will not be available for 48 hours. The Dilantin level obtained on blood is 3.4 mg/L (therapeutic 10–20 mg/L). IV Dilantin is administered and the patient admitted to the pediatric intensive care unit. He does well with no additional seizures. The mother reports that the Dilantin dose has not been increased in four years despite the fact that the boy has grown 11 inches and gained 40 pounds. She has also been buying a less-expensive brand of generic Dilantin.

SUMMARY

In the management of acute head injury, mannitol has proved effective in reducing cerebral edema. Hyperventilation is even more important in minimizing cerebral edema. It is important to remember that stabilization of the cervical spine, maintenance of the airway, and supplemental delivery of oxygen are of primary importance.

In a general motor seizure, as occasionally occurs, the primary treatment is that of protecting the patient from injury. It is important to remember that most epileptic patients are already taking orally one or two anticonvulsant medications. The judicious use of the parenteral agents discussed in this chapter is therefore indicated. It is helpful to the emergency physician to obtain blood samples from seizure patients prior to the administration of an anticonvulsant. Some authorities believe that a significant percentage of patients that have general motor seizures do so because they fail to follow instructions on ordered medications. Blood studies taken before the administration of anticonvulsants will aid the physician in making a diagnosis.

KEY WORDS

amnesia. A loss of memory.

benzodiazepine. A class of drugs frequently used to relieve anxiety and insomnia and to induce sedation.

central nervous system. The central portion of the nervous system, namely the brain and spinal cord.

epilepsy. A group of nervous system disorders characterized by the presence of seizures.

intracranial pressure. The pressure in the intracranial space (skull). Increased intracranial pressure can have a deleterious effect on the brain tissue.

neurogenic shock. A state of inadequate tissue perfusion due to peripheral vasodilation due to loss or interruption of nervous system control.

seizures. A sudden change in nervous function. The symptoms can range from a slight alteration in mental status to violent, generalized uncontrollable contraction of muscles.

status epilepticus. A state of repeated seizures without an intervening period of consciousness.

vertigo. A feeling of faintness or dizziness that may result in an inability to maintain balance.

chapter 11

Drugs Used in the Treatment of Obstetrical and Gynecological Emergencies

OBJECTIVES

1. List three obstetrical and gynecological emergencies that require intervention with pharmacological agents.
2. Define the following terms:
   - abruptio placenta
   - eclampsia
   - ectopic pregnancy
   - placenta previa
   - postpartum hemorrhage
   - preeclampsia
   - spontaneous abortion
3. Describe and list the indications, contraindications, and dosages for oxytocin.
4. List the signs and symptoms of hypertensive disorders of pregnancy.
5. Distinguish between pregnancy-induced hypertension, preeclampsia, and eclampsia.
6. Describe and list the indications, contraindications, and dosages for magnesium sulfate.
7. Describe the management of a patient in preterm labor.

8. Describe and list the indications, contraindications, and dosages for terbutaline.

INTRODUCTION

Prehospital care for most obstetrical and gynecological emergencies is supportive. There are three complications, however, that necessitate intervention with pharmacological agents. These are the hypertensive disorders of pregnancy, severe vaginal bleeding, and preterm labor. *Magnesium sulfate* has proved effective in controlling the convulsions associated with eclampsia. *Pitocin*, a drug chemically identical to the hormone oxytocin, is effective in causing uterine contraction and will control many cases of postpartum vaginal bleeding. *Terbutaline*, a β_2, is effective in suppression of preterm labor.

SEVERE VAGINAL BLEEDING

Vaginal bleeding that occurs during the first trimester of pregnancy is usually due to spontaneous abortion or ectopic pregnancy. During the third trimester of pregnancy, vaginal bleeding is most frequently caused by either abruptio placenta or placenta previa.

Bleeding following childbirth is common. Hypovolemic shock can develop when blood loss is in excess of 500 milliliters. Severe vaginal bleeding can be a life-threatening emergency, necessitating immediate therapy.

The management of severe vaginal bleeding is similar to that employed with any other types of severe hemorrhage. Initial treatment should include airway maintenance, administration of supplemental oxygen, and infusion of intravenous volume expanders. In addition, the IV administration of Pitocin in postpartum hemorrhage can be effective in controlling severe vaginal bleeding.

Oxytocin (Pitocin)

Class: Hormone/Uterine Stimulant

Description

Oxytocin is a naturally occurring hormone that is secreted by the posterior pituitary.

Mechanism of Action

Oxytocin causes contraction of uterine smooth muscle and lactation. Oxytocin is used to induce labor in selected cases and is also effective in inducing uterine contractions following delivery, thereby controlling postpartum hemorrhage.

When a baby is placed on the breast, the sucking action causes the posterior pituitary to release oxytocin. It is important to remember this inherent mechanism whenever confronted by a patient suffering moderate to severe postpartum bleeding.

Indication

- Postpartum hemorrhage

Contraindications

In the prehospital setting, oxytocin should be administered only to patients suffering severe postpartum bleeding. Before administration it is essential to verify that the baby *and the placenta* have been delivered and that there is not an additional fetus in the uterus.

Precautions

Excess oxytocin can cause overstimulation of the uterus and possible uterine rupture. Hypertension, cardiac arrhythmia, and anaphylaxis have been reported in conjunction with the administration of oxytocin. Vital signs and uterine tone should be monitored.

Side Effects

Oxytocin can cause hypotension, arrhythmias, tachycardia, seizures, coma, nausea, and vomiting in the mother. When administered prior to delivery, oxytocin can cause fetal hypoxia, fetal asphyxia, fetal arrhythmias, and possibly fetal intracranial bleeding.

Interactions

Oxytocin can cause hypertension when administered in conjunction with vasoconstrictors such as norepinephrine.

Dosage

The following are two regimens for the administration of oxytocin in the management of patients with postpartum hemorrhage:

3 to 10 units can be administered intramuscularly following delivery of the placenta.

10 to 20 units can be placed in either 500 or 1000 milliliters of D_5W or lactated Ringer's. This should be titrated according to the severity of the bleeding and the uterine response.

Oxytocin should only be administered intramuscularly or by slow IV infusion.

How Supplied

Pitocin is supplied in 0.5- and 1-milliliter ampules containing 10 milligrams per milliliter. A 1-milliliter prefilled syringe containing the same concentration is also available.

HYPERTENSIVE DISORDERS OF PREGNANCY

In addition to vaginal bleeding, you should be aware of several pregnancy-associated problems known collectively as *hypertensive disorders of pregnancy* (formerly called "toxemia of pregnancy"). These disorders are characterized by hypertension, weight gain, edema, protein in the urine, and, in late stages, seizures. Hypertensive disorders of pregnancy occur in approximately 5 percent of pregnancies. They are thought to be caused by abnormal vasospasm in the mother, which results in increased blood pressure and other associated symptoms. The hypertensive disorders of pregnancy generally include:

- *Pregnancy-Induced Hypertension (PIH)*. PIH is characterized by a blood pressure of 140/90 level or greater in pregnancy in a patient who was previously normotensive. PIH is the early stage of the disease process. It is important to remember that blood pressure usually drops in pregnancy, and a blood pressure reading of 130/80 may be elevated.
- *Preeclampsia*. Preeclamptic patients are those that have hypertension, abnormal weight gain, edema, headache, protein in the urine, epigastric pain, and, occasionally, visual disturbances. If untreated, preeclampsia may progress to the next stage, eclampsia.
- *Eclampsia*. Eclampsia is the most serious manifestation of the hypertensive disorders of pregnancy. It is characterized by grand mal seizure activity. Eclampsia is often preceded by visual disturbances, such as flashing lights or spots before the eyes. Also, the development of epigastric pain or pain in the right upper abdominal quadrant often indicates impending seizure. Eclampsia can be distinguished from epilepsy by the history and physical appearance of the patient. Patients who become eclamptic are usually edematous and have markedly elevated blood pressure, while epileptics usually have a prior history of seizures and are taking anticonvulsant medications.

The hypertensive disorders of pregnancy tend to occur most often with a woman's first pregnancy. They also appear to occur more frequently in patients with preexisting hypertension. Diabetes mellitus is also associated with an increased incidence of this disease process.

Patients who develop PIH and preeclampsia are at increased risk for cerebral hemorrhage, the development of renal failure, and pulmonary edema. Patients who are preeclamptic have intravascular volume depletion, since a great deal of their body fluid is in the third space. If eclampsia develops, death of the mother and fetus frequently results.

Eclampsia must be treated aggressively. *Magnesium sulfate* is the drug of choice for controlling convulsions associated with toxemia. In addition, it may be necessary to administer an antihypertensive agent, such as those discussed in Chapter 7, to prevent the complications of hypertensive crisis. The decision to administer an antihypertensive in the prehospital phase of emergency medical care rests with the base station physician. Each case should be treated individually.

Magnesium Sulfate

Class: Electrolyte

Description

Magnesium sulfate is a salt that dissociates into the magnesium cation (Mg^{++}) and the sulfate anion when administered. Magnesium is an essential element in numerous biochemical reactions that occur within the body.

Mechanism of Action

Magnesium sulfate is a central nervous system depressant effective in the management of seizures associated with eclampsia. It is used for the initial therapy of convulsions associated with pregnancy. After cessation of seizure activity, other anticonvulsant agents may be administered.

Indications

- Eclampsia (seizures accompanying pregnancy)
- Preterm labor

Contraindications

Magnesium sulfate should not be administered to any patient with heart block. It should not be administered to patients who are in shock, who have persistent severe hypertension, who routinely undergo dialysis, or who are known to have a decreased calcium level (hypocalcemia).

Precautions

Magnesium sulfate, like other central nervous system depressants, can cause hypotension, circulatory collapse, and depression of cardiac and respiratory function. The most immediate danger is respiratory depression. Calcium chloride should be readily available for IV administration as an antidote in case respiratory depression occurs. Magnesium sulfate should be administered slowly to minimize side effects. Any patient receiving intravenous magnesium sulfate should have continuous cardiac monitoring as well as frequent monitoring of vital signs. If possible, the knee and biceps deep tendon reflexes should be checked prior to magnesium therapy.

Side Effects

Magnesium sulfate can cause flushing, sweating, bradycardia, decreased deep tendon reflexes, drowsiness, respiratory depression, arrhythmias, hypotension, hypothermia, itching, and a rash.

Interactions

Magnesium sulfate can cause cardiac conduction abnormalities if administered in conjunction with digitalis.

Dosage

The standard dosage for the management of convulsions associated with eclampsia is 2–4 grams intravenously. If an IV cannot be started, magnesium sulfate can be administered intramuscularly. Because of the volume of the drug (5–10 ml), the dose should be divided in half and each half administered intramuscularly at a separate site (usually each gluteus.)

How Supplied

Magnesium sulfate is supplied in prefilled syringes containing 5 and 10 milliliters of a 50% solution.

CASE PRESENTATION

An ALS ambulance is called to a rural hospital to transport a maternity patient to a larger city hospital one hour away. Paramedics are asked to bring the monitor in with the stretcher. On arrival at the hospital the nurse attending the patient gives the following information.

The patient is an 18-year-old female, Gravida 1, Para 0, in her third trimester of pregnancy. She came to the hospital by private car after suffering a grand mal seizure at home. She had no prior history of seizures and her pregnancy had been uneventful to date. She evidently was not in labor prior to the seizure. At present the patient is lying on a hospital bed and is not having contractions as based on the external fetal monitor. The fetal heart rate is stable.

Hospital Diagnosis: Eclampsia

Examination

CNS: The patient is conscious but lethargic.

Resp: Respirations are 24 per minute and shallow. There is symmetrical chest wall movement with clear bilateral breath sounds.

CVS: Both carotid and radial pulses are present and strong. A systolic flow murmur can be heard. Minimal blood loss is noted from the vagina. The neck veins are not distended. Her skin color is normal, warm, and diaphoretic to touch. She is very edematous.

ABD: Obviously pregnant with no contractions noted

Extremities: Pedal and finger edema noted

Vital Signs:

Pulse: 100 per minute, regular
Resp: 24 per minute
B/P: 166/112 mmHg
SpO_2: 95
ECG: Normal Sinus Rhythm

Hospital treatment:

The patient is receiving high-flow oxygen. A large bore IV was started in the left forearm. Magnesium sulfate is being infused at a rate of 1 gram per hour. The receiving hospital was notified and is expecting the patient.

Treatment:

The patient is moved to the ambulance stretcher and moved to the ambulance. Oxygen is administered at 12 L/min by nonrebreathing mask. The pulse oximeter is applied and shows an SpO_2 of 96%. The cardiac monitor shows a regular sinus rhythm and is checked frequently by the paramedics watching for any ECG changes. The IV of magnesium sulfate initiated in the hospital is continued at 1 gram per hour. The interior ambulance lights are dimmed to help prevent additional seizure activity. A pre-filled syringe of Valium is removed from the lock box in case the patient again suffers a seizure.

During transport the patient is continually assessed with special attention to the IV of magnesium sulfate. Deep tendon reflexes are periodically checked to assure the magnesium effect is not excessive. The trip to the hospital is uneventful. Upon arrival at the receiving facility, an emergency sonogram is obtained. It shows a fetal age of 37 weeks (+/− 2 weeks). Labor is induced and the patient delivers a healthy female infant 18 hours later.

PRETERM LABOR

Preterm labor is labor that begins before the age of fetal maturity, usually before 36 weeks. If labor begins early, obstetricians will often try to suppress it to allow more time for intrauterine fetal development.

There are three approaches to suppressing preterm labor. The first approach is to sedate the mother. Often, labor begins in response to maternal stress or exhaustion. In these cases, a sedative such as Seconal is given. Alternatively, morphine sulfate can be administered (intramuscularly) for sedation.

The second approach to suppressing preterm labor is administration of a fluid bolus. The hormone oxytocin is manufactured and released from the posterior pituitary. Antidiuretic hormone (ADH) is also manufactured and released from the posterior pituitary. ADH causes the kidneys to retain water. In cases of preterm labor, a fluid bolus (1–2 liters of lactated Ringer's or normal saline) is administered. ADH production and release is inhibited through feedback systems. As ADH and oxytocin come from the same area of the posterior pituitary, suppression of ADH release also suppresses oxytocin release and thus can help suppress preterm labor.

Finally, labor can be suppressed by the use of tocolytics. While there are many tocolytics available, β_2 agonists are frequently used. Stimulation of uterine β_2 receptors causes uterine relaxation and suppression of preterm labor. Common β_2 agonists include terbutaline and ritodrine

(Yutopar). Terbutaline is used more frequently in the emergency setting. Magnesium sulfate, previously discussed, is also effective in suppressing preterm labor.

Terbutaline (Brethine, Bricanyl)

Class: Sympathetic Agonist / Tocolytic

Description

Terbutaline is a synthetic sympathomimetic that is selective for β_2-adrenergic receptors.

Mechanism of Action

Terbutaline, because of its effects on β_2-adrenergic receptors, causes immediate bronchodilation with minimal cardiac effects. It is also used to suppress preterm labor. Stimulation of β_2-adrenergic receptors in the uterus causes uterine relaxation and can suppress labor.

Indication

- Preterm labor

Contraindications

Terbutaline should not be administered to any patient with a history of hypersensitivity to the drug.

Precautions

As with any sympathomimetic, the patient's vital signs must be monitored. Caution should be used when administering terbutaline to elderly patients and those with cardiovascular disease or hypertension.

Side Effects

Terbutaline can cause palpitations, anxiety, dizziness, headache, nervousness, tremor, hypertension, arrhythmias, chest pain, nausea, and vomiting.

Interactions

The possibility of developing unpleasant side effects increases when terbutaline is used with other sympathetic agonists. β blockers may blunt the pharmacological effects of terbutaline.

Dosage

Terbutaline should be initially administered by subcutaneous injection. The initial dose should be 0.25 milligrams subcutaneously. This can be repeated in thirty minutes to one hour as required. A terbutaline drip can be used to provide ongoing suppression of labor. It can be prepared by placing 5 milligrams of terbutaline in 500 mL of lactated Ringer's or normal saline. The drip should be started at 30 ml/hour (5 micrograms per minute). This can be slowly increased to a maximum dose of 80 micrograms per minute as required.

How Supplied

Terbutaline is supplied in vials containing 1 milligram of the drug in 1 milliliter of solvent.

SUMMARY

Most obstetrical and gynecological emergencies are not managed in the field. Prehospital treatment should include stabilization of the airway, administration of supplemental oxygen, and replacement of intravascular volume. In severe postpartum bleeding, the administration of Pitocin is often effective. In the hypertensive disorders of pregnancy, magnesium sulfate may be used during the prehospital phase of emergency medical care to control convulsions. The definitive treatment of preeclampsia and eclampsia is delivery of the fetus.

KEY WORDS

abruptio placenta. A premature separation of the placenta from the uterus before birth. Because it often results in severe bleeding, it is considered to be a serious condition.

eclampsia. The most serious manifestation of the hypertensive disorders of pregnancy. It is characterized by grand mal seizure activity. Eclampsia is often preceded by visual disturbances, such as flashing lights or spots before the eyes. Also, the development of epigastric pain or pain in the right upper abdominal quadrant often indicates impending seizure. Patients who become eclamptic are usually edematous and have markedly elevated blood pressure.

ectopic pregnancy. The implantation of a developing fetus outside the uterus, often in the fallopian tube.

placenta previa. A condition where the placenta partly or completely covers the opening of the cervix. It is the most common cause of painless bleeding in the third trimester.

postpartum hemorrhage. The loss of 500 mL or more blood in the first 24 hours following delivery.

preeclampsia. A manifestation of the hypertensive disorders of pregnancy characterized by hypertension, abnormal weight gain, edema, headache, protein in the urine, epigastric pain, and, occasionally, visual disturbances. If untreated, preeclampsia may progress to the next stage, eclampsia.

spontaneous abortion. A fetal loss, also called a miscarriage, that occurs of its own accord. Most spontaneous abortions occur before the twelfth week of pregnancy. Many occur two weeks after conception and are mistaken for menstrual periods.

chapter 12

Drugs Used in the Treatment of Toxicological Emergencies

OBJECTIVES

1. Discuss the importance of toxicological emergencies in prehospital care.
2. Discuss the role of poison centers within the EMS system.
3. Discuss the importance of obtaining a detailed history in toxicological emergencies.
4. Describe the various entry routes of toxic substances into the body.
5. Describe the general principles of toxicologic management.
6. Define the following terms:
   - allergic reaction
   - anaphylaxis
   - histamine
7. Describe and list the indications, contraindications, and dosages for:
   - epinephrine 1:1,000
   - diphenhydramine
   - methylprednisolone
   - hydrocortisone
8. Define the following terms:
   - overdose
   - poison

9. Explain the first and second steps in the management of any poisoning.
10. Describe and list the indications, contraindications, and dosages for syrup of ipecac and activated charcoal.
11. Describe the pathophysiology and signs and symptoms of organophosphate poisoning.
12. Describe and list the indications, contraindications, and dosages for atropine sulfate and pralidoxime.
13. Describe the signs and symptoms associated with cyanide poisoning.
14. Describe and list the indications, contraindications, and dosages for amyl nitrate.
15. Describe and list the indications, contraindications, and dosages for the following medications used as antidotes in overdoses:
    - naloxone
    - physostigmine
    - flumazenil

INTRODUCTION

The likelihood that one will be exposed to toxins in the home or workplace is increasing. Over-the-counter and prescription medications are common in the home. About two-thirds of visits to physicians result in a prescription. Household chemicals are a hazard and are often designed to have a pleasant odor and color. Industrial chemicals offer another dimension of potential toxic exposures. These chemicals may involve a single victim or create a triage problem in a hazardous materials incident. Overall, most toxic exposures occur in the home.

During recent years, toxicological emergencies have become more prevalent in society. The following figures reveal the high potential for involvement in a toxic substance on an EMS call.

- Over one million persons are poisoned annually.
- Ten percent of all emergency department visits and EMS responses involve toxic exposures.
- Seventy percent of accidental poisonings occur in children under the age of six years.
- A child who has experienced an accidental ingestion has a 25 percent chance of another similar ingestion within one year.
- Eighty percent of all attempted suicides involve a drug overdose.

Intentional toxic exposures tend to have a higher death rate and result in more serious symptoms than accidental exposures or drug reactions. The most commonly encountered route of exposure is by ingestion in the form of an oral drug overdose. The most common prehospital toxicologic problem, but the least likely to be thought of this way, is alcohol intoxication.

POISON CONTROL CENTERS

Poison control centers have been set up across the United States and Canada to assist in the treatment of poison victims and to provide information on new products and new treatment recommendations. They are usually based in major centers and teaching hospitals that serve a large population. Most poison control centers now have computer systems that access information rapidly.

Poison control centers are usually staffed by physicians, pharmacists, nurses, paramedics, or poison control specialists trained in toxicology. These experts provide information to callers 24 hours a day. They update information routinely and offer the most current treatment protocols.

Memorize the number of the nearest poison control center and routinely access it. There are several advantages to this practice. First, the poison control center can help you immediately determine the potential toxicity based on the type of agent, amount and time of exposure, and physical condition of the patient. Second, in about four out of five cases, the most current, definitive treatment can be started in the field. Finally, the poison control center can notify the receiving hospital of current treatment even before arrival of the patient.

History

Obtaining a history from a victim of poisoning may be difficult, and the history you do obtain might not be accurate; the victim may be misinformed, may be deliberately trying to deceive you, or may be subject to a drug-induced confusion. However, to manage the poisoned patient correctly, you need a relevant history. If the patient is a child, other children in the household may have also eaten the poison, so assess all children carefully. Interview family members and witnesses. To begin, look for clues at the scene—overturned or empty medicine bottles, scattered pills or capsules, recently emptied containers, spilled chemicals, spilled cleaning solvents, overturned plants or pieces of plants, and the remains of food or drink or vomitus.

To get as much history as you can, ask the patient or bystanders the following questions:

What was ingested? Ask the patient or bystanders what the patient might have taken. Bring the container and all of its remaining contents, the plant or portions that might have been ingested, or other specimens to the hospital or emergency room. Remember to bring all possible containers—the most obvious open container may not be the one that was used. If a plant was ingested, find out what part was involved (roots, leaves, stem, flower, or fruit). If vomiting has occurred, save a sample of the vomitus in a clean, closed container and transport it with the patient.

How was it taken? Was it ingested, inhaled, absorbed (spilled on skin), or injected?

When was the substance taken? Was the toxin taken all at once? Did the patient take more and more of the substance(s) at repeated intervals? Some patients may inadvertently take a toxic level of pain killers by repeatedly taking medication beyond the prescribed dosage, seeking relief from pain. As well, decisions regarding emesis (inducing vomiting) will depend significantly upon how much time has elapsed since ingestion. Is there a possibility that other substances were taken along with it?

How much was taken? How many pills from each bottle? How many ounces of a liquid substance?

Has an attempt been made to induce vomiting? Has anything been given as an antidote?

Does the patient have a psychiatric history that might suggest a suicide attempt?

Does the patient have an underlying medical illness, allergy, chronic drug use/abuse, or addiction?

Because there are so many types of poisons, the history is especially important. All of the above are critical questions that should be asked of the patient, family, or others present at the scene. In many cases, multiple agents may have been taken.

ROUTES OF TOXIC EXPOSURE

Poisons can enter the body through various routes. These include ingestion, inhalation, injection, and surface absorption.

Ingestion

Ingestion is the most common route of entry for toxic exposures. Frequently ingested poisons include:

- household products
- petroleum-based agents (gasoline, paint)
- cleaning agents (alkalis and soaps)
- cosmetics
- medications (prescribed or illicit)
- plants
- foods

General Principles of Management

Priorities in the management of the poisoned patient are maintenance of airway, breathing, and circulation. Prevention of aspiration is one of the major objectives of prehospital care. Aspiration pneumonia is a serious concern in the definitive care of the toxic patient.

In cases that require more definitive airway management, endotracheal intubation (orally or nasally) may be necessary. Generally, nasotracheal intubation is preferred for patients who have a gag reflex. High-flow oxygen supplementation should be routinely performed.

Induction of Vomiting

If the patient has ingested the toxic substance within 3–6 hours of your arrival, contact the local poison control center.

Inhalation

Inhalation of a poison results in rapid absorption of the toxic agent through the alveolar-capillary membrane. Inhaled toxins can irritate pulmonary passages causing extensive edema and destroying tissue. When these toxins are absorbed, wider systemic effects can occur. Causative agents can appear as gases, vapors, fumes, or aerosols. Commonly inhaled poisons include:

- toxic gases
- carbon monoxide
- ammonia
- chlorine
- freon
- toxic vapors
- fumes or aerosols
- carbon tetrachloride
- tear gas (pepper mace)
- mustard gas
- nitrous oxide

General Principles of Management

The first priority in treating patients who have inhaled toxic gases or powders is safe removal from the source. The following general principles of management apply to most patients exposed to toxic inhalations.

- Safely remove the patient from the poisonous environment. In doing so, take the following essential precautions:
  - Wear protective clothing prior to entry
  - Use appropriate respiratory apparatus
  - Remove patient's contaminated clothing
- Perform the necessary primary and secondary assessments
- Initiate the following treatment procedures:
  - Establish and maintain an airway
  - Administer high-flow oxygen
  - Intubate and assist ventilation, if appropriate
  - Administer CPR, if necessary
  - Use a bag-valve-mask or demand valve
  - Establish IV access
  - Contact poison center

Injection

Injection of a toxic agent under the skin, into a muscle or into the circulatory system, results in both immediate and delayed effects. The immediate local reaction is at the site of the injection. Later, as the toxin is distributed throughout the body by the circulatory system, delayed systemic reactions may occur. In addition, an allergic or anaphylactic reaction may appear. Other than intentional injection of illicit drugs, most poisonings by injection result from bites and stings of insects and animals.

General Principles of Management

In treating a patient who has been bitten or stung, you may have to deal with bacterial contamination introduced by the injection or bodily reaction to any injected substances. As a rule, follow the general principles of field management for bites and stings listed below.

- Protect rescue personnel; the offending life form may still be around.
- Remove the patient from repeated injection, especially in the case of yellow-jackets, wasps, and hornets.
- If possible, identify the insect, reptile, or animal that caused the injury. Bring it along to the emergency department with the patient.
- Perform a primary and secondary assessment.
- Prevent or delay further absorption of poison.
- Watch for anaphylactic reaction.
- Transport the patient as rapidly as possible, if indicated.
- Contact poison center.

Surface Absorption

Surface absorption is the entry of a toxic substance through the skin. This most frequently occurs from contact with poisonous plants, such as poison ivy, poison sumac, and poison oak. Many toxic chemicals may also be absorbed through the skin. The organophosphates, often used as insecticides, are easily absorbed through dermal contact.

The following discussion of prehospital drugs used in the management of toxicological emergencies is divided into three general categories:

Anaphylaxis

Epinephrine
Diphenhydramine (Benadryl)
Methylprednisolone (Solu-Medrol)
Hydrocortisone (Solu-Cortef)

Poisonings

Syrup of ipecac
Activated charcoal
Atropine sulfate
Pralidoxime (Protopam)
Amyl nitrite

Overdoses

Naloxone (Narcan)
Sodium bicarbonate

Physostigmine (Antilirium)
Flumazenil (Romazicon)

ANAPHYLAXIS

In a severe allergic reaction, or anaphylaxis as it is more commonly called, excess release of histamine and other substances can cause severe bronchospasm, dilation of the peripheral blood vessels, and loss of fluid into the tissue spaces. Clinically, anaphylaxis is characterized by restlessness, wheezing, dyspnea, increased heart rate, and diminished blood pressure. If untreated, laryngeal edema, laryngospasm, and respiratory failure can rapidly develop.

Treatment of anaphylaxis is aimed at immediate alleviation of bronchospasm by sympathomimetics. Sustained actions are obtained with the use of a potent antihistamine and, frequently, steroids.

Epinephrine 1:1,000

Class: Sympathetic Agonist

Description

Epinephrine is a naturally occurring catecholamine. It is a potent α and β adrenergic stimulant; however, its effect on β receptors is more profound.

Mechanism of Action

Epinephrine acts directly on α and β adrenergic receptors. Its effect on β receptors is much more profound than its effect on α receptors. The effects of epinephrine include increased heart rate, cardiac contractile force, systemic vascular resistance, and blood pressure. It also causes bronchodilation due to its effects on β_2-adrenergic receptors. It is occasionally used to treat the bronchoconstriction accompanying asthma, COPD, and is also effective in treating bronchoconstriction and the other physiological effects associated with anaphylaxis.

Epinephrine's effects usually appear within 90 seconds of administration, and they are usually of short duration. Occasionally it must be readministered in 15–30 minutes if needed. Epinephrine 1:1,000 is given subcutaneously to ensure a steady and prolonged action. Inhaled β agonists are preferred over epinephrine in the treatment of bronchospasm as they have fewer undesirable side effects.

Indications (Toxicological)

- Anaphylaxis
- Urticaria (hives)
- Asthma/COPD

Contraindications

Because of the cardiac effects seen with the administration of epinephrine, it should not be administered to patients with underlying cardiovascular disease or hypertension. Patients with profound anaphylactic reactions, characterized by hypotension and shock, are usually peripherally vasoconstricted, which will delay absorption of the drug from the subcutaneous site of injection. In these cases, epinephrine 1:10,000 should be administered intravenously.

Precautions

Epinephrine should be protected from light. Also, as with the other catecholamines, it tends to be deactivated by alkaline solutions. Any patient receiving epinephrine 1:1,000 should be carefully monitored for changes in blood pressure, pulse, and EKG. Palpitations, anxiety, nausea, and headache are fairly common side effects.

Side Effects

Epinephrine can cause palpitations, anxiety, tremulousness, headache, dizziness, nausea, and vomiting. Because of its strong inotropic and chronotropic properties, epinephrine increases myocardial oxygen demand. Even in low doses it can cause myocardial ischemia. These effects should be kept in mind when administering epinephrine in the emergency setting.

Interactions

The effects of epinephrine can be intensified in patients who are taking antidepressants.

Dosage

The standard dose of epinephrine 1:1,000 ranges from 0.3 to 0.5 milligram subcutaneously depending on the patient's weight and overall medical condition. Typically, 0.3 milligram is the usual starting dose for adults. The dose for pediatric patients is 0.01 mg/kg subcutaneously. In the prehospital phase of emergency medical care, epinephrine 1:1,000 should only be administered subcutaneously (except in the case of pediatric cardiac arrest).

How Supplied

Epinephrine is supplied in ampules and prefilled syringes containing 1 milligram of the drug in 1 milliliter of solvent.

Diphenhydramine (Benadryl)

Class: Antihistamine

Description

Diphenhydramine is a potent antihistamine that blocks both H_1 and H_2 histamine receptors.

Mechanism of Action

Histamine is released from mast cells following exposure to an antigen to which the body has been previously sensitized. When released into the circulation following an allergic reaction, histamine acts on two different receptors. The first type of receptor, called H_1, when stimulated causes bronchoconstriction and contraction of the gut. The second type of receptor, called H_2, when stimulated causes peripheral vasodilation and secretion of gastric acids.

Antihistamines are administered after epinephrine in the treatment of anaphylaxis. Epinephrine causes immediate bronchodilation by activating β_2 adrenergic receptors, whereas diphenhydramine inhibits histamine release.

Diphenhydramine is also useful in the treatment of dystonic reactions accompanying phenothiazine use. A dystonic, or extrapyramidal, reaction is characterized by an unusual posture, change in muscle tone, drooling, or uncontrolled movements. It is occasionally seen following the administration of antipsychotic medications (Haldol, Thorazine, Mellaril) as well as certain medications used for nausea and vomiting (Phenergan, Compazine, Reglan). Diphenhydramine, when administered, causes marked improvement, if not total resolution of the symptoms.

Indications

- Anaphylaxis
- Allergic reactions
- Dystonic (extrapyramidal) reactions

Contraindications

Diphenhydramine should not be used in the management of lower respiratory diseases such as asthma.

Precautions

The primary drug for the treatment of severe allergic reactions, anaphylaxis, and urticaria is epinephrine. Epinephrine will reverse many of the effects of histamine. Diphenhydramine will block histamine receptors preventing subsequent stimulation by circulating histamine.

Side Effects

Diphenhydramine can cause hypotension, headache, palpitations, tachycardia, sedation, drowsiness, and disturbed coordination.

Interactions

The sedative effects of diphenhydramine can be potentiated by the administration of CNS depressants, other antihistamines, narcotics, and alcohol.

Dosage

The standard dosage of diphenhydramine is 25 to 50 milligrams, either intravenously or intramuscularly.

How Supplied

Diphenhydramine is supplied in ampules and prefilled syringes containing 50 milligrams of the drug in 1 milliliter of solvent.

CASE PRESENTATION

At 9:45 P.M. you are dispatched to a local restaurant for a "medical problem." En route the dispatcher provides further information. The patient is a 42-year-old male who is experiencing difficulty breathing. On arrival you are met by a waiter who takes you to a booth in the restaurant. You approach the man who is in obvious respiratory distress. He is gasping for air and using accessory muscles.

Examination

CNS: The patient is conscious, but unable to speak and in obvious distress.

Resp: Respirations are 40 per minute, gasping and shallow. His lung sounds reveal diffuse wheezes throughout. The trachea is midline. There is prominent accessory muscles usage. There are no signs of trauma.

CVS: The carotid pulse is present and weak, but the radial pulse is absent. His skin is red and hot.

ABD: The abdomen is soft and non-tender in all 4 quadrants.

Musc/Skel: No injuries are noted.

Vital Signs:

Pulse: 112 per minute

Resp: 40 per minute, shallow

B/P: 84/48 mmHg

SpO_2: 68%

ECG: Sinus Tachycardia

Past Hx: According to the patient's wife, the patient has a severe allergy to peanuts. The waiter states that some of the food is cooked in peanut oil, and it states that on the menu. The patient's wife states that her husband is in good health and does not take any medications.

Treatment:

The paramedics recognize the serious nature of the patient's condition. Oxygen is administered by non-rebreather at 12 l/min, but is not well tolerated by the patient. 0.5 mg of epinephrine 1:1,000 is administered subcutaneously. (Intravenous administration of 0.5 mg [5 ml] of epinephrine 1:10,000 is also acceptable in severe anaphylaxis). An intravenous line is established. Albuterol (Proventil or Ventolin) is administered using a small-volume nebulizer. 2.5 mg in 2.5 ml of normal saline is given to the patient with the assistance of the paramedic.

The combination of epinephrine and albuterol begins to relieve the patient's symptoms, his vital signs stabilize, and he is transported to the hospital in improved condition. At the hospital, 50 milligrams of diphenhydramine (Benadryl) is administered IV push. The patient is released from the hospital 6 hours later.

Methylprednisolone (Solu-Medrol)

Class: Corticosteroid/Anti-Inflammatory

Description

Methylprednisolone is a synthetic steroid with potent anti-inflammatory properties.

Mechanism of Action

The pharmacological actions of the steroids are vast and complex. In general medical practice, steroids have a wide range of uses. Effective as anti-inflammatory agents, they are used in the management of allergic reactions, asthma, and anaphylaxis. Methylprednisolone is considered an intermediate-acting steroid with a plasma half-life of about 3 to 4 hours.

Indications

- Severe anaphylaxis
- Asthma/COPD
- Urticaria

Contraindications

There are no major contraindications to the use of methylprednisolone in the acute management of severe anaphylaxis.

Precautions

A single dose of methylprednisolone is all that should be given in the prehospital phase of care. Long-term steroid therapy can cause gastrointestinal bleeding, prolonged wound healing, and suppression of adrenocortical steroids.

Side Effects

Methylprednisolone can cause fluid retention, congestive heart failure, hypertension, abdominal distention, vertigo, headache, nausea, malaise, and hiccups.

Interactions

Few in the prehospital setting

Dosage

The standard dosage of methylprednisolone in the management of severe anaphylaxis is 125 to 250 milligrams intravenously. Methylprednisolone may be administered intravenously or intramuscularly. The intravenous route is preferred in emergency medicine.

How Supplied

Methylprednisolone is supplied in Mix-O-Vials containing 125 milligrams of the drug. Methylprednisolone is supplied in powder form that must be reconstituted in the supplied Mix-O-Vial system. Once reconstituted, it should be used within 48 hours.

Hydrocortisone (Solu-Cortef)

Class: Corticosteroid/Anti-Inflammatory

Description

Hydrocortisone is a potent corticosteroid with anti-inflammatory properties.

Mechanism of Action

The pharmacological actions of the steroids are vast and complex. Hydrocortisone is considered a short-acting steroid with a plasma half-life of 90 minutes. Like the other adrenocorticosteroids, it is effective as an adjunct in the management of severe anaphylaxis.

Indications

- Severe anaphylaxis
- Asthma/COPD
- Urticaria (hives)

Contraindications

There are no major contraindications to the use of hydrocortisone in the acute management of anaphylaxis.

Precautions

A single dose of hydrocortisone is all that should be given in the prehospital phase of care. Long-term steroid therapy can cause gastrointestinal bleeding, prolonged wound healing, and suppression of adrenocortical steroids.

Side Effects

Hydrocortisone can cause fluid retention, congestive heart failure, hypertension, abdominal distention, vertigo, headache, nausea, malaise, and hiccups.

Interactions

Few in the prehospital setting

Dosage

The standard dosage of hydrocortisone in the management of severe anaphylaxis is 40 to 250 milligrams intravenously.

Route

The IV route is preferred in emergency medicine. However, hydrocortisone can be administered intramuscularly when an IV cannot be started.

How Supplied

Hydrocortisone is supplied in Mix-O-Vials containing 100 and 250 milligrams of the drug.

POISONING

The term *poisoning* is used to describe the accidental or inadvertent ingestion of a substance that causes a destructive effect on the body. *Overdose*, although actually a form of poisoning, is used to describe the intentional ingestion of a substance by a patient during an attempt at self-destruction or by inadvertent ingestion of the wrong medication. In this discussion of toxicological emergencies, overdose and poisoning will be addressed separately.

The first step in the management of any poisoning is to locate and identify the poison. Although this is not always possible, when known it can aid in definitive treatment of the patient. Treatment of the patient is divided into two stages. The first stage is to prevent or reduce absorption of the toxin into the body. This can be done by inducing vomiting in conscious patients. Vomiting is effectively induced by the drug *syrup of ipecac*. *Activated charcoal* is a common and effective adsorbent.

If indicated, the second phase of management involves the administration of an *antidote*. Antidotes are drugs that tend to counteract the toxic effects of a poison. Usually, prehospital administration of antidotes is not indicated, but *organophosphate* or *cyanide* poisonings require prehospital administration of antidotes. *Atropine sulfate* and *pralidoxime* (2-PAM) can be effective in the management of organophosphate poisonings. *Amyl nitrite* is of use in reversing some of the toxic effects associated with cyanide poisoning.

Syrup of Ipecac

Class: Emetic

Description

Syrup of ipecac is a potent and effective emetic used in the management of poisonings where the induction of vomiting is indicated.

Mechanism of Action

Syrup of ipecac is used to remove the stomach contents in cases of poisoning. Syrup of ipecac acts as a local irritant on the enteric tract and on emetic centers within the brain thus causing emesis. To assure complete evacuation of the stomach, the administration of ipecac is usually followed by several glasses of warm water. Recently, some studies have advocated the use of carbonated beverages instead of warm water. Carbonated beverages may cause emesis sooner. Emesis, following administration, usually occurs within 5 to 10 minutes.

Indications

- Poisoning
- Overdose

Contraindications

Vomiting should not be induced in any patient with impaired consciousness. It should also not be induced when the ingested substance is a strong acid base (that is, caustic ingestion) or petroleum distillate.

In addition, administration of syrup of ipecac is not indicated when the ingested agent was an antiemetic, especially of the phenothiazine type.

The trend in the management of toxicological emergencies has been to use activated charcoal alone without ipecac. This is primarily because of the increased risk of aspiration associated with ipecac usage.

Precautions

It is important to monitor constantly the patient's airway during and following emesis. Activated charcoal should only be administered after vomiting has occurred. Ipecac should be used with caution in patients with heart disease.

Side Effects

Ipecac can cause arrhythmias, hypotension, diarrhea, depression, and bleeding from Mallory-Weiss tears and esophageal varices.

Interactions

Syrup of ipecac should not be given with activated charcoal as the activated charcoal can nullify the effects of the ipecac.

Dosage

The standard dose of syrup of ipecac is 15 to 30 milliliters orally followed by several glasses of warm water or carbonated soda.

Route

Syrup of ipecac should only be administered orally.

How Supplied

Syrup of ipecac is supplied in bottles containing 1 ounce (approximately 30 milliliters).

Activated Charcoal

Class: Adsorbent

Description

Activated charcoal is a fine black powder that binds and adsorbs ingested toxins still present in the gastrointestinal tract following emesis.

Mechanism of Action

Activated charcoal has a tremendous surface area. It binds and adsorbs ingested toxins present in the gastrointestinal tract. Once bound to the activated charcoal, the combined complex is excreted from the body.

Indication

- Poisoning (following emesis, or in cases in which emesis may be contraindicated)

Contraindications

There are no major contraindications to the use of activated charcoal in severe poisoning.

Precautions

Activated charcoal should not be administered to the patient who has an altered level of consciousness unless administered by nasogastric tube and the airway protected by an endotracheal tube. If emesis is to be induced with ipecac, it is often best to wait until the patient has vomited to administer activated charcoal.

Side Effects

Activated charcoal can cause nausea, vomiting, abdominal cramping, abdominal bloating, and constipation.

Interactions

Activated charcoal should not be given with syrup of ipecac as the activated charcoal can nullify the effects of the ipecac.

Dosage

The standard dosage in the management of poisoning is 50–75 grams mixed with a glass of water to form a slurry. This is administered orally or through a nasogastric tube. Activated charcoal is often mixed with a cathartic, commonly sorbitol, to promote elimination of the ingested poison from the GI tract and to prevent the constipation associated with activated charcoal usage. Activated charcoal should only be administered orally in a slurry solution made with water as described earlier.

How Supplied

Activated charcoal is supplied in bottles containing 25 and 50 grams of the drug.

ORGANOPHOSPHATE POISONING

Organophosphates serve as the active agents in many insecticides and nerve gases. Common insecticide preparations that employ organophosphates include Parathion, Malathion, and EPN. These insecticides are widely used in agriculture and are occasionally found within the home. They are easily absorbed through the skin, lungs, and by ingestion. Patients suspected of suffering organophosphate poisoning should have their clothes removed immediately to prevent continued absorption. Organophosphates deactivate, by phosphorylation, the enzyme cholinesterase. Cholinesterase is vital to normal body function as it deactivates the neurotransmitter acetylcholine. Acetylcholine is the neurotransmitter used by both the voluntary and the parasympathetic nervous system.

Signs and symptoms of organophosphate poisoning include ocular pain, watery nasal discharge, diaphoresis, bradycardia, abdominal cramps, and vomiting. Advanced organophosphate poisoning is characterized by involuntary muscle twitching, generalized weakness, paralysis, and respiratory depression.

In the advanced stage, the prompt administration of atropine and possibly 2-PAM is essential. Atropine binds to acetylcholine receptors, thus diminishing the actions of acetylcholine. Cholinesterase is reactivated by 2-PAM.

Atropine Sulfate

Class: Parasympatholytic

Description

Atropine sulfate is a potent parasympatholytic (anticholinergic). It blocks acetylcholine receptors, thus aiding the management of organophosphate poisonings. Organophosphate poisonings inhibit the enzyme cholinesterase, causing an increase and accumulation of the neurotransmitter acetylcholine. Often, large doses are required to achieve atropinization. Severe poisonings, especially those characterized by paralysis and muscle twitching, require pralidoxime (2-PAM), in addition to atropine.

Indications

- Organophosphate poisoning
- Bradycardias that are hemodynamically significant
- Asystole

Contraindications

There are no contraindications to atropine when used in the management of severe organophosphate poisoning.

Precautions

It is important to remove all clothing from a patient who has suffered organophosphate poisoning. The patient must then be completely bathed to remove all residual organophosphate present on the skin. Always be sure to protect the rescuer. Atropine may actually worsen the bradycardia associated with second-degree Mobitz II and third-degree AV blocks. In these cases, go straight to transcutaneous pacing instead of trying atropine.

Side Effects

Atropine sulfate can cause blurred vision, dilated pupils, dry mouth, tachycardia, drowsiness, and confusion.

Interactions

Few in the prehospital setting

Dosage

One milligram of atropine should be administered initially to determine whether or not the patient is tolerant to atropine. If the patient responds to the diagnostic dose, then most likely he or she is not severely poisoned or is not tolerant to atropine. If there is no improvement, a second dose of 2 to 5 milligrams may be indicated for an adult (0.05 milligrams per kilogram for a child). Doses exceeding 100 milligrams are sometimes required to treat severe organophosphate poisoning. In prehospital care, following the initial administration of atropine, prompt transportation to an emergency department is indicated. In severe organophosphate poisoning, atropine sulfate is administered intravenously.

How Supplied

Atropine sulfate is supplied in prefilled syringes containing 1 milligram of the drug in 10 milliliters of solvent.

Pralidoxime (2-PAM) (Protopam)

Class: Cholinesterase Reactivator

Description

Pralidoxime is a cholinesterase reactivator.

Mechanism of Action

Pralidoxime is an antidote for severe organophosphate poisonings. It chemically removes the phosphate group from cholinesterase that was transferred from an organophosphate poison. Once cholinesterase is reactivated, it can deactivate acetylcholine. Pralidoxime also detoxifies some organophosphates by direct chemical reaction. It reverses respiratory depression and skeletal muscle paralysis resulting from organophosphate poisoning.

Pralidoxime should be reserved for severe organophosphate poisonings characterized by muscle twitching and paralysis. It should follow atropinization.

Indication

- Severe organophosphate poisoning

Contraindications

Pralidoxime should not be used in cases of poisoning resulting from inorganic phosphates or the carbamate class of insecticides.

Precautions

Always protect yourself and other rescuers when caring for the victim of organophosphate poisoning.

Intravenous administration should be carried out slowly as tachycardia, laryngospasm, and muscle rigidity have been seen with rapid administration. When used in conjunction with atropine, the effects of atropinization may be seen much earlier than expected. This is especially true if the atropine dose has been large. Excitement and manic behavior have been known to occur immediately following recovery from unconsciousness in a few cases.

Side Effects

Pralidoxime can cause tachycardia, increased salivation, headache, altered mental status, dizziness, blurred vision, nausea, and vomiting.

Interactions

Patients who have sustained organophosphate poisonings should not receive respiratory depressants as these can potentiate the effects of the organophosphates. These drugs include narcotics, phenothiazines (antiemetics), antihistamines, and alcohol. Pralidoxime should not be used with theophylline preparations (including aminophylline).

Dosage

One to two grams of pralidoxime should be placed in 250 to 500 milliliters of normal saline and infused over 30 minutes. Pralidoxime should be administered by IV infusion or slow IV bolus only.

How Supplied

Pralidoxime is supplied in 20-milliliter vials with 1 gram of the drug. The drug must be reconstituted with 20 milliliters of sterile water, which is supplied.

CYANIDE POISONING

Cyanide is one of the most rapidly acting and deadly poisons known to humans. It has been used in executions, in the mass suicides in Guyana, and was responsible for several deaths after it was placed into capsules of a popular over-the-counter analgesic.

Cyanide reacts with iron, thus inhibiting cellular respiration, causing cellular hypoxia, and finally death. Clinically, the patient with cyanide poisoning exhibits a rapid respiratory rate, severe headache, and, finally, convulsions and death. Cyanide poisoning may produce the peculiar smell of "bitter almonds" on the patient's breath. Treatment, if it is to be effective, must be initiated immediately. Amyl nitrite, administered by inhalation, causes hemoglobin to be converted to methemoglobin. Methemoglobin reacts with the toxic cyanide-ion to form cyanomethemoglobin, which is enzymatically degraded.

Amyl Nitrite

Class: Vasodilator/Cyanide Antidote

Description

Amyl nitrite is a potent vasodilator and an antidote for cyanide poisoning.

Mechanism of Action

Amyl nitrite, which is chemically related to nitroglycerin, has been used for many years in the treatment and symptomatic relief of angina. It is also effective in the emergency management of cyanide poisoning. It is supplied in a glass inhalant that can be broken and inhaled immediately. Amyl nitrite causes the oxidation of hemoglobin to a compound called *methemoglobin*. Methemoglobin reacts with the toxic cyanide ion to form *cyanomethemoglobin*, which can be enzymatically degraded. This serves to remove cyanide from the blood.

Indication

- Cyanide poisoning

Contraindications

There are no contraindications to the use of amyl nitrite in the management of cyanide poisoning.

Precautions

Headache and hypotension have been known to occur following the inhalation of amyl nitrite. Amyl nitrite is a drug of abuse and should be kept in a secure place with the narcotics. It has a horrible odor resembling dirty sweat socks.

Side Effects

Amyl nitrite can cause severe headache, weakness, dizziness, flushing, cold sweats, tachycardia, syncope, orthostatic hypotension, nausea, and vomiting.

Interactions

The hypotensive effects of amyl nitrite can be potentiated by antihypertensive agents, β blockers, and certain antiemetics (phenothazines).

Dosage

One to two inhalants of amyl nitrite should be crushed and inhaled. This should be maintained until the patient has reached an emergency department. Therapeutic effects diminish after approximately 20 minutes. Amyl nitrite should be administered by inhalation only.

How Supplied

Amyl nitrite is supplied in inhalants containing 0.3 milliliters of the drug.

OVERDOSE

Overdose with both prescribed and nonprescribed medications is common. Prehospital management of the overdose patient is aimed primarily at supportive care. In some cases, however, the administration of antidotes may be indicated.

The principal problem with medication overdose is depression of the central nervous system. Diminished level of consciousness and respiratory depression are commonly seen. Prehospital care should include immediate management of the airway, supplemental administration of oxygen, and placement of an intravenous line. If the suspected drug is a narcotic or narcotic-like agent, *naloxone* may be effective in reversing the respiratory depression. If the agent was atropine or one of the drugs with anticholinergic properties, like the tricyclic antidepressants, then *physostigmine* may be effective. *Sodium bicarbonate* is occasionally used in tricyclic antidepressant overdoses. It is used to alkalinize the urine, which promotes elimination of the drug from the body. *Flumazenil*, a benzodiazepine antagonist, can be used to reverse respiratory depression in severe cases of benzodiazepine poisoning.

Naloxone (Narcan)

Class: Narcotic Antagonist

Description

Naloxone is an effective narcotic antagonist. It has proved effective in the management and reversal of overdoses caused by narcotics or synthetic narcotic agents.

Mechanism of Action

Naloxone is chemically similar to the narcotics. However, it has only antagonistic properties. Naloxone competes for opiate receptors in the brain. It also displaces narcotic molecules from opiate receptors. It can reverse respiratory depression associated with narcotic overdose.

Indications

- For the complete or partial reversal of depression caused by narcotics including the following agents:

  morphine *Demerol* *heroin*
  paregoric *Dilaudid* *codeine*
  Percodan *Fentanyl* *methadone*
- For the complete or partial reversal of depression caused by synthetic narcotic analgesic agents including the following drugs:

  Nubain *Talwin* *Stadol*
  Darvon
- Treatment of coma of unknown origin

Contraindications

Naloxone should not be administered to a patient with a history of hypersensitivity to the drug.

Precautions

Naloxone should be administered cautiously to patients who are known or suspected to be physically dependent on narcotics. Abrupt and complete reversal by naloxone can cause withdrawal-type effects. This includes newborn infants of mothers with known or suspected narcotic dependence.

Side Effects

Side effects associated with naloxone are rare. However, hypotension, hypertension, ventricular arrhythmias, nausea, and vomiting have been reported.

Interactions

Naloxone may cause narcotic withdrawal in the narcotic-dependent patient. In cases of suspected narcotic dependence, administer only enough of the drug to reverse respiratory depression.

Dosage

The standard dosage for suspected or confirmed narcotic or synthetic narcotic overdoses is 1 to 2 milligrams IV. If unsuccessful, then a second dose may be administered 5 minutes later. Failure to obtain reversal after 2 to 3 doses indicates another disease process or overdosage on non-opioid drugs.

Larger than average doses (2 to 5 milligrams) have been used in the management of Darvon overdoses and alcoholic coma.

An intravenous infusion can be prepared by placing 2 milligrams of naloxone in 500 milliliters of D_5W. This gives a concentration of 4 micrograms per milliliter. One hundred milliliters per hour should be infused, thus delivering 0.4 milligrams per hour. In the emergency setting, naloxone should be administered intravenously only. When an IV line cannot be established, intramuscular or subcutaneous administration can be performed.

Naloxone can be administered endotracheally. The dose should be increased to 2.0–2.5 times the intravenous dose. Furthermore, naloxone should be diluted in enough normal saline to provide a total of 10 milliliters of fluid.

How Supplied

Naloxone is supplied in ampules and prefilled syringes containing 2 milligrams in 2 milliliters of solvent. In addition, vials containing 10 milliliters of the 1 milligram per milliliter concentration are also available.

CASE PRESENTATION

Early one evening Waterville EMS is called to a residence in an upscale area of the city. Dispatch informs them that they are responding to a "man down," unconscious, unresponsive, and not breathing. On arrival the paramedics are met by a woman in her twenties who states that her boyfriend is not breathing. Paramedics are led to the living room where they find a male in his mid-twenties lying supine on the floor. There is emesis near the patient.

Examination

CNS: The patient is unresponsive. The Glasgow Coma Scale is 3. Both pupils are pinpoint, yet equal.

RESP: Respirations are 6 per minute and very shallow. The airway has residue from vomiting.

CVS: The carotid pulse is slow and weak. The radial pulse is absent. His skin is pale. Lips are blue.

ABD: Soft and non-tender in all 4 quadrants. The patient has vomited.

Musc/Skel: No other injuries present.

Vital Signs:

Pulse: 56 per minute

Resp: 6 per minute

B/P: 70/52 mmHg

SpO_2: 72

ECG: Sinus bradycardia

Past Hx: Initially the patient's girlfriend states that she doesn't know what happened. She states that her boyfriend is very healthy, has no medical problems, and does not take any medication. Paramedics specifically ask about alcohol or recreational drugs. The girlfriend emphatically states, "No."

Treatment:

Police backup is requested. The initial treatment begins with the ABCs. The airway is suctioned and an oropharyngeal airway is placed. Ventilation by bag-valve-mask and 100% oxygen by reservoir bag is initiated at 24 breaths per minute. Airway compliance is good. An IV of normal saline is prepared and paramedics perform venipuncture with a 16 gauge catheter. Blood is drawn for a "red top" tube and the hub of the needle is used to obtain a blood sample for glucose testing. The IV of normal saline is connected to the catheter, and the fluid is administered at 100 ml/hr.

As one paramedic was starting the IV, she looked for previous needle marks and did not find any. The absence of needle marks did not change the paramedic's assessment. Based on the age of the patient (male in the mid-twenties does not just stop breathing), the slow respirations, and the pinpoint pupils, the paramedic was fairly certain that the patient had taken a narcotic or some designer drug.

The patient's girlfriend is questioned once again as to whether her boyfriend uses any drugs. The paramedic tells her that her boyfriend's condition is very serious and that she must be absolutely honest with her. Finally the girlfriend states that her boyfriend does use heroin. She found him on the floor when she came home and then called for the ambulance after she hid the drugs and syringes.

At this point the police arrive and assist the paramedics. The patient is moved to the stretcher and restrained. The paramedics are concerned for their safety since the patient may be aggressive or violent as he comes out of the coma. His airway is still patent and intubation is not required at this time. Narcan is administered intravenously in 1.0 mg dosages. The paramedics carefully titrate the dose to increase the respiratory rate. The stretcher and patient are moved to the ambulance and a police officer agrees to accompany the paramedics to the hospital. The patient is not fighting against the bag-valve-mask or straining against the restraints. The patient's girlfriend gives the paramedics the rest of the drugs and the syringe.

En route to the hospital a paramedic monitors the patient's vital signs closely. Respirations increase to 20/min and the patient is placed on oxygen by non-rebreather mask at 12 l/min. The pulse rate increases to 112/min and blood pressure increases to 124/82. The blood glucose reading is 125mg/dl (7.0 mmol/L). The half-life of Narcan is likely to be less than that of the narcotic. Thus, the patient's level of consciousness may decrease. On arrival at the hospital, the patient is conscious, verbally abusive, and has stable vital signs. While awaiting the results of laboratory tests, the patient gets up, sneaks out the back door, and leaves the ED unseen.

Sodium Bicarbonate

Class: Alkalinizing Agent

Description

Sodium bicarbonate is a salt that provides bicarbonate to buffer metabolic acidosis, which can accompany several disease processes.

Mechanism of Action

For many years sodium bicarbonate was the cornerstone of advanced cardiac life support care. Controlled studies have shown that sodium bicarbonate was ineffective in the treatment of cardiac arrest. In many instances it has been actually associated with many adverse reactions.

Sodium bicarbonate is occasionally used in the treatment of certain types of drug overdose. The most common example is drugs in the tricyclic class of antidepressants. Overdosage of these drugs has serious effects including life-threatening cardiac arrhythmias. Tricyclic antidepressant excretion from the body is enhanced by making the urine more alkaline (raising the pH). Sodium bicarbonate is sometimes administered to increase the pH of the urine to speed excretion of the drug from the body.

Indications

- Late in the management of cardiac arrest, if at all. Hyperventilation, prompt defibrillation, and the administration of epinephrine and lidocaine should always precede use of sodium bicarbonate. Because these therapies take at least 10 minutes to carry out, sodium bicarbonate should rarely be administered in the first 10 minutes of a resuscitation.
- Tricyclic antidepressant overdose
- Phenobarbital overdose
- Severe acidosis refractory to hyperventilation
- Known hyperkalemia (elevated potassium levels)

Contraindications

When used in the management of the situations described earlier, there are no absolute contraindications.

Precautions

Sodium bicarbonate can cause metabolic alkalosis when administered in large quantities. It is important to calculate the dosage based on patient weight and size.

Side Effects

Few when used in the emergency setting

Interactions

Most catecholamines and vasopressors (i.e., dopamine and epinephrine) can be deactivated by alkaline solutions like sodium bicarbonate. Sodium bicarbonate should not be administered in conjunction with calcium chloride. A precipitate can form, which may clog the IV line.

Dosage

The usual dose of sodium bicarbonate is 1 milliequivalent per kilogram of body weight initially followed by 0.5 milliequivalent per kilogram of body weight every 10 minutes. When possible, the dosage of sodium bicarbonate should be based on the results of arterial blood gas studies. Sodium bicarbonate should be administered only as an IV bolus.

How Supplied

Sodium bicarbonate comes in prefilled syringes containing 50 milliequivalents of the drug in 50 milliliters of solvent.

CASE PRESENTATION

Paramedics are called to meet the police at a residence where there is a reported party. The police dispatcher states that partiers found an unconscious, yet breathing person in the bedroom. Upon arrival with two police cruisers you are escorted into the house where a loud party continues in progress. You are led to a back bedroom where you find a 24-year-old female lying on the bed. With the heavy metal beat of Metallica in the background you complete your assessment.

Examination

CNS: The patient is unresponsive. Her pupils are equal, dilated, and unresponsive to light.

Resp: Respirations are 32 per minute and shallow. Her lungs are clear bilaterally with equal air entry. The trachea is midline and there are no signs of trauma.

CVS: The carotid pulse is present, but weak. The radial pulse is absent. Her skin is warm, flushed, and dry with dry mucous membranes.

ABD: Soft and non-tender in all 4 quadrants. There are no signs of vomiting or diarrhea.

Musc/Skel: No injuries are noted.

Vital Signs:

Pulse: 136 per minute

Resp: 32 per minute and shallow

B/P: 70/44 mmHg

SpO_2: 84%

ECG: Sinus Tachycardia

Past Hx: The patient's friends state that the patient is a loner and often moody and depressed. They don't know when she came into this room. When they came into the room, they found her lying on the bed unresponsive with a pill bottle next to her. An empty bottle of amitriptyline (Elavil) is shown to the paramedics.

Treatment:

The patient's respirations are assisted by a bag-valve-mask device with 100% oxygen via a reservoir bag. The patient is placed on a cardiac monitor, which shows a sinus tachycardia with widened QRS complexes (greater than 0.12 mm). An intravenous line with a 16 gauge catheter is initiated and a solution of normal saline run at a 100 ml bolus and then 150 ml/hour. Sodium bicarbonate, two 50 ml ampules, is administered. The patient is prepared for transport to the hospital with the assistance of the police. Following the administration of the sodium bicarbonate, the QRS complexes eventually narrow to 0.08mm. However, the patient's level of consciousness does not change. Once in the ambulance, the patient is intubated. The patient's condition remains unchanged during transport to the hospital. On arrival at the hospital, the patient is treated with gastric lavage and activated charcoal and then admitted to ICU. She slowly regains consciousness and is transferred from the ICU to psychiatry 48 hours later.

Physostigmine (Antilirium)

Class: Cholinesterase Inhibitor

Description

Physostigmine is a potentially effective antidote for the management of poisonings resulting from atropine-type drugs and overdoses of tricyclic-type antidepressants.

Mechanism of Action

Physostigmine inhibits the breakdown of acetylcholine. This causes an increase in acetylcholine and an accumulation of acetylcholine at the cholinergic synapses. Atropine-type poisonings and tricyclic antidepressant overdoses block acetylcholine receptors and cause an increase in cholinesterase activity, thus inhibiting the action of acetylcholine in both parasympathetic and voluntary nerves. Physostigmine inhibits the destructive action of cholinesterase, thus exaggerating the effect of acetylcholine.

Atropine-type poisonings can result from an overdose of atropine or scopolamine. Several plants contain atropine-type chemicals. Ingestion of parts of these plants can cause anticholinergic poisoning.

Tricyclic poisoning occurs only following an overdose of the drugs within the tricyclic class. Tricyclic drugs are frequently prescribed for the management of depression and as muscle relaxants. They are also used in the management of chronic pain. Overdoses of tricyclics are particularly dangerous because of the serious effects they have on the heart. Cardiac arrhythmias, especially those indicative of conduction system disturbances, are common. Toxic doses of tricyclics result in cholinesterase inhibition. The administration of physostigmine is often effective in reversing the ill effects.

The administration of physostigmine to tricyclic overdose is controversial. Most authorities agree that alkalinization is the primary treatment. Local protocols should be followed regarding physostigmine usage.

Indications

- To reverse the toxic effects of the tricyclic class of antidepressants including the following:

  Tofranil *Adapin* *Norpramin*

  Sinequan *Elavil* *Triavil*

- To reverse the toxic effects of atropine and atropine-like drugs including the following plants with belladonna agents present:

  Pyrocantha *Lantana* *Jimsonweed*

  Angel's Trumpet

Contraindications

Physostigmine should not be administered in the presence of asthma, gangrene, diabetes, narrow-angle glaucoma, or cardiovascular disease.

Precautions

If excessive parasympathetic actions are seen, such as increased salivation, or if emesis or bradycardia occurs, then the dosage of the drug should be reduced. IV administration should be at a slow and controlled rate. No more than 1 milligram per minute should be administered. Atropine sulfate should be on hand for use as an antagonist.

Side Effects

Physostigmine can cause bradycardia, hypotension, excessive salivation, nausea, vomiting, increased urination, and defecation.

Interactions

Anticholinergic drugs, such as atropine, antidepressants, antihistamines, and phenothiazines can antagonize the effects of physostigmine.

Dosage

The usual adult dosage is 0.5 to 2 milligrams slow IV bolus. It may be necessary to repeat the dose 5 minutes later if life-threatening signs occur. Physostigmine should be given via slow IV bolus. When an IV line cannot be started, then intramuscular injection can be used.

How Supplied

Antilirium is supplied in 2-milliliter ampules containing 2 milligrams (1 milligram per milliliter).

Flumazenil (Romazicon)

Class: Benzodiazepine Antagonist

Description

Flumazenil is a benzodiazepine antagonist. It is used to reverse the sedative effects of benzodiazepines, especially respiratory depression.

Mechanism of Action

Flumazenil antagonizes the actions of the benzodiazepines in the central nervous system. Particularly, it inhibits their actions on the GABA/benzodiazepine complex. It is used to reverse the sedative effects of the benzodiazepines.

Indications

- For complete and partial reversal of CNS and respiratory depression caused by benzodiazepines including the following agents:

Valium	*Versed*	*Ativan*
Halcion	*Restoril*	*Dalmane*
Tranxene	*Serax*	*Klonopin*
Ambien	*Doral*	*ProSom*
Centrax	*Xanax*	

Flumazenil should NOT be used as a diagnostic agent for benzodiazepine overdose in the manner naloxone is used for narcotic overdose. The potential of inducing a life-threatening benzodiazepine withdrawal reaction in patients addicted to benzodiazepines with flumazenil is not worth the perceived benefits.

Contraindications

Flumazenil is contraindicated in patients with a known hypersensitivity to the drug or to benzodiazepines. It should not be administered to patients who have received benzodiazepines to control life-threatening conditions such as status epilepticus. It should not be used in patients with tricyclic antidepressant overdoses.

Precautions

Flumazenil should be administered with caution to patients dependent on benzodiazepines. Benzodiazepine withdrawal can be life-threatening. Signs and symptoms of benzodiazepine withdrawal include tachycardia, hypertension, anxiousness, confusion, and seizures.

The effects of flumazenil can wear off resulting in the return of sedation. Following administration, patients should be monitored for signs of re-sedation and respiratory depression.

Side Effects

Flumazenil can cause fatigue, headache, agitation, nervousness, dizziness, flushing, confusion, convulsions, arrhythmias, nausea, and vomiting.

Interactions

Few in the emergency setting

Dose

The standard dose of flumazenil is 0.2 milligram intravenously administered over 30 seconds. This can be repeated, as required, up to a maximum dose of 1.0 milligram. Flumazenil should only be given intravenously in the emergency setting.

How Supplied

Flumazenil (Romazicon) is supplied in 5- and 10- milliliter multi-dose vials containing 0.1 milligram per milliliter.

SUMMARY

Treatment of toxicological emergencies is usually only supportive in the prehospital phase of emergency medical care. Several agents are effective in alleviation of the life-threatening effects of anaphylaxis, however. The primary drug in managing anaphylaxis is epinephrine. Benadryl and the common steroid preparations, Solu-Medrol and Solu-Cortef, may also be effective, however. Poisoning and overdoses should be treated symptomatically. Essential care includes airway maintenance, administration of supplemental oxygen, and establishment of an IV infusion. In addition, it is often necessary to reduce or prohibit the adsorption of the drug into the body. Syrup of ipecac and activated charcoal are often effective in accomplishing this. In addition, several antidotes are available to reverse the systemic effects of a great many agents.

KEY WORDS

allergic reaction. A hypersensitivity to a given antigen. A reaction more pronounced than would occur in the general population.

anaphylaxis. An acute, generalized, and violent antigen-antibody reaction that can be rapidly fatal.

antidote. A substance that neutralizes a poison or the effects of a poison.

histamine. A chemical released by mast cells and basophils upon stimulation. It is one of the most powerful vasodilators known and a major mediator of anaphylaxis.

overdose. A dose of a drug in excess of that usually prescribed. An overdose can adversely affect the patient's health.

poisoning. The process of taking a substance into the body that interferes with normal physiological functions.

chapter 13

Drugs Used in the Treatment of Behavioral Emergencies

OBJECTIVES

1. Define the term *behavioral emergency.*
2. List the intrapsychic causes of altered behavior.
3. Explain interpersonal and environmental causes of behavioral emergencies.
4. Explain organic causes of behavioral emergencies.
5. Describe and list the indications, contraindications, and dosages for the following drugs used in behavioral emergencies:
   - haloperidol
   - chlorpromazine
   - diazepam
   - hydroxyzine

INTRODUCTION

Behavioral emergencies rarely require pharmacological intervention during the prehospital phase of emergency medical care. There are situations, however, in which emergency personnel may be called on to administer a sedative or similar agent. Among these are acute anxiety reactions and paranoid psychoses. Occasionally, it may be necessary to administer a sedative to friends or family of a patient who has been severely injured or who has recently died.

UNDERSTANDING BEHAVIORAL EMERGENCIES

A *behavioral emergency* is an intrapsychic, environmental, situational, or organic alteration that results in behavior that cannot be tolerated by the patient or other members of society. It usually requires immediate attention.

Intrapsychic Causes

Intrapsychic causes of altered behavior arise from problems within the person. Such behavior usually results from an acute stage of an underlying psychiatric condition. A wide range of behaviors can be manifested. These include:

> depression, withdrawal, catatonia, violence, suicidal acts, homicidal acts, paranoid reactions, phobias, hysterical conversion, disorientation, and disorganization.

In the field, behavioral emergencies resulting from intrapsychic causes are less common than those resulting from other causes, such as alcohol or drug abuse.

Interpersonal/Environmental Causes

Interpersonal and *environmental causes* of behavioral emergencies result from reactions to stimuli outside the person. They often result from overwhelming and stressful incidents, such as the death of a loved one, rape, or a disaster. The change in behavior can frequently be linked to a specific incident or series of incidents. The range of behavior manifested is broad, and a patient's specific symptoms often relate to the type of incident that precipitated them.

Organic Causes

An *organic cause* of altered behavior results from a disturbance in the patient's physical or biochemical state. Such disturbances include drug abuse/substance abuse, alcohol abuse, trauma, medical illness, and dementia. The area of the brain affected by the disturbance determines the type of behavior change.

It is important to consider the possibility of organic disease in *ALL* behavioral emergencies. As a result, physical assessment of patients with aberrant behavior is extremely important. It may uncover unsuspected causes of the altered behavior, such as drug/alcohol abuse, hypoxia, hypoglycemia, head injury, or meningitis.

Common agents used in the acute treatment of behavioral emergencies include haloperidol (Haldol), chlorpromazine (Thorazine), diazepam (Valium), and hydroxyzine (Vistaril).

Haloperidol (Haldol)

Class: Major Tranquilizer

Description

Haloperidol is a frequently used major tranquilizer.

Mechanism of Action

Haloperidol is a major tranquilizer that has proved effective in the management of acute psychotic episodes. It has pharmacological properties similar to those of the phenothiazine class of drugs (for example, Thorazine). Haloperidol appears to block dopamine receptors in the brain associated with mood and behavior. However, its precise mechanism of action is not clearly understood. Haloperidol has weak anticholinergic properties.

Indication

- Acute psychotic episodes

Contraindications

Haloperidol should not be administered in cases in which other drugs, especially sedatives, may be present. Haloperidol should not be used in the management of dysphoria caused by Talwin as it may promote sedation and anesthesia.

Precautions

Haloperidol may impair mental and physical abilities. Occasionally, orthostatic hypotension may be seen in conjunction with haloperidol use. Caution should be used when administering haloperidol to patients on anticoagulants.

Extrapyramidal, or Parkinson-like, reactions have been known to occur following the administration of haloperidol, especially in children. Diphenhydramine (Benadryl) should be readily available.

Side Effects

Haloperidol can cause extrapyramidal symptoms (EPS), insomnia, restlessness, sedation, seizures, respiratory depression, dry mouth, constipation, increased salivation, hypotension, and tachycardia.

Interactions

Antihypertensive medications may increase the likelihood of a patient developing hypotension with haloperidol administration. Haloperidol should be used with caution in patients taking lithium, as irreversible brain damage (encephalopathic syndrome) has been reported when these two drugs are used together.

Dosage

Doses of 2 to 5 milligrams intramuscularly are fairly standard in the management of an acute psychotic episode with severe symptoms. Haloperidol should be given intramuscularly only.

How Supplied

Haloperidol is supplied in 1-milliliter ampules containing 5 milligrams of the drug.

CASE PRESENTATION

Early on Sunday morning you are dispatched to a local nursing home for an elderly gentleman who is "causing problems." On arrival you are met by a member of the nursing home staff who explains the situation. This gentleman has been causing a fuss at breakfast. It seems he thinks he is back in World War II and is telling everyone to "hit the floor" and is shouting "incoming." Staff have tried to calm him but have had no success. You call dispatch and ask them to send police backup.

When the police arrive a few minutes later, you approach the patient. He is sitting in a chair carefully watching your every move. You introduce yourself as a paramedic and introduce your partner and the police. The patient smiles at you and says, "I know who you are. You aren't going to take me alive. I won't tell you anything." The patient then looks over his shoulder and says, "Jim, get away. Don't worry about me. Save yourself. I won't tell them anything."

Examination

(You are unable to physically assess the patient at this time. A visual survey reveals the following:)

CNS: The patient is conscious, able to speak, and appears in good physical health.

Resp: His respirations are 20 per minute. His trachea is midline. There are no signs of trauma.

CVS: His skin is pink in color.

ABD: Unable to assess

Musc/Skel: No injuries noticed

Vitals Signs: Unable to assess

Past Hx: Over the past three months the patient has experienced these episodes more frequently. Usually they last only 10–15 minutes. This time it has been over an hour. He is scaring the other residents. Staff at the nursing home are afraid to approach him. He has hit staff in the past.

Treatment:

The paramedics realize that there are several factors to recognize here. First, the patient's age. The patient is 72 years old and, while he appears to be in good physical health, an attempt to physically restrain him for a prolonged period of time would not be wise. Second, there is his history of violence. To what extent that is, the paramedics are not sure. Finally, there is the history that this is the longest such incident yet. Paramedics feel that the patient truly believes he has been captured in World War II.

Medical control was contacted. An order for Haldol (Haloperidol), 5 mg IM, was given. Advice from the medical director was for the paramedics and police to restrain the patient long enough to give the Haldol, and then release the patient and give the medication time to work. The patient was then to be brought to the hospital with vital signs monitored en route.

A paramedic explained the situation to the police officers and with a coordinated effort they were able to restrain the patient and give the Haloperidol. Fifteen minutes later the patient was placed on the stretcher, and restrained. An uneventful trip to the hospital followed. At the hospital he was admitted to the psychiatric service with a diagnosis of multi-infarct dementia. He was started on chronic Haldol therapy and had no additional flashbacks to World War II.

Chlorpromazine (Thorazine, Largactil)

Class: Major Tranquilizer

Description

Chlorpromazine is a major tranquilizer used in the management of severe psychotic episodes.

Mechanism of Action

Chlorpromazine is a member of the phenothiazine class of drugs. Phenothiazine drugs are thought to block dopamine receptors in the brain associated with behavior and mood. Chlorpromazine is also effective in the management of mild alcohol withdrawal and intractable hiccoughs. It is also effective in treating nausea and vomiting, although better agents are available.

Indications

- Acute psychotic episodes
- Mild alcohol withdrawal
- Intractable hiccoughs
- Nausea and vomiting

Contraindications

Chlorpromazine should not be administered to patients in comatose states or who have recently taken a large amount of sedatives. Chlorpromazine should not be administered to patients who may have recently taken hallucinogens as it tends to promote seizures.

Precautions

Chlorpromazine may impair mental and physical abilities. Occasionally, orthostatic hypotension may be seen in conjunction with chlorpromazine use. Extrapyramidal, or Parkinson-like, reactions have been known to occur following the administration of chlorpromazine, especially in children. Diphenhydramine should be readily available.

Side Effects

Chlorpromazine can cause dry mouth, constipation, blurred vision, dry eyes, sedation, headache, drowsiness, hypotension, and tachycardia.

Interactions

Antihypertensive medications may increase the likelihood of a patient developing hypotension with chlorpromazine administration.

Dosage

The standard dose of chlorpromazine in the management of an acute psychotic episode is 25–50 milligrams intramuscularly. Intractable hiccoughs will usually respond to a 25-milligram dose of chlorpromazine. Chlorpromazine should only be administered intramuscularly.

How Supplied

Chlorpromazine is supplied in 1- and 2-milliliter ampules containing 25 milligrams per milliliter.

Diazepam (Valium)

Class: Sedative/Anticonvulsant

Description

Diazepam is a benzodiazepine that is frequently used as a sedative, hypnotic, and anticonvulsant.

Mechanism of Action

Diazepam, one of the most frequently prescribed medications in the United States, is used in the management of anxiety and stress. It is effective in treating the tremors and anxiety associated with alcohol withdrawal. It is also an effective skeletal muscle relaxant, which makes it an effective adjunct in orthopedic injuries. It is a good premedication for minor operative procedures and cardioversion because it induces amnesia, which diminishes the patient's recall of such procedures.

In emergency medicine, diazepam is principally used for its anticonvulsant properties. It suppresses the spread of seizure activity through the motor cortex of the brain. It does not appear to abolish the abnormal discharge focus, however.

Indications

- Acute anxiety states
- Premedication before cardioversion
- Skeletal muscle relaxant
- Major motor seizures
- Status epilepticus

Contraindications

Diazepam should not be administered to any patient with a history of hypersensitivity to the drug.

Precautions

Because diazepam is a relatively short-acting drug, seizure activity may recur. In such cases, an additional dose may be required. Flumazenil (Romazicon), a benzodiazepine antagonist, should be available to use as an antidote if required.

Injectable diazepam can cause local venous irritation. To minimize this, it should only be injected into relatively large veins and should not be given faster than 1 milliliter per minute.

Side Effects

Diazepam can cause hypotension, drowsiness, headache, amnesia, respiratory depression, blurred vision, nausea, and vomiting.

Interactions

Diazepam is incompatible with many medications. Any time diazepam is given intravenously in conjunction with other drugs, the IV line should be adequately flushed. The effects of diazepam can be additive when used in conjunction with other CNS depressants and alcohol.

Dosage

In acute anxiety reactions, the standard dosage is 2 to 5 milligrams intramuscularly or intravenously.

To induce amnesia prior to cardioversion, a dosage of 5 to 15 milligrams of diazepam is given intravenously. Peak effects are seen in 5 to 10 minutes.

Diazepam should be given intravenously by slow IV push. It can be injected intramuscularly, but absorption via this route is variable. When an IV line cannot be started, parenteral diazepam can be administered rectally with a similar onset of action.

In the management of seizures, the usual dose of diazepam is 5 to 10 milligrams IV. In many instances it may be necessary to give diazepam directly into the vein, as the seizure activity will prevent the insertion of an indwelling catheter. When given directly into a vein, it is essential that a large vein, preferably in the antecubital fossa, is used.

How Supplied

Valium is supplied in ampules and prefilled syringes containing 10 milligrams in 2 milliliters of solvent.

Hydroxyzine (Vistaril, Atarax)

Class: Antihistamine

Description

Hydroxyzine is an antihistamine with sedative properties. It is a versatile drug used frequently in emergency medicine.

Mechanism of Action

Hydroxyzine is chemically unrelated to the phenothiazines. Because of its antihistamine properties, hydroxyzine has been shown to exert a calming effect during acute psychotic states. It is an effective antiemetic and muscle relaxant. When administered concurrently with many analgesics, it tends to potentiate their effects.

Indications

- To potentiate the effects of narcotics and synthetic narcotics
- Nausea and vomiting
- Anxiety reactions

Contraindications

Hydroxyzine should not be administered to any patient with a history of hypersensitivity to the drug.

Precautions

Hydroxyzine is given by intramuscular injection only. When administered concomitantly with analgesics, the potentiating effects of hydroxyzine should be kept in mind, and the total analgesic dose should be adjusted accordingly.

Side Effects

Hydroxyzine can cause sedation, dizziness, headache, dry mouth, and nausea.

Interactions

The sedative effects of hydroxyzine can be potentiated by CNS depressants such as narcotics, other antihistamines, sedatives, hypnotics, and alcohol.

Dosage

The standard dosage of hydroxyzine in the management of an acute anxiety reaction is 50 to 100 milligrams intramuscularly. The standard antiemetic dose is 25 to 50 milligrams. Hydroxyzine should be administered by intramuscular injection. Localized burning is a common complaint following an injection of hydroxyzine.

How Supplied

Hydroxyzine is supplied in single-dose vials containing 25 or 50 milligrams in 1 milliliter. Because the vials resemble each other, it is important to recheck the label to assure the correct dose is delivered to the patient.

SUMMARY

It is important to consider and rule out physical causes for bizarre behavior before determining that a patient's disorder is of a psychiatric origin. Disorders such as diabetes, head injury, and alcohol intoxication can cause bizarre behavior easily mistaken for psychosis. The psychotic patient is best handled in an emergency department by personnel skilled in psychiatric intervention. However, some patients may require pharmacological intervention before transport is possible.

chapter 14

Drugs Used in the Treatment of Gastrointestinal Emergencies

OBJECTIVES

1. Define the term *antiemetic.*
2. Describe and list the indications, contraindications, and dosages for:
   - promethazine
   - dimenhydrinate
   - prochlorperazine
   - metoclopramide
   - trimethobenzamide

GASTROINTESTINAL MEDICATIONS

While there are many medications for use in the treatment of gastrointestinal problems, few are used in prehospital care. The majority of gastrointestinal drugs used in prehospital care are antiemetics. These drugs are effective in treating nausea and vomiting. Many of these medications are used concomitantly with narcotics both to potentiate their effects and to reduce the likelihood of side effects commonly associated with narcotic usage. Antiemetics commonly used in emergency medicine include promethazine (Phenergan), dimenhydrinate (Gravol, Dramamine), prochlorperazine (Compazine), hydroxyzine (Vistaril), metoclopramide (Reglan), and trimethobenzamide (Tigan). Hydroxyzine was discussed in Chapter 13.

Promethazine (Phenergan)

Class: Antihistamine/Antiemetic

Description

Promethazine is a phenothiazine derivative with potent antihistamine properties and anticholinergic properties.

Mechanism of Action

Promethazine possesses sedative, antihistamine, antiemetic, and anticholinergic properties. It competitively blocks histamine receptors. The duration of action of promethazine is 4–6 hours. It is an effective and frequently used antiemetic. Promethazine, unlike hydroxyzine, can be given intravenously. It is often administered with analgesics, particularly narcotics, to potentiate their effect.

Indications

- Nausea and vomiting
- Motion sickness
- To potentiate the effects of analgesics
- Sedation

Contraindications

Promethazine is contraindicated in comatose states and in patients who have received a large amount of depressants. Also, it should not be administered to any patient with a history of hypersensitivity to the drug.

Precautions

Promethazine may impair mental and physical abilities. Care must be taken to avoid accidental intra-arterial injection. It should never be administered subcutaneously. Extrapyramidal symptoms (EPS) have been reported following promethazine use. Diphenhydramine (Benadryl) should be available.

Side Effects

Promethazine can cause drowsiness, sedation, blurred vision, tachycardia, bradycardia, and dizziness.

Interactions

The CNS-depressant effect of narcotics, sedative/hypnotics, and alcohol is potentiated by promethazine. An increased incidence of extrapyramidal symptoms has been reported when promethazine is administered to patients taking monamine oxidase inhibitors (MAOI).

Dosage

The standard dosage of promethazine in the management of nausea and vomiting is 12.5 to 25 milligrams either intravenously or intramuscularly.

The standard dosage in adjunctive use with analgesics is 25 milligrams. Promethazine should be given by IV or deep intramuscular injection only. Care must be taken to avoid accidental intra-arterial injection.

How Supplied

Promethazine is supplied in ampules and Tubex syringes containing 25 milligrams of the drug in 1 milliliter of solvent.

Dimenhydrinate (Gravol, Dramamine)

Class: Antiemetic

Description

Dimenhydrinate belongs to the antihistamine class of drugs although it is not commonly used for this action. Its site and action are not precisely known.

Mechanism of Action

The mechanism of action of dimenhydrinate is not precisely known. There is evidence that it acts to depress hyperstimulated labyrinthine functions or associated neural pathways. It is an effective and frequently used antiemetic in Canada. It is often used with analgesics, particularly narcotics.

Indications

- Prevention/relief of nausea and vomiting
- Prevention/relief of motion sickness
- Prevention/relief of drug induced nausea and vomiting (particularly narcotics)

Contraindications

No significant contraindications in the emergency setting

Precautions

Dimenhydrinate should be used with caution in patients with seizure disorders and asthma. Users should be cautioned against operating motor vehicles or dangerous machinery because of drowsiness associated with the drug.

Side Effects

Dimenhydrinate can cause drowsiness, dizziness, blurred vision, dry mouth, dry nose and bronchi, and tinnitus.

Interactions

The CNS-depressant effect of narcotics, sedative/hypnotics, and alcohol is potentiated by dimenhydrinate.

Dosage

The standard dose of dimenhydrinate in the management of nausea and vomiting is 12.5–25 mg (diluted) slow IV or 50–100 mg IM or PO. This can be repeated every 4 hours as needed.

How Supplied

Dimenhydrinate is supplied as 50 mg/5 ml vials/ampules (10 mg/ml), 50 mg/1 ml ampule (50 mg/ml), and 50 mg/2 ml (25 mg/ml).

Prochlorperazine (Compazine)

Class: Antiemetic

Description

Prochlorperazine is a phenothiazine derivative. It is highly effective in the treatment of severe nausea and vomiting.

Mechanism of Action

Prochlorperazine is an effective and frequently used antiemetic. It does not prevent vertigo and motion sickness like many of the other phenothiazines. Prochlorperazine blocks dopaminergic receptors in the brain. It also has weak anticholinergic properties.

Indications

- Severe nausea and vomiting
- Acute psychosis

Contraindications

Prochlorperazine should not be used in patients with a history of hypersensitivity to the drug or the phenothiazine class of medications. It should not be administered to comatose patients or those who have received large amounts of CNS depressants.

Precautions

Prochlorperazine may impair mental and physical abilities. It should never be administered subcutaneously because of local tissue irritation. The incidence of extrapyramidal symptoms (EPS) appears to be higher with prochlorperazine than with many of the other phenothiazines. Diphenhydramine (Benadryl) should be available.

Side Effects

Prochlorperazine can cause drowsiness, sedation, blurred vision, tachycardia, bradycardia, dizziness, and hypotension.

Interactions

The CNS-depressant effect of narcotics, sedative/hypnotics, and alcohol is potentiated by prochlorperazine.

Dosage

The standard dose of prochlorperazine is 5–10 milligrams intramuscularly or intravenously. The intravenous route is preferred with severe nausea and vomiting because the onset of action is much more rapid. Often, 10 milligrams of prochlorperazine is placed into 1 liter of normal saline or lactated Ringer's and administered.

How Supplied

Prochlorperazine (Compazine) is supplied in 2-milliliter vials containing 5 milligrams per milliliter of the drug.

Metoclopramide (Reglan)

Class: Antiemetic

Description

Metoclopramide is a medication used in the treatment of gastroesophageal reflux and nausea and vomiting.

Mechanism of Action

Metoclopramide is an effective antiemetic. It stimulates motility of the upper gastrointestinal tract and promotes emptying of the stomach. It increases the tone of the valve between the esophagus and the stomach (lower esophageal sphincter). This reduces reflux of stomach contents into the distal esophagus. Metoclopramide's antiemetic effects appear to result from its blockade of central and peripheral dopamine receptors.

Indications

- Severe nausea and vomiting
- Gastroesophageal reflux

Contraindications

Metoclopramide should not be used in patients with possible gastrointestinal hemorrhage, bowel obstruction, or perforation. It is also contraindicated in patients with a history of hypersensitivity to the drug.

Precautions

Metoclopramide may impair mental and physical abilities. Mental depression has occurred in patients with and without a prior history of depression following metoclopramide therapy. Extrapyramidal symptoms (EPS) can occur following metoclopramide administration. Diphenhydramine (Benadryl) should be available.

Side Effects

Metoclopramide can cause drowsiness, fatigue, sedation, dizziness, mental depression, hypertension, hypotension, tachycardia, bradycardia, and diarrhea.

Interactions

The effects of metoclopramide on gastric motility can be antagonized by anticholinergic drugs such as atropine. The CNS-depressant effect of narcotics, sedative/hypnotics, and alcohol can be potentiated by metoclopramide. Hypertension can result when metoclopramide is administered to patients receiving monamine oxidase inhibitors (MAOI).

Dosage

The standard dose of metoclopramide is 10–20 milligrams intramuscularly. Metoclopramide can be administered intravenously for severe or intractable nausea and vomiting. The standard intravenous dose is 10 milligrams administered by slow IV push over 1–2 minutes. Alternatively, 10 milligrams of metoclopramide can be diluted in 50 milliliters of normal saline and administered over 15 minutes. The intravenous route is preferred in severe nausea and vomiting because the onset of action is much more rapid.

How Supplied

Metoclopramide (Reglan) is supplied in 2-milliliter vials containing 5 milligrams per milliliter of the drug.

Trimethobenzamide (Tigan)

Class: Antiemetic

Description

Trimethobenzamide is an antiemetic that does not have the sedative effects of other commonly used antiemetic drugs.

Mechanism of Action

The mechanism of action of trimethobenzamide is unclear. It appears to work on the chemoreceptor trigger zone in the medulla oblongata.

Indication

- Severe nausea and vomiting

Contraindications

The injectable form of trimethobenzamide should not be used in children. Trimethobenzamide should not be administered to patients with a history of hypersensitivity to the drug.

Precautions

The antiemetic effects of trimethobenzamide may render diagnosis more difficult in conditions such as appendicitis. Extrapyramidal symptoms (EPS) have been reported following administration of trimethobenzamide. However, the incidence of this appears to be much less than with other antiemetics. Diphenhydramine (Benadryl) should be available. Trimetho–benzamide should not be administered intravenously.

Side Effects

Trimethobenzamide can cause blurred vision, diarrhea, dizziness, headache, muscle cramps, and allergic symptoms.

Interactions

The CNS-depressant effects of alcohol may be potentiated by trimethobenzamide.

Dosage

The standard dose of trimethobenzamide is 200 milligrams intramuscularly. Trimethobenzamide should not be administered intravenously.

How Supplied

Trimethobenzamide (Tigan) is supplied in 2-milliliter ampules and vials containing 100 milligrams per milliliter of the drug.

SUMMARY

Medications are rarely required in the prehospital management of gastrointestinal emergencies. However, many EMS systems utilize antiemetics for severe or intractable nausea and vomiting. Prehospital administration of antiemetics decreases the potential for dehydration, improves patient comfort, and reduces exposure of EMS personnel to body fluids. The antiemetics are often used to potentiate the effects of the narcotics. Paramedics are encouraged to be familiar with antiemetics used in their system.

chapter 15

Drugs Used in Pain Management

OBJECTIVES

1. Discuss the history of pain management in prehospital care.
2. Explain the characteristics of the ideal analgesic agent for prehospital care.
3. Define the terms *analgesic* and *narcotic*.
4. Describe the analgesics available for use in prehospital care.
5. Describe and list the indications, contraindications, and dosages for the following medications used in pain management: morphine sulfate, meperidine, fentanyl citrate, nitrous oxide, nalbuphine, butorphanol, and ketorolac.

INTRODUCTION

Emergency Medical Services and the prehospital care of patients have made significant advances over the past decade. The focus of these efforts has been primarily the overall reduction of death and disability in the critically ill or injured patient. However, controversy continues around the extent of prehospital intervention and the influence these efforts have on the outcome of these patients. Through these advances, very little attention has been given to the relief of pain and anxiety.

In the early 1970s the focus of prehospital care in the United States and Canada was directed at the treatment of cardiac arrest and myocardial infarction. Because of the importance of pain relief in the treatment of acute myocardial infarction, a narcotic (usually morphine) was included in the treatment protocol for prehospital advanced life support. However, the use of analgesics for pain relief has not been universally accepted beyond its use in myocardial infarction.

Meanwhile, British clinicians took a different view. Baskett introduced the use of fixed-ratio mixture (50:50) of nitrous oxide and oxygen to the ambulance service in 1969. During the next decade, use of the gas mixture became widespread for both basic and advanced life support systems in Australia, Canada, and the United States.

However, during the past decade there has been a lack of interest in providing adequate pain relief for patients in the prehospital care setting. *"In every medical study of analgesia in hospital settings, pain relief in patients was found to be inconsistent, inadequate and revealing of serious misconceptions or frank ignorance on the part of the physician or nursing staff. Add to this the fact that the uncontrolled prehospital environment argued against the safe administration of any medication, and there is little wonder that relief of pain in patients got a short shrift."*[1] And despite the advances made in prehospital care and medical control over the past decade, very little progress has been made in the area of pain relief.

"There has been the suggestion (albeit an old chestnut, seemingly resuscitated) that field analgesics will complicate in-hospital management and confuse diagnosis. This attitude, a variation on the old dictum with origins in the 19th and early 20th centuries, appears to have a new lease on life when applied to the prehospital setting. The availability of newer agents given in appropriate doses by appropriate routes should relegate this formerly sound medical truism to the scrap heap of medical myths.[1]

Is the relief of pain in the prehospital setting important? This question can be put to rest by patients who have suffered in agony while trapped in a motor vehicle or by patients with compound fractures who have been bounced around while being moved out of ditches and transported across rural or urban roads. What about the pain experienced by patients with extensive body surface burns? Not only is it humanitarian to provide pain relief in prehospital care, but the relief of pain can be of physiologic benefit to seriously ill and injured patients.

Perhaps it is time we paid more attention to managing the most common complaint faced in prehospital care today—pain. The ideal analgesic agent for prehospital care must have characteristics that are not easily met by one agent. First, the safety of the analgesic must be of prime concern. Second, it must be rapid in onset and short in duration. Rapidity of onset is the function of the route of administration, and that implies the intravenous route. Third, the ease with which an agent is stored and administered is important in prehospital care. For example, the relative bulk and weight of double- or single-tank nitrous oxide/oxygen mixtures have been more inhibiting to their frequent use in the prehospital setting than is generally appreciated. Perhaps then, the ideal agent has yet to be discovered.

Still, much can be done in the prehospital setting to relieve pain and anxiety. In the prehospital care setting, basic measures should consist of gentle handling, splinting, and compassionate caring rapport with the patient. Other factors, such as exposure to the cold, may occur during extrication or other prehospital procedures. Exposure may cause shivering and movement of fractures or other painful parts, increasing the patient's discomfort and negating the effect of almost any analgesic agent.

The good news is that pain relief is being reexamined as an important element of prehospital care. Not only is this interest focused on agents previously used, but new drugs and routes of administration are being explored. This chapter will prepare you to provide prehospital patients with relief from pain and freedom from fear and anxiety. Many agents appropriate for prehospital care are discussed on the following pages.

Reference

1. Stewart RD: "Analgesia in the Field." *Prehospital and Disaster Medicine.* 4(1). 1989

ANALGESICS

Drugs that have proved to be effective in alleviating pain are referred to as "analgesics." Although they may be administered in many different types of emergencies, they are usually reserved for the treatment of emergencies involving the cardiovascular system, especially myocardial infarction.

As a rule, undiagnosed pain is usually not treated. Early administration of analgesics to these patients may alter physical findings and impair subsequent evaluation by the emergency physician. Some types of pain may be easy to distinguish and are sometimes treated in the prehospital setting. These include chest pain associated with acute myocardial infarction, severe burns, and kidney stones.

Analgesics used in prehospital care include the following:

- morphine sulfate
- meperidine (Demerol)
- fentanyl (Sublimaze)
- nitrous oxide (Nitronox)
- nalbuphine (Nubain)
- butorphanol tartrate (Stadol)
- ketorolac (Toradol)

Morphine is derived from the opium plant. It has impressive analgesic and hemodynamic effects. Meperidine, although similar to morphine in its analgesic effects, is considerably different chemically and is synthetically derived. Nalbuphine (Nubain) is also a potent synthetic analgesic. It does not have the hemodynamic effects that morphine does, yet it is often used in emergency medicine because it does not cause respiratory depression and has a low tendency for abuse. Stadol, another of the new breed of synthetic analgesics, is similar to Nubain but is rarely used in treating cardiovascular emergencies. Nitronox, a 50% mixture of oxygen and nitrous oxide that can be easily inhaled by the patient, is entirely different from the other analgesic agents discussed. Its analgesic effects are also very potent yet disappear within a few minutes after the cessation of administration. Thus, Nitronox can be given for many types of pain in the field without fear of impairing subsequent physical examination in the emergency department. In addition to its analgesic effects, Nitronox delivers oxygen to the patient, which makes it useful in cardiac emergencies. Ketorolac (Toradol) is the first injectable nonsteroidal anti-inflammatory agent. It is often used in emergency medicine as an analgesic as it does not affect the patient's mental status.

Morphine Sulfate

Class: Narcotic Analgesic

Description

Morphine is a central nervous system depressant and a potent analgesic. Although morphine sulfate is one of the most potent analgesics known to humans, it also has hemodynamic properties that make it extremely useful in emergency medicine.

Mechanism of Action

Morphine sulfate is a central nervous system depressant that acts on opiate receptors in the brain providing both analgesia and sedation. It increases peripheral venous capacitance and decreases venous return. This effect is sometimes called a "chemical phlebotomy." Morphine also decreases myocardial oxygen demand. This action is due to both the decreased systemic vascular resistance and the sedative effects of the drug. Patient apprehension and fear can significantly increase myocardial oxygen demand and in some cases can conceivably increase the size of myocardial infarction. The hemodynamic properties of morphine make it one of the most important drugs used in the treatment of pulmonary edema. Morphine is frequently administered to patients with signs and symptoms of pulmonary edema who are not having chest pain.

Indications

- Severe pain associated with myocardial infarction, kidney stones, etc.
- Pulmonary edema either with or without associated pain

Contraindications

Because of the hemodynamic effects described earlier, morphine should not be used in patients who are volume depleted or severely hypotensive. Morphine should not be administered to any patient with a history of hypersensitivity to the drug or to patients with undiagnosed head injury or abdominal pain.

Precautions

Morphine is a narcotic derivative of opium. It has a high tendency for addiction and abuse and is thus covered under the Controlled Substances Act of 1970. It is classified as a Schedule II drug. Because of this, there are special considerations involved in the handling of the drug. Many emergency medical services (EMS) systems have opted to use the synthetic analgesics, like nalbuphine and pentazocine instead of morphine and meperidine because of these problems.

Morphine causes severe respiratory depression in higher doses. This is especially true in patients who already have some form of respiratory impairment. The narcotic antagonist naloxone (Narcan) should be readily available whenever the drug is administered.

Side Effects

Morphine can cause nausea, vomiting, abdominal cramps, blurred vision, constricted pupils, altered mental status, headache, and respiratory depression.

Interactions

The CNS depression associated with morphine can be enhanced when administered with antihistamines, antiemetics, sedatives, hypnotics, barbiturates, and alcohol.

Dosage

There are many different approaches to the administration of morphine. An initial dose in the range of 2 to 10 milligrams intravenously is standard. This can be augmented with additional doses of 2 milligrams every few minutes and can be continued until the pain is relieved or until signs of respiratory depression occur.

Intramuscular injection usually requires 5 to 15 milligrams, based on the patient's weight, to attain desired effects. However, morphine is routinely given intravenously in emergency medicine and is often administered with an antiemetic agent such as promethazine (Phenergan). This helps prevent the nausea and vomiting that often accompany morphine administration. The antiemetics also tend to potentiate morphine's effects. Morphine can also be given intramuscularly and subcutaneously.

How Supplied

Morphine comes in tamper-proof ampules and Tubex prefilled cartridges. To ease administration, the 10 milligrams in 1-milliliter dilution is preferred.

CASE PRESENTATION

At 1130 hours paramedics are called to a gravel pit for a man who is pinned in some gravel crushing equipment. En route the dispatcher tells the paramedics that the 26-year-old male is no longer trapped, is conscious and breathing, and has a large laceration and possible fracture of his left leg. On arrival paramedics are directed to a gravel crusher. They find their patient lying on the ground with a bloody torn left pant leg. The patient is moaning in pain. He is heavily dressed in coveralls. His left leg is severely angulated, and he complains of pain in his left leg and ankle.

On Examination

CNS:	The patient is conscious, alert, and oriented × 4; in extreme pain
Resp:	Respirations are 24, trachea is midline, no signs of trauma, lung sound clear bilaterally
CVS:	Carotid and radial pulses are present and weak, skin is pale and cool
ABD:	Soft and non-tender
Extremities:	Arms and right leg intact with good pulses, sensation, and strength. Left leg angulated 30 degrees laterally with obvious fractures and bleeding. No distal pulse palpable in left leg. Left foot cooler than right. No injuries above the knee.

Vitals:

Pulse:	76/min, regular, strong except for left foot, absent
Resp:	24/min, shallow
BP:	112/80
SpO_2:	94%
ECG:	Regular sinus rhythm
Hx:	The patient is not taking any medications, has no known allergies, and states he is a healthy person.

Treatment:

Paramedics give the patient oxygen by non-rebreather at 12 l/min. SpO_2 increases to 99%. They expose the patient's injuries. His leg is severely angulated mid-tib-fib with 4 inches of tibia protruding. Further assessment reveals that the left leg is rotated 270 degrees, not 30 degrees. His left foot is pulseless and becoming cyanosed. An IV is initiated using a 16 gauge catheter in the antecubital fossa. The IV of normal saline is run wide open. Paramedics give the patient 5.0 mg of morphine IV over 3 minutes as per standing order. The paramedics and the co-workers immobilize the leg in a pillow splint. The patient is moved to the ambulance.

In the ambulance contact is made with the base hospital, and the physician directs paramedics to straighten the leg. The patient is still in considerable pain and another 5.0 mg of morphine is administered. The patient's vital signs, especially respirations and SpO_2, are closely monitored. The leg is straightened and placed in a rigid splint. A pulse is detected in the foot and color begins to return. The trip to the hospital is uneventful. On arrival at the hospital, the patient is quickly assessed and sent to the operating theater.

Meperidine (Demerol)

Class: Narcotic Analgesic

Description

Meperidine is a central nervous system depressant and a potent analgesic. It is used extensively in medicine in the treatment of moderate to severe pain. It is less potent than morphine sulfate. Sixty to 80 milligrams of meperidine are roughly equivalent in action to 10 milligrams of morphine.

Mechanism of Action

Meperidine is a central nervous system depressant that acts on opiate receptors in the brain providing both analgesia and sedation. It does not have the same hemodynamic properties as morphine but has the same tendency for physical dependence and abuse. Because it causes respiratory depression, naloxone should be available whenever meperidine is administered. The rate of onset is slightly faster than morphine yet its effects are much shorter in duration. Like morphine, meperidine is a Schedule II drug regulated under the Controlled Substances Act of 1970.

Indication

- Moderate to severe pain

Contraindications

Meperidine should not be administered to patients with known hypersensitivity to the drug. In addition, it should not be administered to patients with undiagnosed abdominal pain or head injury.

Meperidine should not be administered to patients who are receiving, or who have recently received, monoamine oxidase inhibitors (for example, Nardil, Parnate, and Eutron). Therapeutic doses of meperidine have occasionally caused severe, and sometimes fatal, reactions in patients receiving these agents.

Precautions

Meperidine can cause respiratory depression. Naloxone (Narcan) should always be available to reverse the effects of the drug if respiratory depression ensues. Like morphine, meperidine should be kept in a secure locked box.

Side Effects

Meperidine can cause nausea, vomiting, abdominal cramps, blurred vision, constricted pupils, altered mental status, hallucinations, headache, and respiratory depression.

Interactions

Meperidine should not be administered to patients who are receiving, or who have recently received, monoamine oxidase inhibitors (for example, Nardil, Parnate, and Eutron). These agents are used for certain types of depression and behavioral disorders. Therapeutic doses of meperidine have occasionally caused severe, and sometimes fatal, reactions in patients receiving these agents.

Dosage

The usual dose used in the treatment of severe pain is 25 to 50 milligrams intravenously. When administered intramuscularly, 50 to 100 milligrams is a standard dose. Meperidine is often administered with an antiemetic agent such as promethazine (Phenergan). This helps prevent the nausea and vomiting that often accompany meperidine administration. Meperidine can be administered either intravenously or intramuscularly.

How Supplied

Meperidine (Demerol) is supplied in ampules and Tubex prefilled cartridges containing 25, 50, or 100 milligrams of the drug in 1 milliliter of solvent.

Fentanyl Citrate (Sublimaze)

Class: Narcotic Analgesic

Description

Fentanyl, although chemically unrelated to morphine, produces pharmacologic effects and a degree of analgesia similar to morphine. On a weight basis, however, fentanyl is 50 to 100 times more potent than morphine, but its duration of action is shorter than that of meperidine or morphine. A parenteral dose of 100 mcg of fentanyl is approximately equivalent in analgesic activity to 10 mg of morphine or 75 mg of meperidine.

Mechanism of Action

The principal actions of therapeutic value are analgesic and sedation. Fentanyl is a narcotic analgesic with a rapid onset and a short duration of action. Alterations in respiratory rate and alveolar ventilation, associated with narcotic analgesics, may last longer than the analgesic effect. Large doses may produce apnea. Fentanyl appears to have less emetic activity than other narcotic analgesics.

Indications

- Maintenance of analgesia
- Adjunct in rapid sequence induction intubation
- Severe pain

Contraindications

- Severe hemorrhage
- Shock
- Known hypersensitivity

Precautions

Vital signs should be monitored routinely. Fentanyl may produce bradycardia, which may be treated with atropine. However, fentanyl should be used with caution in patients with cardiac bradydysrhythmias.

Fentanyl should be administered with caution to patients with liver and kidney dysfunction because of the importance of these organs in the metabolism and excretion of drugs.

As with other CNS depressants, patients who have received fentanyl should have appropriate surveillance. Resuscitation equipment and a narcotic agonist such as naloxone should be readily available to manage apnea.

Side Effects

As with other narcotic analgesics, the most common serious reactions reported to occur with fentanyl are:

- respiratory depression
- apnea
- muscle rigidity
- bradycardia

If the above remain untreated, respiratory arrest, circulatory depression, or cardiac arrest could occur.

Interactions

Other CNS depressant drugs (e.g., barbiturates, tranquilizers, narcotics, and general anesthetics) will have an additive or potentiating effect with fentanyl. When patients have received such drugs, the dose of fentanyl required will be less than usual. Likewise, following the administration of fentanyl, the dose of other CNS depressant drugs should be reduced.

Severe and unpredictable potentiation by MAO inhibitors has been reported with narcotic analgesics. Since the safety of fentanyl in this regard has not been established, its use in patients who have received MAO inhibitors within 14 days is not recommended.

Dosage

Adult

- IV—25 to 100 mcg (0.025 to 0.1 mg)
- Direct IV—slowly over at least 1 minute, preferably over 2–3 minutes (not necessary to dilute—may be diluted to facilitate administration)
- Dilute 100 mcg/2 ml in 3 ml of NS for a concentration of 20 mcg/ml

Pediatric

- 2–12 years—1.7 to 3.3 mcg/kg
- Reduce dose in very young or elderly or poor-risk patients

How Supplied

Fentanyl is supplied in 2-ml ampules containing 50 mcg/ml.

Protect from light during storage.

Nitrous Oxide (Nitronox, Entonox)

Class: Analgesic/Anesthetic Gas

Description

Nitronox is a blended mixture of 50 percent nitrous and 50 percent oxygen, which has potent analgesic effects.

Mechanism of Action

Nitrous oxide is a CNS depressant with analgesic properties. In the prehospital setting it is delivered in a fixed mixture of 50% nitrous oxide and 50% oxygen. When inhaled, it has potent analgesic effects. These quickly dissipate, however, within 2 to 5 minutes after cessation of administration.

The Nitronox unit consists of one oxygen and one nitrous oxide cylinder. The gases are fed into a blender that combines them at the appropriate concentration. The mixture is then delivered to a modified demand valve for administration to the patient.

Nitronox must be self-administered. It is effective in treating many varieties of pain encountered in the prehospital setting including pain from many types of trauma. The high concentration of oxygen delivered along with the nitrous oxide will increase the oxygen tension in the blood, thus reducing hypoxia.

Indications

- Pain of musculoskeletal origin, particularly fractures
- Burns
- Suspected ischemic chest pain
- States of severe anxiety including hyperventilation

Contraindications

Nitronox should not be used in any patient who cannot comprehend verbal instructions or who is intoxicated with alcohol or other drugs. It should not be administered to any patient with a head injury who exhibits an altered mental status. Nitronox should not be administered to any patient with COPD where the high concentration of oxygen (50 percent) might result in respiratory depression. Nitrous oxide tends to diffuse into closed spaces more readily than either carbon dioxide or oxygen. Many COPD patients have air-containing blebs in their lungs, and nitrous oxide can concentrate in these blebs causing them to swell. Swollen blebs may rupture causing a pneumothorax.

Nitronox should not be administered to patients with a thoracic injury suspicious of pneumothorax, as the gas may accumulate in the pneumothorax increasing its size. Also, patients with severe abdominal pain and distention, suggestive of bowel obstruction, should not receive Nitronox. Nitrous oxide can concentrate in pockets of an obstructed bowel possibly leading to rupture.

Precautions

Nitronox should only be used in areas that are well ventilated. When the gas is used in the patient compartment of an ambulance, it is recommended that a scavenging system be in place.

Nitrous oxide exists in a liquid state inside the gas cylinder. Heat present in the air, in the cylinder wall, or in the various regulators and lines causes the liquid to vaporize. This vaporization process makes the cylinder tank and lines cool to touch. Following prolonged use, frost may develop on the cylinder, regulator, or lines. In very cold environments, generally less than 21°F (6°C), the liquid may be slow to vaporize, and administration may be impossible.

Side Effects

Nitrous oxide/oxygen mixture can cause dizziness, light-headedness, altered mental status, hallucinations, nausea, and vomiting.

Interactions

Nitrous oxide can potentiate the effects of other CNS depressants such as narcotics, sedatives, hypnotics, and alcohol.

Dosage

Nitronox should only be self-administered. Continuous administration may take place until the pain is significantly relieved or until the patient drops the mask. The patient care record should document the duration of drug administration.

How Supplied

Nitrous oxide/oxygen mixture is supplied in a cylinder system where both gases are fed into a blender that delivers a fixed 50%/50% mixture to the patient. The blender is designed to shut off if the oxygen cylinder becomes depleted. It will allow continued administration of oxygen if the nitrous oxide cylinder becomes depleted.

In several countries (England, Canada, Australia) the nitrous oxide/oxygen mixture (Entonox, Dolonox) is premixed and supplied in a single cylinder. This setup is much lighter than the system used in the United States.

CASE PRESENTATION

At 1900 hours on a fall evening paramedics are called to the high school football stadium for a football player who has injured his shoulder. On arrival they are directed to the sidelines where the coaches are attending to a player. The player is not wearing shoulder pads and is slouched to his right side.

On Examination

CNS: The patient is conscious, alert, and oriented × 4; in moderate pain

Resp: Respirations are 24, trachea is midline

CVS: Carotid and radial pulses are present, skin is warm and dry

ABD: Soft and non-tender

Extremities: Dislocation of right shoulder

Vitals:

Pulse: 88/min, regular

Resp: 18/min, shallow

BP: 118/72

SpO_2: 96%

Hx: The patient is not taking any medications, has no known allergies, and states he is a healthy person.

The coaches tell the paramedics that the football player is the team quarterback. He was sacked on a play and landed heavily on his shoulder.

Treatment:

On assessment paramedics find that the shoulder is dislocated anteriorly. They give the patient nitrous oxide to self-administer. After several minutes of breathing the nitrous oxide, the patient states that the pain is not as intense. Paramedics sling and swathe the arm and shoulder and move the patient to the ambulance. Once in the unit, they administer 75 mg of meperidine IM in the left deltoid. The combination of nitrous oxide and meperidine give the patient almost total pain relief. The transport to the hospital is uneventful.

Nalbuphine (Nubain)

Class: Synthetic Analgesic

Description

Nalbuphine is a synthetic analgesic agent with a potency equivalent to morphine on a milligram to milligram basis.

Mechanism of Action

Like the narcotics, nalbuphine is a centrally acting analgesic that binds to the opiate receptors in the central nervous system. Its onset of action is considerably faster than morphine, occurring within 2 to 3 minutes after intravenous administration. Its duration of effect is reported to be 3 to 6 hours. Although nalbuphine causes some respiratory depression in doses up to 10 milligrams, these effects do not seem to get worse in doses that exceed 10 milligrams. Naloxone (Narcan) is an effective antagonist and should be available when nalbuphine is administered.

In addition to its effects on opiate receptors, nalbuphine also has antagonistic effects similar to naloxone. This feature minimizes the abuse potential of the drug and appears to lessen the chances of significant respiratory depression. At this time, nalbuphine is not regulated under the Controlled Substances Act. Current studies show that it has a minimal tendency for physical dependence and abuse. This property has made nalbuphine increasingly popular in prehospital care.

Indication

- Moderate to severe pain

Contraindications

Nalbuphine should not be administered to patients with head injury or undiagnosed abdominal pain.

Precautions

The primary precaution in using nalbuphine is in patients with impaired respiratory function. Small doses of nalbuphine may cause significant respiratory depression. Naloxone should be readily available. Nalbuphine also has narcotic antagonistic properties. Thus, it should be administered with caution to patients dependent on narcotics, as it may cause withdrawal effects.

The dosage of nalbuphine should be reduced in older patients since the effects are less predictable in this age group. Small repeated boluses are often safer than a single large dose.

Side Effects

Nalbuphine can cause headache, altered mental status, hypotension, bradycardia, blurred vision, rash, respiratory depression, nausea, and vomiting.

Interactions

Nalbuphine can potentiate the CNS depression associated with narcotics, sedatives, hypnotics, and alcohol. Because of its antagonistic properties, nalbuphine can cause withdrawal symptoms in patients addicted to narcotics. Nalbuphine can interfere with certain types of anesthesia (nitrous/narcotic techniques) because of its antagonistic properties.

Dosage

The general regimen for nalbuphine administration is 5 milligrams intravenously initially. This may be augmented with additional 2-milligram doses if necessary. Nalbuphine is often administered with an antiemetic agent such as promethazine (Phenergan). This helps prevent the nausea and vomiting that often accompany morphine administration. Nalbuphine can be administered intravenously or intramuscularly.

How Supplied

Nalbuphine is supplied in 1-milliliter ampules containing 10 milligrams of the drug.

Butorphanol Tartrate (Stadol)

Class: Synthetic Analgesic

Description

Butorphanol is a synthetic analgesic used frequently in emergency medicine. It is quite potent with the analgesic effects of 2 milligrams of butorphanol being roughly equivalent to 10 milligrams of morphine.

Mechanism of Action

Butorphanol is a centrally acting analgesic that binds to the opiate receptors in the central nervous system causing CNS depression and analgesia. Like nalbuphine, it has some antagonistic (naloxone-like) properties.

Although butorphanol can cause respiratory depression, this effect usually plateaus following administration of approximately 4 milligrams. Currently, butorphanol is not restricted under the Controlled Substances Act. This makes it quite attractive for use in the prehospital phase of emergency medical care.

Indication

- Moderate to severe pain

Contraindications

Butorphanol should not be administered to any patient with a history of hypersensitivity to the drug. Also, it should not be given to patients dependent on narcotics as it may well cause some reversal of the narcotic effects. It should not be administered to patients with head injury or undiagnosed abdominal pain.

Precautions

If butorphanol causes marked respiratory depression, then Narcan can be administered to reverse its effects. Remember, when administering any potent analgesic, it is possible to mask other signs and symptoms, thus delaying the complete physical examination and determination of a diagnosis. All analgesics should be administered only after a thorough physical examination. Butorphanol should not be administered to any patient with head injury as it may well cause an increase in cerebrospinal pressure.

The dosage of nalbuphine should be reduced in older patients because the effects are less predictable in this age group. Small repeated boluses are often safer than a single large dose.

Side Effects

Butorphanol can cause headache, altered mental status, hypotension, bradycardia, blurred vision, rash, respiratory depression, nausea, and vomiting.

Interactions

Like nalbuphine, butorphanol has some narcotic antagonistic properties. Caution should be used when administering butorphanol to patients already dependent on narcotics as it may precipitate withdrawal.

Dosage

The standard dose of butorphanol is 1 milligram intravenously every 3 to 4 hours. When given intramuscularly, the standard dose is 2 milligrams. Butorphanol should only be administered intravenously or intramuscularly.

How Supplied

Butorphanol is supplied in 2-milliliter vials containing 2 milligrams of the drug.

Ketorolac (Toradol)

Class: Non-Steroidal Anti-Inflammatory Agent

Description

Ketorolac is the first injectable non-steroidal anti-inflammatory drug to become available in the United States. It is useful in treating mild to moderate pain.

Mechanism of Action

Ketorolac is a non-steroidal anti-inflammatory drug (NSAID). It has analgesic, anti-inflammatory, and antipyretic effects. Unlike narcotics, which act on the central nervous system, ketorolac is considered a peripherally acting analgesic. Because of this, it does not have the sedative properties of the narcotics. Ketorolac has been used concomitantly with morphine and meperidine without adverse effects. In dental studies, ketorolac was found to be quite effective as an analgesic.

Indication

- Mild to moderate pain

Contraindications

Ketorolac should not be used in patients with a known hypersensitivity to the drug. It should not be administered to patients who report allergies to aspirin or the non-steroidal anti-inflammatory drugs.

Precautions

Gastrointestinal irritation and hemorrhage can result from therapy with NSAIDs. Long term usage increases the incidence of serious GI side effects. Ketorolac is cleared through the kidneys. Long term usage can result in renal impairment.

Side Effects

Ketorolac can cause edema, hypertension, rash, itching, nausea, heartburn, constipation, diarrhea, drowsiness, and dizziness.

Interactions

Ketorolac, when administered with other NSAIDS (including aspirin), can worsen the side effects associated with the use of drugs in this class. Intramuscular ketorolac has been found to reduce the diuretic response to furosemide (Lasix).

Dosage

The typical dose of ketorolac is 30–60 milligrams intramuscularly. Half the original dose can be repeated every 6 hours. Recently approved for IV use by the FDA, many emergency departments use ketorolac intravenously to obtain more prompt analgesia. The typical intravenous dose is 30 milligrams. Some practitioners will use 60 milligrams intravenously. Few adverse reactions have been reported with intravenous ketorolac.

How Supplied

Ketorolac is supplied in prefilled syringes containing 15, 30, and 60 milligrams of the drug.

KEY WORDS

analgesic. A drug used in the relief of pain.

narcotic. A substance that works on the central nervous system to decrease or relieve the sensation of pain. Narcotic pain killers (analgesics) are made from opium or made artificially.

appendix A

American Heart Association Advanced Cardiac Life Support Protocols

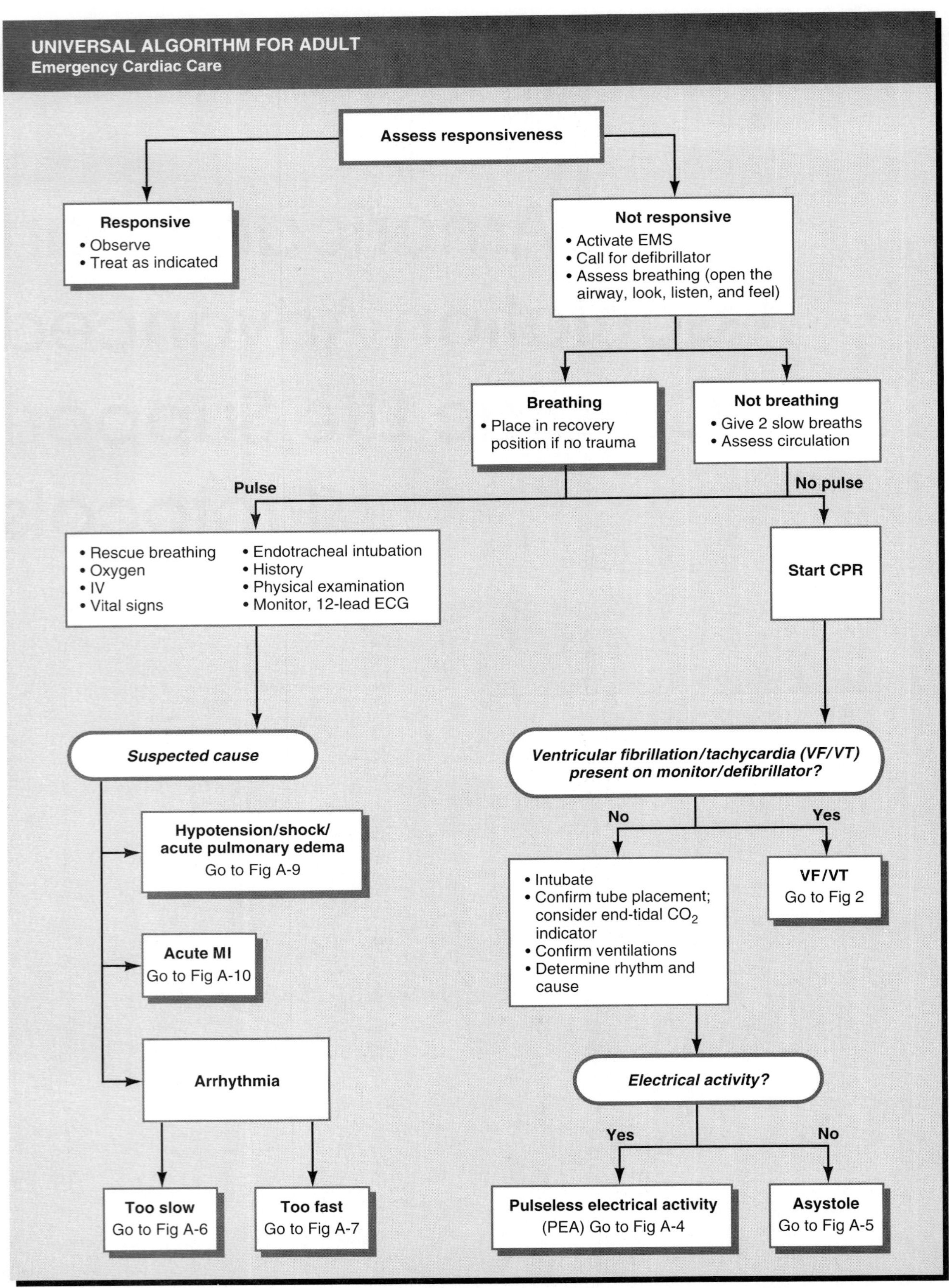

Figure A-1 *Journal of the American Medical Association (JAMA),* October 28, 1992. Volume 268, Number 16 (pages 2171–2302). Copyright 1992, American Medical Association. Reproduced with permission.

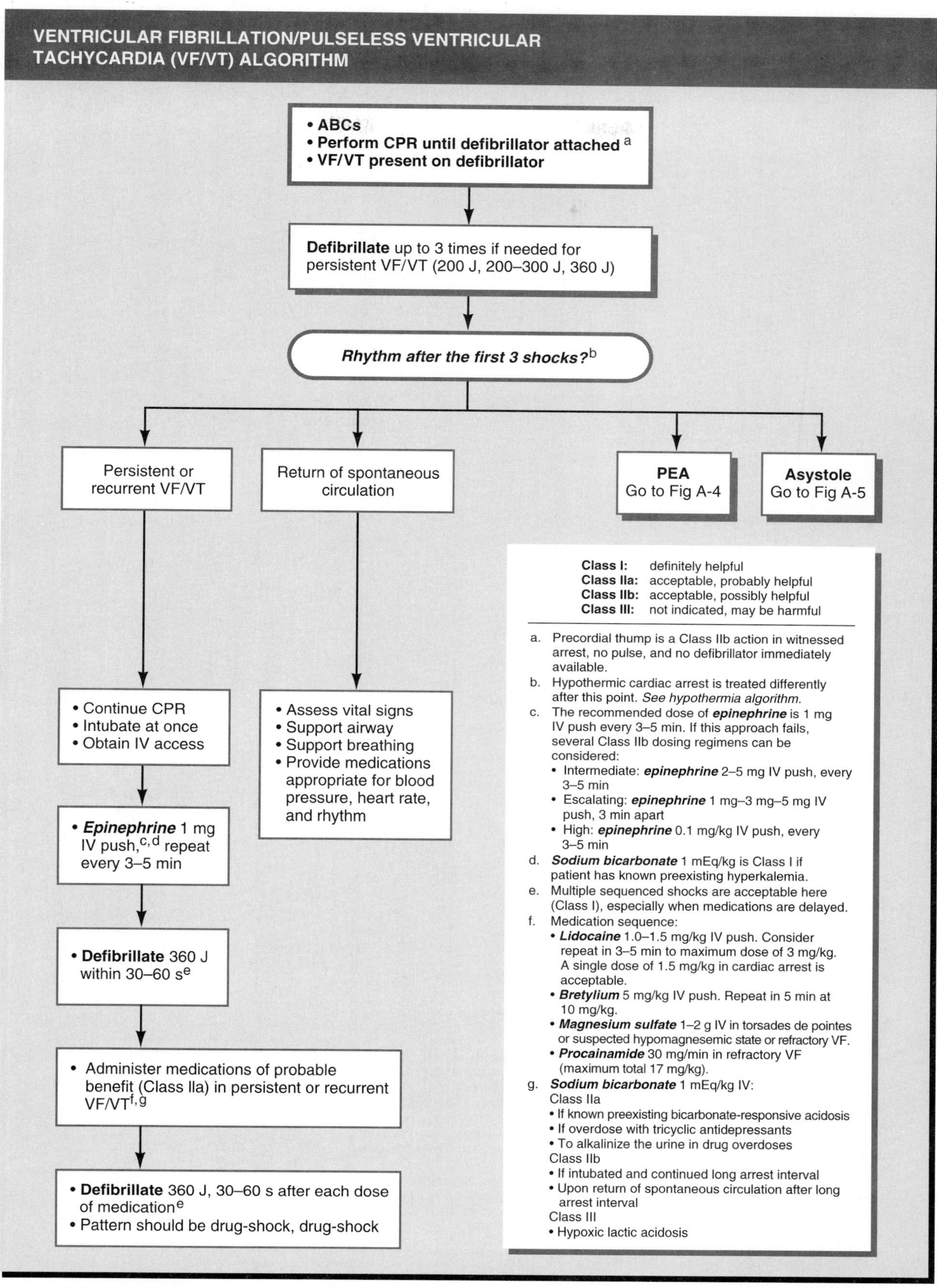
VENTRICULAR FIBRILLATION/PULSELESS VENTRICULAR TACHYCARDIA (VF/VT) ALGORITHM
• ABCs
• Perform CPR until defibrillator attached [a]
• VF/VT present on defibrillator
Defibrillate up to 3 times if needed for persistent VF/VT (200 J, 200–300 J, 360 J)
Rhythm after the first 3 shocks? [b]
Persistent or recurrent VF/VT
Return of spontaneous circulation
PEA Go to Fig A-4
Asystole Go to Fig A-5
• Continue CPR
• Intubate at once
• Obtain IV access
• Epinephrine 1 mg IV push,[c,d] repeat every 3–5 min
• Defibrillate 360 J within 30–60 s[e]
• Administer medications of probable benefit (Class IIa) in persistent or recurrent VF/VT[f,g]
• Defibrillate 360 J, 30–60 s after each dose of medication[e]
• Pattern should be drug-shock, drug-shock
• Assess vital signs
• Support airway
• Support breathing
• Provide medications appropriate for blood pressure, heart rate, and rhythm
Class I: definitely helpful
Class IIa: acceptable, probably helpful
Class IIb: acceptable, possibly helpful
Class III: not indicated, may be harmful
a. Precordial thump is a Class IIb action in witnessed arrest, no pulse, and no defibrillator immediately available.
b. Hypothermic cardiac arrest is treated differently after this point. See hypothermia algorithm.
c. The recommended dose of epinephrine is 1 mg IV push every 3–5 min. If this approach fails, several Class IIb dosing regimens can be considered:
• Intermediate: epinephrine 2–5 mg IV push, every 3–5 min
• Escalating: epinephrine 1 mg–3 mg–5 mg IV push, 3 min apart
• High: epinephrine 0.1 mg/kg IV push, every 3–5 min
d. Sodium bicarbonate 1 mEq/kg is Class I if patient has known preexisting hyperkalemia.
e. Multiple sequenced shocks are acceptable here (Class I), especially when medications are delayed.
f. Medication sequence:
• Lidocaine 1.0–1.5 mg/kg IV push. Consider repeat in 3–5 min to maximum dose of 3 mg/kg. A single dose of 1.5 mg/kg in cardiac arrest is acceptable.
• Bretylium 5 mg/kg IV push. Repeat in 5 min at 10 mg/kg.
• Magnesium sulfate 1–2 g IV in torsades de pointes or suspected hypomagnesemic state or refractory VF.
• Procainamide 30 mg/min in refractory VF (maximum total 17 mg/kg).
g. Sodium bicarbonate 1 mEq/kg IV:
Class IIa
• If known preexisting bicarbonate-responsive acidosis
• If overdose with tricyclic antidepressants
• To alkalinize the urine in drug overdoses
Class IIb
• If intubated and continued long arrest interval
• Upon return of spontaneous circulation after long arrest interval
Class III
• Hypoxic lactic acidosis

Figure A-2 *Journal of the American Medical Association (JAMA),* October 28, 1992. Volume 268, Number 16 (pages 2171–2302). Copyright 1992, American Medical Association. Reproduced with permission.

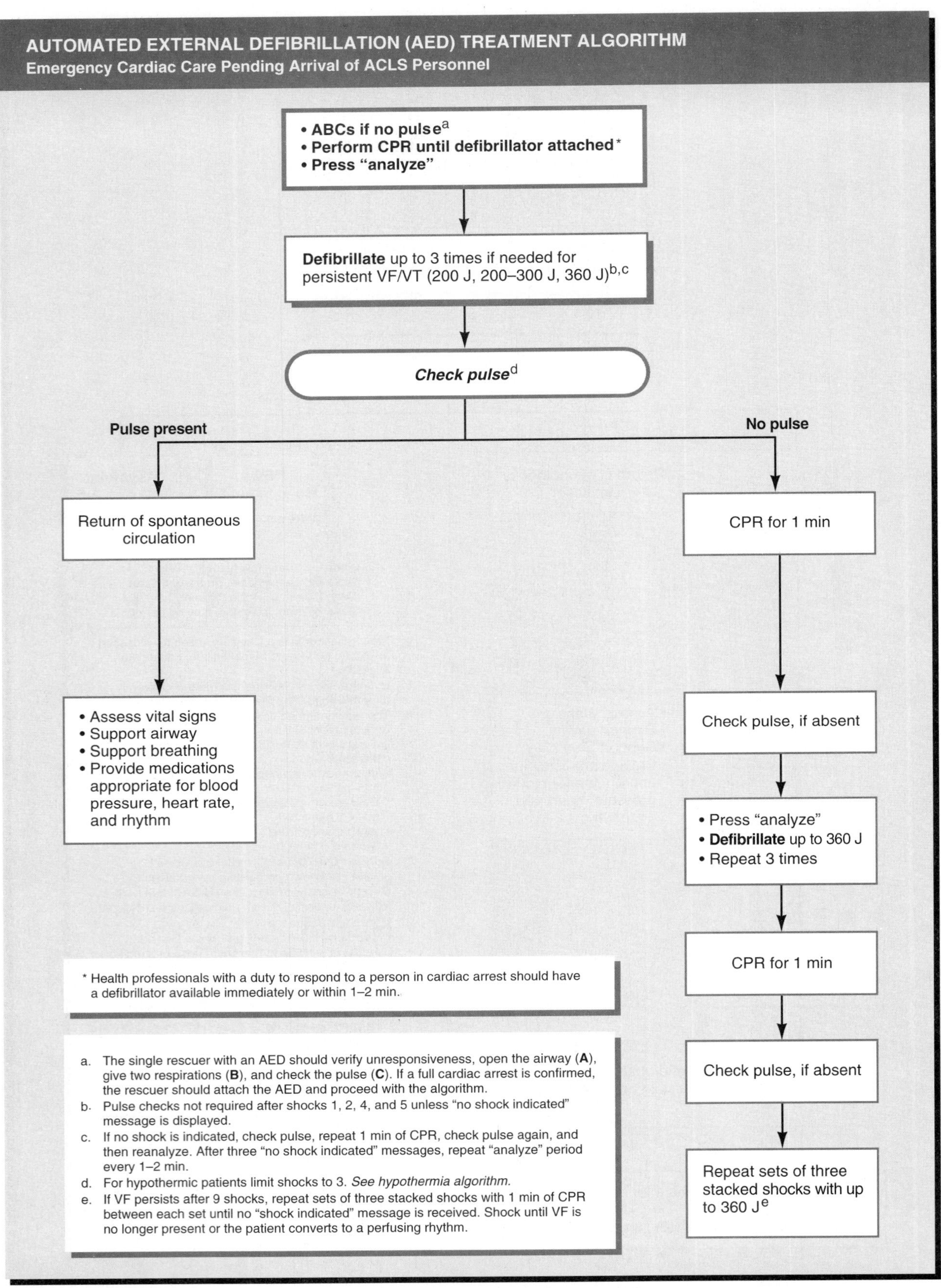

Figure A-3 *Journal of the American Medical Association (JAMA),* October 28, 1992. Volume 268, Number 16 (pages 2171–2302). Copyright 1992, American Medical Association. Reproduced with permission.

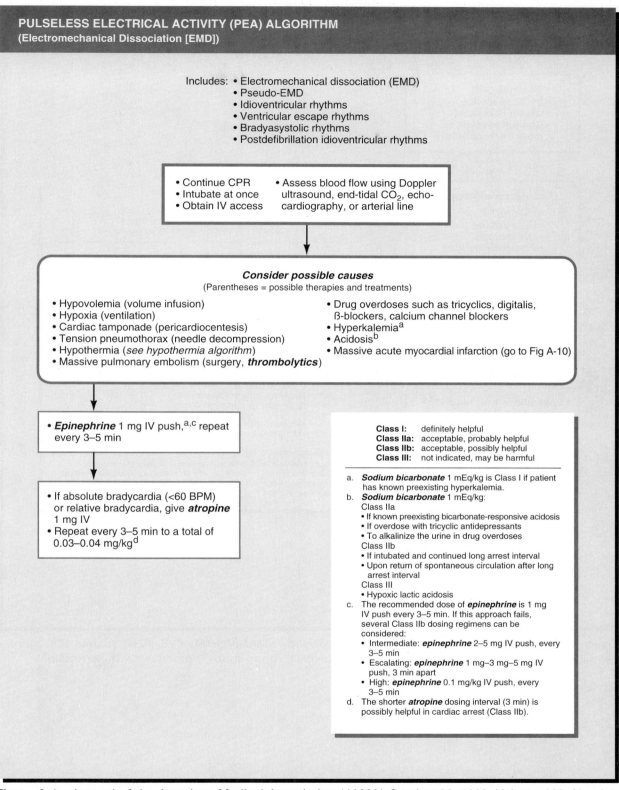

PULSELESS ELECTRICAL ACTIVITY (PEA) ALGORITHM
(Electromechanical Dissociation [EMD])

Includes:
- Electromechanical dissociation (EMD)
- Pseudo-EMD
- Idioventricular rhythms
- Ventricular escape rhythms
- Bradyasystolic rhythms
- Postdefibrillation idioventricular rhythms

- Continue CPR
- Intubate at once
- Obtain IV access
- Assess blood flow using Doppler ultrasound, end-tidal CO_2, echocardiography, or arterial line

↓

Consider possible causes

(Parentheses = possible therapies and treatments)

- Hypovolemia (volume infusion)
- Hypoxia (ventilation)
- Cardiac tamponade (pericardiocentesis)
- Tension pneumothorax (needle decompression)
- Hypothermia (*see hypothermia algorithm*)
- Massive pulmonary embolism (surgery, ***thrombolytics***)
- Drug overdoses such as tricyclics, digitalis, ß-blockers, calcium channel blockers
- Hyperkalemia[a]
- Acidosis[b]
- Massive acute myocardial infarction (go to Fig A-10)

↓

- ***Epinephrine*** 1 mg IV push,[a,c] repeat every 3–5 min

↓

- If absolute bradycardia (<60 BPM) or relative bradycardia, give ***atropine*** 1 mg IV
- Repeat every 3–5 min to a total of 0.03–0.04 mg/kg[d]

Class I: definitely helpful
Class IIa: acceptable, probably helpful
Class IIb: acceptable, possibly helpful
Class III: not indicated, may be harmful

a. ***Sodium bicarbonate*** 1 mEq/kg is Class I if patient has known preexisting hyperkalemia.

b. ***Sodium bicarbonate*** 1 mEq/kg:
Class IIa
- If known preexisting bicarbonate-responsive acidosis
- If overdose with tricyclic antidepressants
- To alkalinize the urine in drug overdoses

Class IIb
- If intubated and continued long arrest interval
- Upon return of spontaneous circulation after long arrest interval

Class III
- Hypoxic lactic acidosis

c. The recommended dose of ***epinephrine*** is 1 mg IV push every 3–5 min. If this approach fails, several Class IIb dosing regimens can be considered:
- Intermediate: ***epinephrine*** 2–5 mg IV push, every 3–5 min
- Escalating: ***epinephrine*** 1 mg–3 mg–5 mg IV push, 3 min apart
- High: ***epinephrine*** 0.1 mg/kg IV push, every 3–5 min

d. The shorter ***atropine*** dosing interval (3 min) is possibly helpful in cardiac arrest (Class IIb).

Figure A-4 *Journal of the American Medical Association (JAMA),* October 28, 1992. Volume 268, Number 16 (pages 2171–2302). Copyright 1992, American Medical Association. Reproduced with permission.

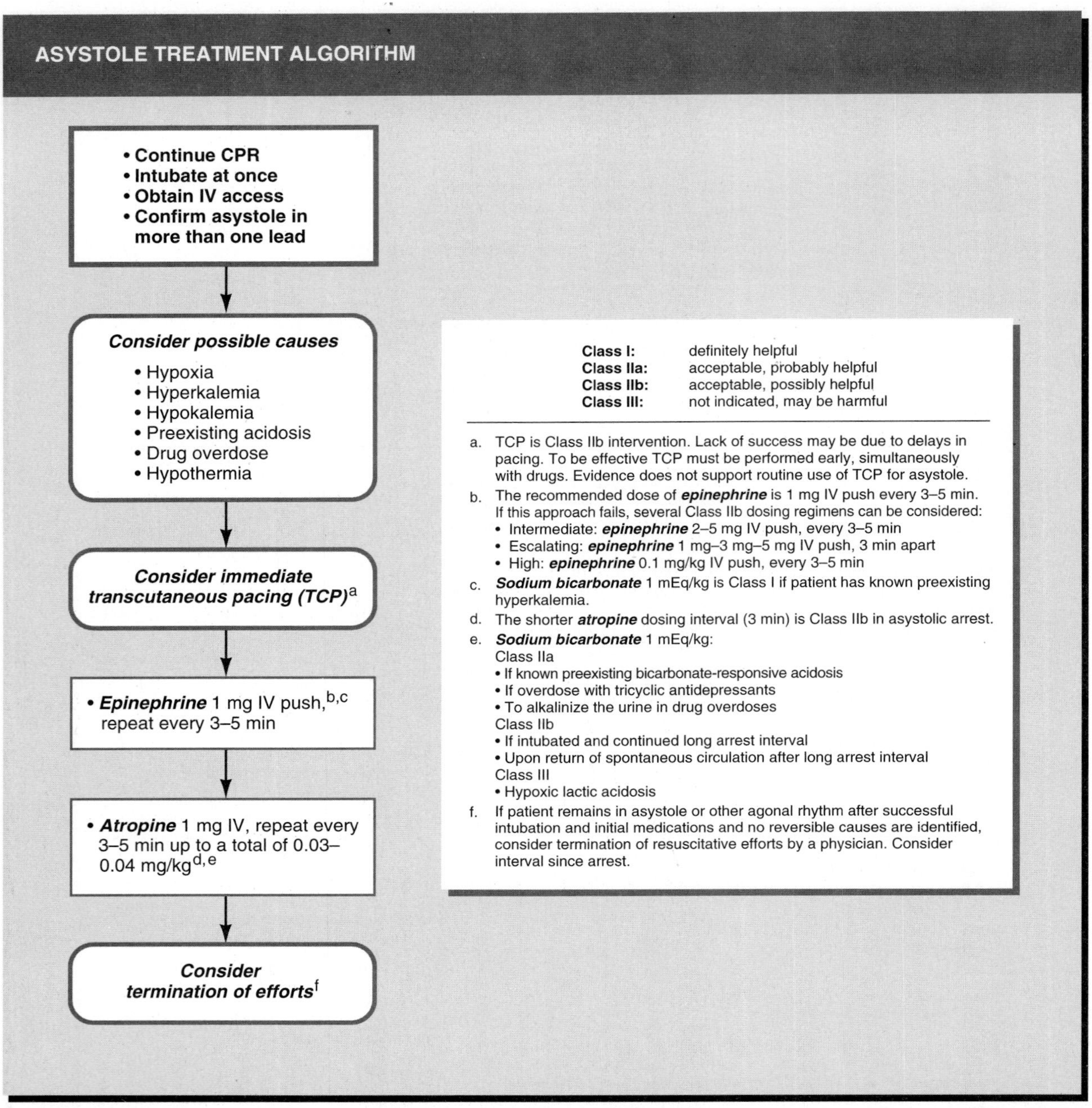

ASYSTOLE TREATMENT ALGORITHM
• Continue CPR
• Intubate at once
• Obtain IV access
• Confirm asystole in more than one lead
Consider possible causes
• Hypoxia
• Hyperkalemia
• Hypokalemia
• Preexisting acidosis
• Drug overdose
• Hypothermia
Consider immediate transcutaneous pacing (TCP)[a]
• Epinephrine 1 mg IV push,[b,c] repeat every 3–5 min
• Atropine 1 mg IV, repeat every 3–5 min up to a total of 0.03–0.04 mg/kg[d,e]
Consider termination of efforts[f]
Class I: definitely helpful
Class IIa: acceptable, probably helpful
Class IIb: acceptable, possibly helpful
Class III: not indicated, may be harmful
a. TCP is Class IIb intervention. Lack of success may be due to delays in pacing. To be effective TCP must be performed early, simultaneously with drugs. Evidence does not support routine use of TCP for asystole.
b. The recommended dose of epinephrine is 1 mg IV push every 3–5 min. If this approach fails, several Class IIb dosing regimens can be considered:
• Intermediate: epinephrine 2–5 mg IV push, every 3–5 min
• Escalating: epinephrine 1 mg–3 mg–5 mg IV push, 3 min apart
• High: epinephrine 0.1 mg/kg IV push, every 3–5 min
c. Sodium bicarbonate 1 mEq/kg is Class I if patient has known preexisting hyperkalemia.
d. The shorter atropine dosing interval (3 min) is Class IIb in asystolic arrest.
e. Sodium bicarbonate 1 mEq/kg:
Class IIa
• If known preexisting bicarbonate-responsive acidosis
• If overdose with tricyclic antidepressants
• To alkalinize the urine in drug overdoses
Class IIb
• If intubated and continued long arrest interval
• Upon return of spontaneous circulation after long arrest interval
Class III
• Hypoxic lactic acidosis
f. If patient remains in asystole or other agonal rhythm after successful intubation and initial medications and no reversible causes are identified, consider termination of resuscitative efforts by a physician. Consider interval since arrest.

Figure A-5 *Journal of the American Medical Association (JAMA),* October 28, 1992. Volume 268, Number 16 (pages 2171–2302). Copyright 1992, American Medical Association. Reproduced with permission.

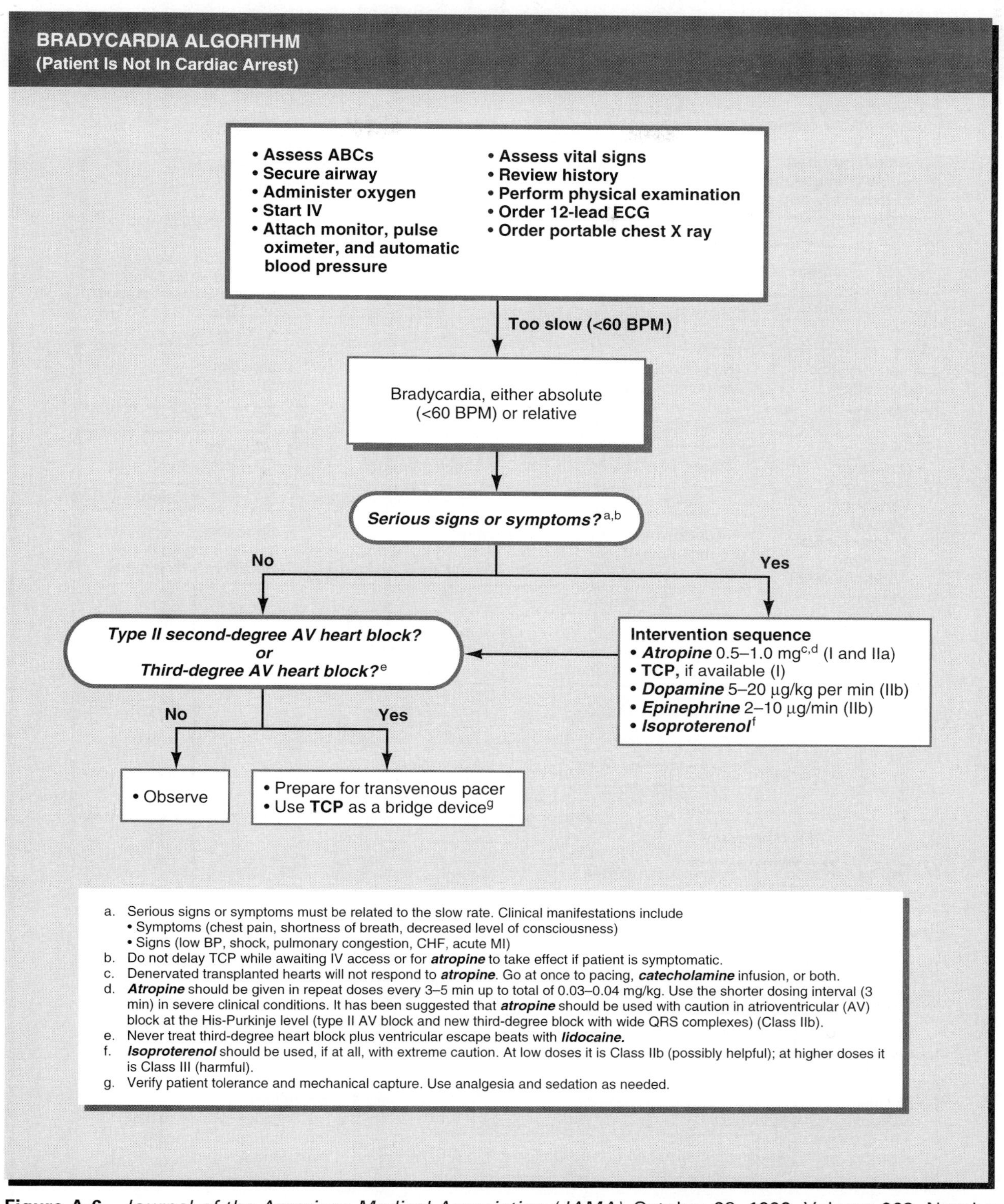

BRADYCARDIA ALGORITHM
(Patient Is Not In Cardiac Arrest)
• Assess ABCs
• Secure airway
• Administer oxygen
• Start IV
• Attach monitor, pulse oximeter, and automatic blood pressure
• Assess vital signs
• Review history
• Perform physical examination
• Order 12-lead ECG
• Order portable chest X ray
Too slow (<60 BPM)
Bradycardia, either absolute (<60 BPM) or relative
Serious signs or symptoms?[a,b]
No
Yes
Type II second-degree AV heart block? or Third-degree AV heart block?[e]
Intervention sequence
• Atropine 0.5–1.0 mg[c,d] (I and IIa)
• TCP, if available (I)
• Dopamine 5–20 μg/kg per min (IIb)
• Epinephrine 2–10 μg/min (IIb)
• Isoproterenol[f]
No
Yes
• Observe
• Prepare for transvenous pacer
• Use TCP as a bridge device[g]
a. Serious signs or symptoms must be related to the slow rate. Clinical manifestations include
• Symptoms (chest pain, shortness of breath, decreased level of consciousness)
• Signs (low BP, shock, pulmonary congestion, CHF, acute MI)
b. Do not delay TCP while awaiting IV access or for atropine to take effect if patient is symptomatic.
c. Denervated transplanted hearts will not respond to atropine. Go at once to pacing, catecholamine infusion, or both.
d. Atropine should be given in repeat doses every 3–5 min up to total of 0.03–0.04 mg/kg. Use the shorter dosing interval (3 min) in severe clinical conditions. It has been suggested that atropine should be used with caution in atrioventricular (AV) block at the His-Purkinje level (type II AV block and new third-degree block with wide QRS complexes) (Class IIb).
e. Never treat third-degree heart block plus ventricular escape beats with lidocaine.
f. Isoproterenol should be used, if at all, with extreme caution. At low doses it is Class IIb (possibly helpful); at higher doses it is Class III (harmful).
g. Verify patient tolerance and mechanical capture. Use analgesia and sedation as needed.

Figure A-6 *Journal of the American Medical Association (JAMA),* October 28, 1992. Volume 268, Number 16 (pages 2171–2302). Copyright 1992, American Medical Association. Reproduced with permission.

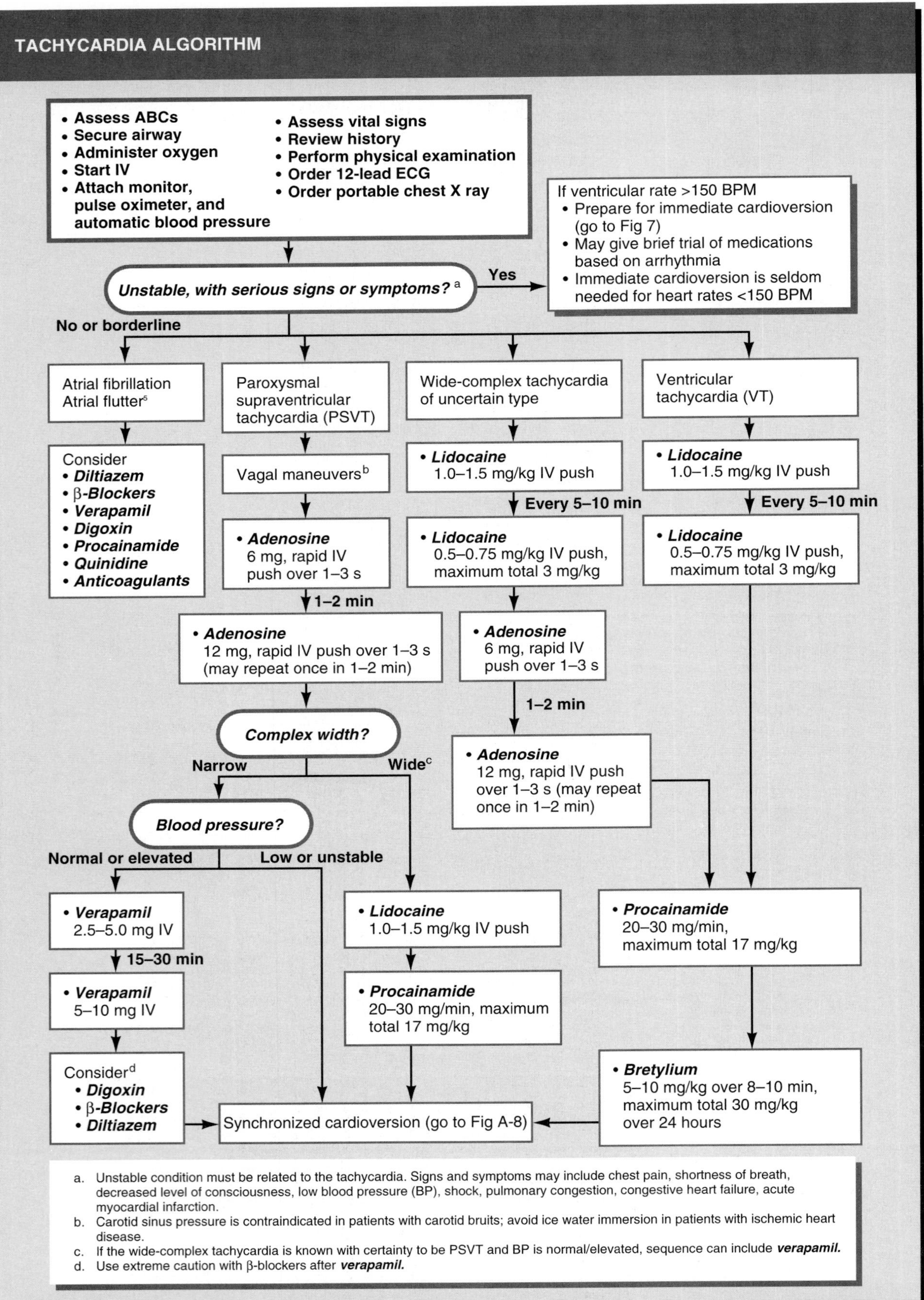
TACHYCARDIA ALGORITHM
• Assess ABCs
• Secure airway
• Administer oxygen
• Start IV
• Attach monitor, pulse oximeter, and automatic blood pressure
• Assess vital signs
• Review history
• Perform physical examination
• Order 12-lead ECG
• Order portable chest X ray
Unstable, with serious signs or symptoms? a
Yes
If ventricular rate >150 BPM
• Prepare for immediate cardioversion (go to Fig 7)
• May give brief trial of medications based on arrhythmia
• Immediate cardioversion is seldom needed for heart rates <150 BPM
No or borderline
Atrial fibrillation
Atrial flutter5
Consider
• Diltiazem
• β-Blockers
• Verapamil
• Digoxin
• Procainamide
• Quinidine
• Anticoagulants
Paroxysmal supraventricular tachycardia (PSVT)
Vagal maneuvers b
• Adenosine 6 mg, rapid IV push over 1–3 s
1–2 min
• Adenosine 12 mg, rapid IV push over 1–3 s (may repeat once in 1–2 min)
Complex width?
Narrow
Wide c
Blood pressure?
Normal or elevated
Low or unstable
• Verapamil 2.5–5.0 mg IV
15–30 min
• Verapamil 5–10 mg IV
Consider d
• Digoxin
• β-Blockers
• Diltiazem
Wide-complex tachycardia of uncertain type
• Lidocaine 1.0–1.5 mg/kg IV push
Every 5–10 min
• Lidocaine 0.5–0.75 mg/kg IV push, maximum total 3 mg/kg
• Adenosine 6 mg, rapid IV push over 1–3 s
1–2 min
• Adenosine 12 mg, rapid IV push over 1–3 s (may repeat once in 1–2 min)
Ventricular tachycardia (VT)
• Lidocaine 1.0–1.5 mg/kg IV push
Every 5–10 min
• Lidocaine 0.5–0.75 mg/kg IV push, maximum total 3 mg/kg
• Lidocaine 1.0–1.5 mg/kg IV push
• Procainamide 20–30 mg/min, maximum total 17 mg/kg
• Procainamide 20–30 mg/min, maximum total 17 mg/kg
• Bretylium 5–10 mg/kg over 8–10 min, maximum total 30 mg/kg over 24 hours
Synchronized cardioversion (go to Fig A-8)
a. Unstable condition must be related to the tachycardia. Signs and symptoms may include chest pain, shortness of breath, decreased level of consciousness, low blood pressure (BP), shock, pulmonary congestion, congestive heart failure, acute myocardial infarction.
b. Carotid sinus pressure is contraindicated in patients with carotid bruits; avoid ice water immersion in patients with ischemic heart disease.
c. If the wide-complex tachycardia is known with certainty to be PSVT and BP is normal/elevated, sequence can include verapamil.
d. Use extreme caution with β-blockers after verapamil.

Figure A-7 *Journal of the American Medical Association (JAMA),* October 28, 1992. Volume 268, Number 16 (pages 2171–2302). Copyright 1992, American Medical Association. Reproduced with permission.

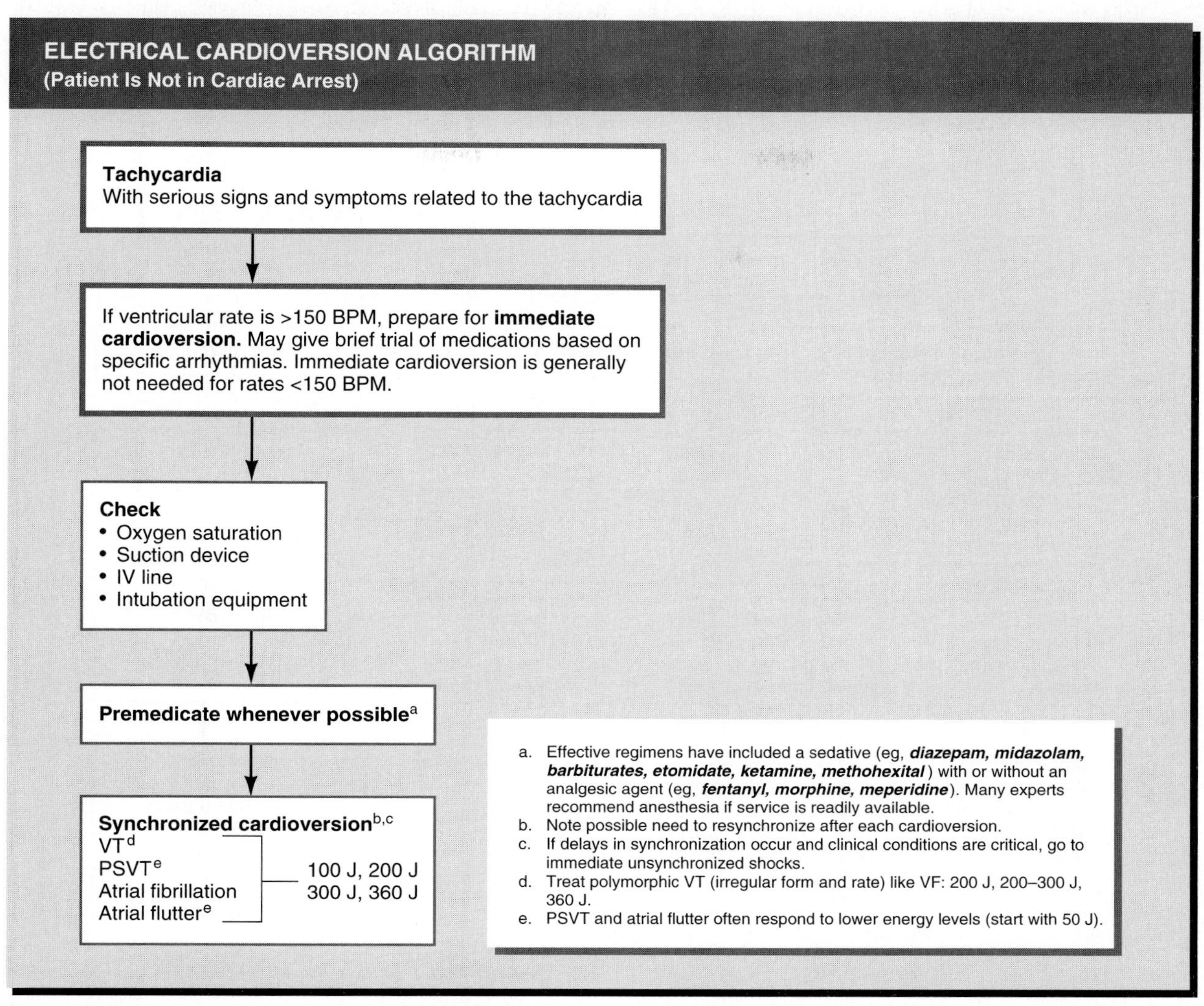

ELECTRICAL CARDIOVERSION ALGORITHM
(Patient Is Not in Cardiac Arrest)
Tachycardia
With serious signs and symptoms related to the tachycardia
If ventricular rate is >150 BPM, prepare for immediate cardioversion. May give brief trial of medications based on specific arrhythmias. Immediate cardioversion is generally not needed for rates <150 BPM.
Check
• Oxygen saturation
• Suction device
• IV line
• Intubation equipment
Premedicate whenever possible[a]
Synchronized cardioversion[b,c]
VT[d]
PSVT[e]
Atrial fibrillation
Atrial flutter[e]
100 J, 200 J
300 J, 360 J
a. Effective regimens have included a sedative (eg, diazepam, midazolam, barbiturates, etomidate, ketamine, methohexital) with or without an analgesic agent (eg, fentanyl, morphine, meperidine). Many experts recommend anesthesia if service is readily available.
b. Note possible need to resynchronize after each cardioversion.
c. If delays in synchronization occur and clinical conditions are critical, go to immediate unsynchronized shocks.
d. Treat polymorphic VT (irregular form and rate) like VF: 200 J, 200–300 J, 360 J.
e. PSVT and atrial flutter often respond to lower energy levels (start with 50 J).

Figure A-8 *Journal of the American Medical Association (JAMA),* October 28, 1992. Volume 268, Number 16 (pages 2171–2302). Copyright 1992, American Medical Association. Reproduced with permission.

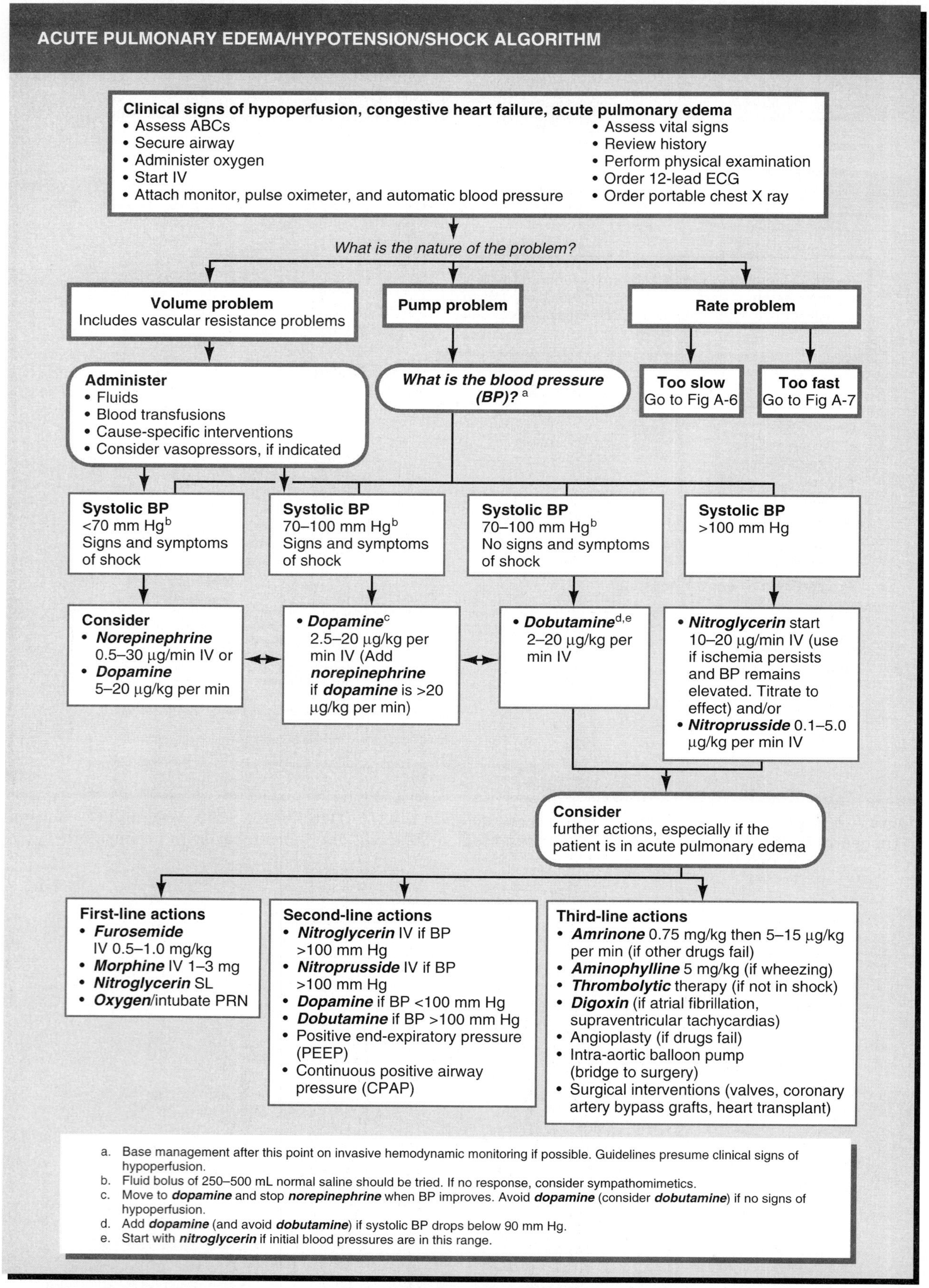

ACUTE PULMONARY EDEMA/HYPOTENSION/SHOCK ALGORITHM

Clinical signs of hypoperfusion, congestive heart failure, acute pulmonary edema

- Assess ABCs
- Secure airway
- Administer oxygen
- Start IV
- Attach monitor, pulse oximeter, and automatic blood pressure
- Assess vital signs
- Review history
- Perform physical examination
- Order 12-lead ECG
- Order portable chest X ray

What is the nature of the problem?

Volume problem
Includes vascular resistance problems

Administer
- Fluids
- Blood transfusions
- Cause-specific interventions
- Consider vasopressors, if indicated

Pump problem

What is the blood pressure (BP)? [a]

Rate problem

Too slow
Go to Fig A-6

Too fast
Go to Fig A-7

Systolic BP
<70 mm Hg[b]
Signs and symptoms of shock

Consider
- ***Norepinephrine*** 0.5–30 μg/min IV or
- ***Dopamine*** 5–20 μg/kg per min

Systolic BP
70–100 mm Hg[b]
Signs and symptoms of shock

- ***Dopamine***[c] 2.5–20 μg/kg per min IV (Add ***norepinephrine*** if ***dopamine*** is >20 μg/kg per min)

Systolic BP
70–100 mm Hg[b]
No signs and symptoms of shock

- ***Dobutamine***[d,e] 2–20 μg/kg per min IV

Systolic BP
>100 mm Hg

- ***Nitroglycerin*** start 10–20 μg/min IV (use if ischemia persists and BP remains elevated. Titrate to effect) and/or
- ***Nitroprusside*** 0.1–5.0 μg/kg per min IV

Consider
further actions, especially if the patient is in acute pulmonary edema

First-line actions
- ***Furosemide*** IV 0.5–1.0 mg/kg
- ***Morphine*** IV 1–3 mg
- ***Nitroglycerin*** SL
- ***Oxygen***/intubate PRN

Second-line actions
- ***Nitroglycerin*** IV if BP >100 mm Hg
- ***Nitroprusside*** IV if BP >100 mm Hg
- ***Dopamine*** if BP <100 mm Hg
- ***Dobutamine*** if BP >100 mm Hg
- Positive end-expiratory pressure (PEEP)
- Continuous positive airway pressure (CPAP)

Third-line actions
- ***Amrinone*** 0.75 mg/kg then 5–15 μg/kg per min (if other drugs fail)
- ***Aminophylline*** 5 mg/kg (if wheezing)
- ***Thrombolytic*** therapy (if not in shock)
- ***Digoxin*** (if atrial fibrillation, supraventricular tachycardias)
- Angioplasty (if drugs fail)
- Intra-aortic balloon pump (bridge to surgery)
- Surgical interventions (valves, coronary artery bypass grafts, heart transplant)

a. Base management after this point on invasive hemodynamic monitoring if possible. Guidelines presume clinical signs of hypoperfusion.
b. Fluid bolus of 250–500 mL normal saline should be tried. If no response, consider sympathomimetics.
c. Move to ***dopamine*** and stop ***norepinephrine*** when BP improves. Avoid ***dopamine*** (consider ***dobutamine***) if no signs of hypoperfusion.
d. Add ***dopamine*** (and avoid ***dobutamine***) if systolic BP drops below 90 mm Hg.
e. Start with ***nitroglycerin*** if initial blood pressures are in this range.

Figure A-9 *Journal of the American Medical Association (JAMA)*, October 28, 1992. Volume 268, Number 16 (pages 2171–2302).

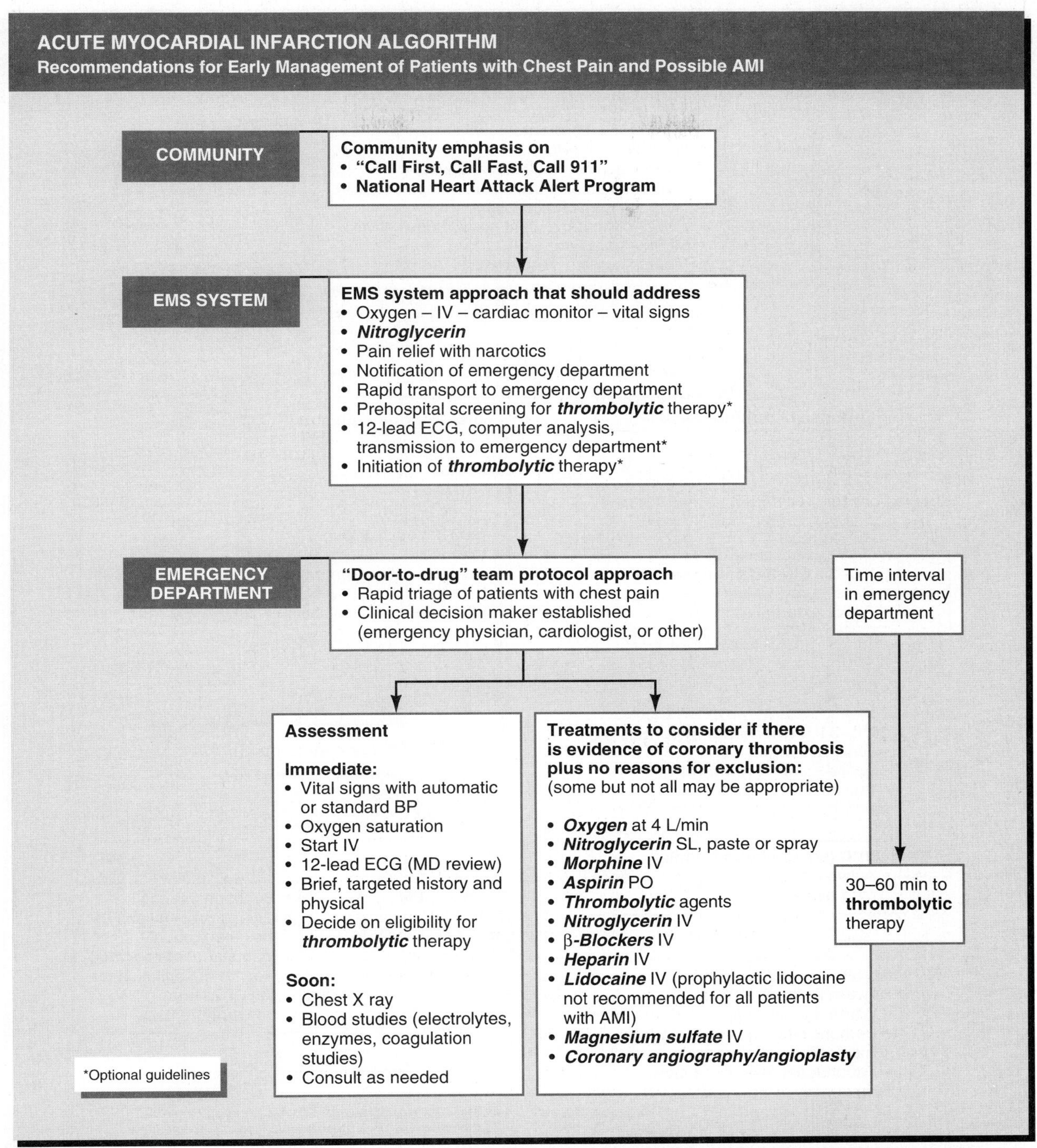

ACUTE MYOCARDIAL INFARCTION ALGORITHM
Recommendations for Early Management of Patients with Chest Pain and Possible AMI
COMMUNITY
Community emphasis on
• "Call First, Call Fast, Call 911"
• National Heart Attack Alert Program
EMS SYSTEM
EMS system approach that should address
• Oxygen – IV – cardiac monitor – vital signs
• Nitroglycerin
• Pain relief with narcotics
• Notification of emergency department
• Rapid transport to emergency department
• Prehospital screening for thrombolytic therapy*
• 12-lead ECG, computer analysis, transmission to emergency department*
• Initiation of thrombolytic therapy*
EMERGENCY DEPARTMENT
"Door-to-drug" team protocol approach
• Rapid triage of patients with chest pain
• Clinical decision maker established (emergency physician, cardiologist, or other)
Time interval in emergency department
Assessment
Immediate:
• Vital signs with automatic or standard BP
• Oxygen saturation
• Start IV
• 12-lead ECG (MD review)
• Brief, targeted history and physical
• Decide on eligibility for thrombolytic therapy
Soon:
• Chest X ray
• Blood studies (electrolytes, enzymes, coagulation studies)
• Consult as needed
Treatments to consider if there is evidence of coronary thrombosis plus no reasons for exclusion:
(some but not all may be appropriate)
• Oxygen at 4 L/min
• Nitroglycerin SL, paste or spray
• Morphine IV
• Aspirin PO
• Thrombolytic agents
• Nitroglycerin IV
• β-Blockers IV
• Heparin IV
• Lidocaine IV (prophylactic lidocaine not recommended for all patients with AMI)
• Magnesium sulfate IV
• Coronary angiography/angioplasty
30–60 min to thrombolytic therapy
*Optional guidelines

Figure A-10 *Journal of the American Medical Association (JAMA),* October 28, 1992. Volume 268, Number 16 (pages 2171–2302). Copyright 1992, American Medical Association. Reproduced with permission.

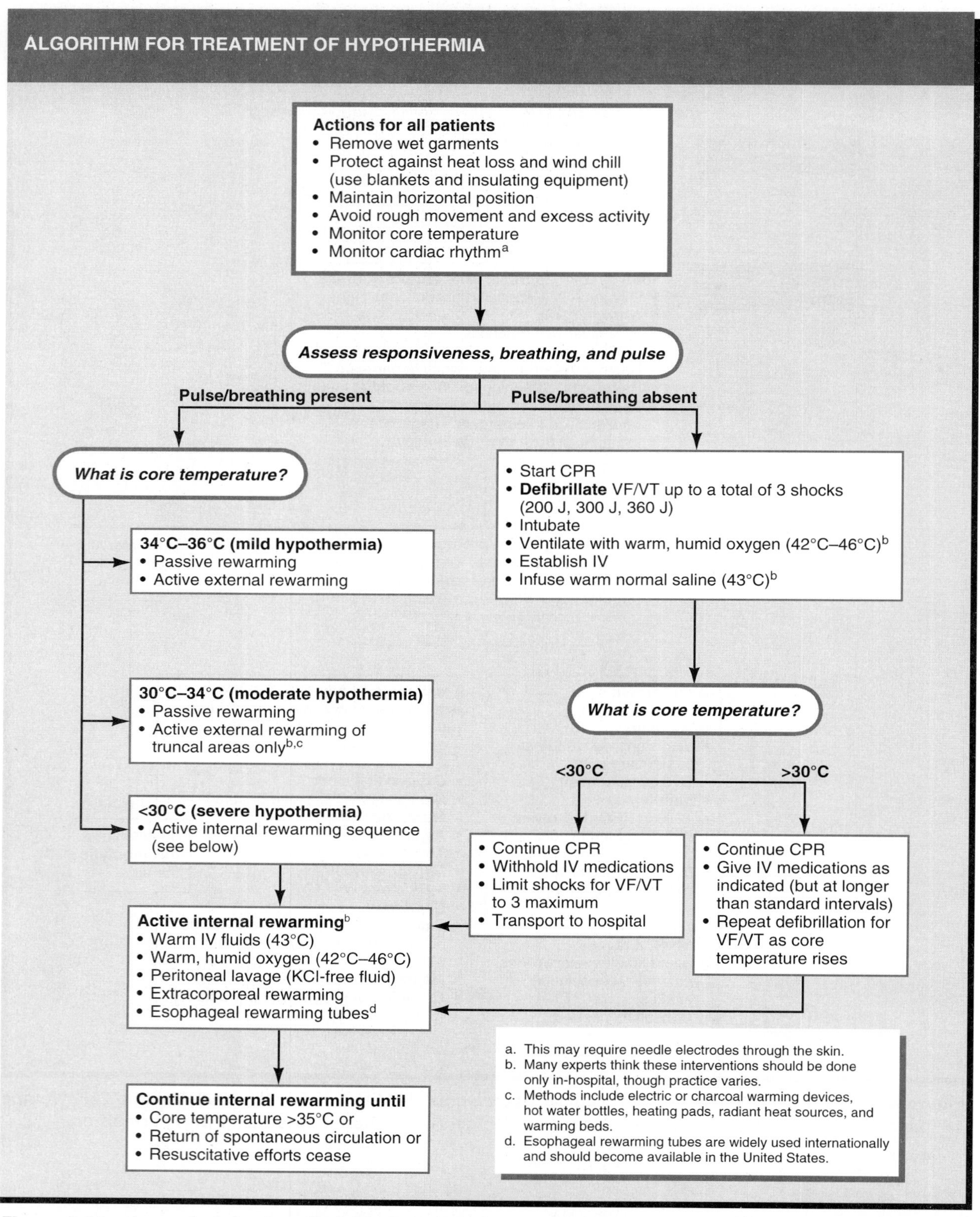
ALGORITHM FOR TREATMENT OF HYPOTHERMIA
Actions for all patients
• Remove wet garments
• Protect against heat loss and wind chill (use blankets and insulating equipment)
• Maintain horizontal position
• Avoid rough movement and excess activity
• Monitor core temperature
• Monitor cardiac rhythm[a]
Assess responsiveness, breathing, and pulse
Pulse/breathing present
Pulse/breathing absent
What is core temperature?
34°C–36°C (mild hypothermia)
• Passive rewarming
• Active external rewarming
30°C–34°C (moderate hypothermia)
• Passive rewarming
• Active external rewarming of truncal areas only[b,c]
<30°C (severe hypothermia)
• Active internal rewarming sequence (see below)
• Start CPR
• Defibrillate VF/VT up to a total of 3 shocks (200 J, 300 J, 360 J)
• Intubate
• Ventilate with warm, humid oxygen (42°C–46°C)[b]
• Establish IV
• Infuse warm normal saline (43°C)[b]
What is core temperature?
<30°C
>30°C
• Continue CPR
• Withhold IV medications
• Limit shocks for VF/VT to 3 maximum
• Transport to hospital
• Continue CPR
• Give IV medications as indicated (but at longer than standard intervals)
• Repeat defibrillation for VF/VT as core temperature rises
Active internal rewarming[b]
• Warm IV fluids (43°C)
• Warm, humid oxygen (42°C–46°C)
• Peritoneal lavage (KCl-free fluid)
• Extracorporeal rewarming
• Esophageal rewarming tubes[d]
Continue internal rewarming until
• Core temperature >35°C or
• Return of spontaneous circulation or
• Resuscitative efforts cease
a. This may require needle electrodes through the skin.
b. Many experts think these interventions should be done only in-hospital, though practice varies.
c. Methods include electric or charcoal warming devices, hot water bottles, heating pads, radiant heat sources, and warming beds.
d. Esophageal rewarming tubes are widely used internationally and should become available in the United States.

Figure A-11 *Journal of the American Medical Association (JAMA),* October 28, 1992. Volume 268, Number 16 (pages 2171–2302). Copyright 1992, American Medical Association. Reproduced with permission.

appendix B

Emergency IV Fluids Quick Reference Guide

Plasma Protein Fraction (Plasmanate)

Class: Protein colloid

Action: Plasma volume expander

Indication: Hypovolemic states (especially burn shock)

Contraindications: None when used in the management of lifethreatening situations

Precautions: Hypertension
Short shelf life

Side Effect: Edema

Dosage: Dosage should be titrated according to patient's hemodynamic response; follow accepted resuscitation formulas in the management of burn shock

Route: IV infusion

Pediatric Dosage: Same as adult

Dextran

Class: Imitation protein (sugar) colloid

Action: Plasma volume expander

Indication: Hypovolemic shock

Contraindications: Patients with known hypersensitivity to the drug
Patients receiving anticoagulants

Precautions: Severe anaphylactic reactions have been known to occur
Monitor for circulatory overload
Can impede accurate blood typing as dextran molecule coats the erythrocytes; draw tube of blood for blood typing before administering Dextran

Side Effects: Nausea
Vomiting

Dosage: Dosage should be titrated according to patient's hemodynamic response

Route: IV infusion

Pediatric Dosage: Same as adult

Hetastarch (Hespan)

Class: Artificial colloid

Action: Plasma volume expander

Indication: Hypovolemic shock

Contraindication: Patients receiving anticoagulants

Precautions: Monitor for circulatory overload
Large volumes of hetastarch may alter the coagulation mechanism

Side Effects: Nausea
Vomiting

Dosage: Dosage should be titrated according to patient's hemodynamic response

Route: IV infusion

Pediatric Dosage: Safety in children has not been established

Lactated Ringer's

Class: Isotonic crystalloid

Action: Approximates the electrolyte concentration of the blood

Indication: Hypovolemic shock

Contraindications: Congestive heart failure
Renal failure

Precaution: Monitor for circulatory overload

Side Effects: Rare

Dosage: *Hypovolemic Shock (systolic less than 90 mmHg)*
Infuse "wide open" until a systolic of 100 mmHg is attained; once a systolic of 100 mmHg has been attained, infusion should be slowed to 100 ml/hr

Other

As indicated by the patient's condition and situation being treated

Route: IV infusion

Pediatric Dosage: 20 ml/kg repeated as required based on hemodynamic response

5% Dextrose in Water (D_5W)

Class: Sugar solution

Action: Glucose nutrient solution

Indications: IV access for emergency drugs
For dilution of concentrated drugs for IV infusion

Contraindication: Should not be used as a fluid replacement for hypovolemic states

Precautions: Monitor for circulatory overload
Draw tube of blood before administering to diabetics

Side Effects: Rare

Dosage: Generally administered TKO

Route: IV infusion

Pediatric Dosage: Same as adult

10% Dextrose in Water ($D_{10}W$)

Class: Hypertonic sugar solution

Action: Replaces blood glucose

Indications: Hypoglycemia
Neonatal resuscitation

Contraindication: Should not be used as fluid replacement for hypovolemic states

Precautions: Monitor for circulatory overload
Draw tube of blood before administering $D_{10}W$ to diabetics

Side Effects: Rare

Dosage: Dependent on patient's condition and condition being treated

Route: IV infusion

Pediatric Dosage: Same as adult

0.9% Sodium Chloride (Normal Saline)

Class: Isotonic electrolyte

Action: Fluid and sodium replacement

Indications:	Heat-related problems (heat exhaustion and heat stroke) Freshwater drowning Hypovolemia Diabetic ketoacidosis
Contraindication:	Congestive heart failure
Precaution:	Electrolyte depletion (K^+, Mg^{++}, Ca^{++}, among others) can occur following administration of large amounts of normal saline
Side Effect:	Thirst
Dosage:	Dependent on patient's condition and situation being treated; in freshwater drowning and heat emergencies, the administration is usually rapid
Route:	IV infusion
Pediatric Dosage:	Dose is dependent on patient's size and condition

0.45% Sodium Chloride (1/2 Normal Saline)

Class:	Hypotonic electrolyte
Action:	Slow rehydration
Indications:	Patients with diminished renal or cardiovascular function for which rapid rehydration is not indicated
Contraindications:	Cases in which rapid rehydration is indicated
Precaution:	Electrolyte depletion can occur following administration of large amounts of 1/2 normal saline
Side Effects:	Rare
Dosage:	Dependent on patient's condition and situation being treated
Route:	IV infusion
Pediatric Dosage:	Dose is based on patient's size and condition

5% Dextrose in 0.9% Sodium Chloride (D_5NS)

Class:	Hypertonic sugar and electrolyte solution
Action:	Provides electrolyte and sugar replacement
Indications:	Heat-related disorders Freshwater drowning Hypovolemia Peritonitis
Contraindications:	Should not be administered to patients with impaired renal or cardiovascular function
Precaution:	Draw tube of blood before administering to diabetics
Side Effects:	Rare
Dosage:	Dependent on patient's condition and situation being treated

Route: IV infusion
Pediatric Dosage: Dose is dependent on patient's size and condition

5% Dextrose in 0.45% Sodium Chloride ($D_5$1/2NS)

Class: Slightly hypertonic sugar and electrolyte solution
Action: Provides electrolyte and sugar replacement
Indications: Heat exhaustion
Diabetic disorders
For use as a TKO solution in patients with impaired renal or cardiovascular function
Contraindications: Situations in which rapid fluid replacement is indicated
Precaution: Draw tube of blood before administering to diabetics
Side Effects: Rare
Dosage: Dependent on patient's condition and situation being treated
Route: IV infusion
Pediatric Dosage: Dose is dependent on patient's size and condition

5% Dextrose in Lactated Ringer's (D_5LR)

Class: Hypertonic sugar and electrolyte solution
Action: Provides electrolyte and sugar replacement
Indications: Hypovolemic shock
Hemorrhagic shock
Certain cases of acidosis
Contraindications: Should not be administered to patients with decreased renal or cardiovascular function
Precautions: Monitor for signs of circulatory overload
Draw tube of blood before administering to diabetics
Side Effects: Rare
Dosage: Dependent on patient's condition and situation being treated
Route: IV infusion
Pediatric Dosage: Dose is dependent on patient's size and condition

appendix C

Quick Drug Reference

INTRODUCTION

This section provides a quick reference to the most commonly used emergency medications. The dosages and indications have been taken from the most recent Advanced Cardiac Life Support (ACLS) standards of the American Heart Association. Drugs not covered in ACLS are taken from the American Medical Association's *Drug Evaluation.* It is important to remember that specific drugs, dosages, indications, and routes may vary in your particular area. It is essential to be familiar with these variations and follow the guidelines established by the medical director of the system in which you work.

Activated Charcoal

Class: Adsorbent

Action: Adsorbs toxins by chemical binding and prevents gastrointestinal adsorption

Indications: Poisoning following emesis or when emesis is contraindicated

Contraindications: None in severe poisoning

Precautions: Should only be administered following emesis in cases in which it is so indicated

	Use with caution in patients with altered mental status May absorb ipecac before emesis; if ipecac is administered, wait at least 10 minutes to administer activated charcoal
Side Effects:	Nausea, vomiting, and constipation
Dosage:	1 g/kg (typically 50–75 grams) mixed with a glass of water to form a slurry
Route:	Oral
Pediatric Dosage:	1 g/kg mixed with a glass of water to form a slurry

Adenosine (Adenocard)

Class:	Antiarrhythmic
Action:	Slows AV conduction
Indication:	Symptomatic PSVT
Contraindications:	Second- or third-degree heart block Sick-sinus syndrome Known hypersensitivity to the drug
Precautions:	Arrhythmias, including blocks, are common at the time of cardioversion Use with caution in patients with asthma
Side Effects:	Facial flushing, headache, shortness of breath, dizziness, and nausea
Dosage:	6 mg given as a rapid IV bolus over a 1–2 second period; if, after 1–2 minutes, cardioversion does not occur, administer a 12-mg dose over 1–2 seconds
Route:	IV; should be administered directly into a vein or into the medication administration port closest to the patient and followed by flushing of the line with IV fluid
Pediatric Dosage:	Safety in children has not been established

Albuterol (Proventil) (Ventolin)

Class:	Sympathomimetic (β_2 selective)
Action:	Bronchodilation
Indications:	Asthma Reversible bronchospasm associated with COPD
Contraindications:	Known hypersensitivity to the drug Symptomatic tachycardia
Precautions:	Blood pressure, pulse, and EKG should be monitored Use caution in patients with known heart disease
Side Effects:	Palpitations, anxiety, headache, dizziness, and sweating
Dosage:	*Metered-Dose Inhaler* 1–2 sprays (90 micrograms per spray) *Small-Volume Nebulizer* 0.5 ml (2.5 mg) in 2.5 ml normal saline over 5–15 minutes

Rotohaler
One 200-microgram Rotocap should be placed in the inhaler and breathed by the patient

Route: Inhalation

Pediatric Dosage: 0.15 mg (0.03 ml)/kg in 2.5 ml normal saline by small-volume nebulizer

Aminophylline

Class: Xanthine bronchodilator

Actions:
Smooth muscle relaxant
Causes bronchodilation
Has mild diuretic properties
Increases heart rate

Indications:
Bronchial asthma
Reversible bronchospasm associated with chronic bronchitis and emphysema
Congestive heart failure
Pulmonary edema

Contraindications:
Patients with history of hypersensitivity to the drug
Hypotension
Patients with peptic ulcer disease

Precautions:
Monitor for arrhythmias
Monitor blood pressure
Do not administer to patients on chronic theophylline preparations until the theophylline blood level has been determined

Side Effects:
Convulsions, tremor, anxiety, and dizziness
Vomiting, palpitations, PVCs, and tachycardia

Dosages:
Method 1
250–500 mg in 90 or 80 ml of D_5W, respectively, infused over 20–30 minutes (approximately 5–10 mg/kg/hr)
Method 2
250–500 mg (5–7 mg/kg) in 20 ml of D_5W infused over 20–30 minutes

Route: Slow IV infusion

Pediatric Dosage: 6 mg/kg loading dose to be infused over 20–30 minutes; maximum dose not to exceed 12 mg/kg per 24 hours

Amrinone (Inocor)

Class: Cardiac inotrope

Actions:
Increases cardiac contractility
Vasodilator

Indication: Short-term management of severe congestive heart failure

Contraindication: Patients with history of hypersensitivity to the drug

Precautions:	May increase myocardial ischemia Blood pressure, pulse, and EKG should be constantly monitored Amrinone should only be diluted with normal saline or 1/2 normal saline; no dextrose solutions should be used Furosemide (Lasix) should not be administered into an IV line delivering amrinone
Side Effects:	Reduction in platelets Nausea and vomiting Cardiac arrhythmias
Dosage:	0.75 mg/kg bolus given slowly over 2–5 minute interval followed by maintenance infusion of 2–15 μg/kg minute
Route:	IV bolus and infusion as described earlier
Pediatric Dosage:	Safety in children has not been established

Amyl Nitrite

Class:	Nitrate
Actions:	Causes coronary vasodilation Removes cyanide-ion via complex mechanism
Indication:	Cyanide poisoning (bitter almond smell to breath)
Contraindications:	None when used in the management of cyanide poisoning
Precautions:	Hypotension common Has tendency for abuse
Side Effects:	Headache Hypotension, reflex tachycardia Nausea
Dosage:	Inhalant should be broken and inhaled, repeated as needed until patient is delivered to emergency department; effects diminish after 20 minutes
Route:	Inhalation
Pediatric Dosage:	Inhalant should be broken and inhaled, repeated until patient is delivered to emergency department

Anistreplase (Eminase)

Class:	Thrombolytic
Action:	Dissolves blood clots
Indication:	Acute MI
Contraindications:	Persons with internal bleeding Suspected aortic dissection Traumatic CPR Severe persistent hypertension Recent head trauma or known intracranial tumor History of stroke in the last 6 months Pregnancy

Precautions: May be ineffective if administered within 12 months of prior streptokinase of anistreplase therapy
Antiarrhythmic and resuscitative drugs should be available

Side Effects: Bleeding
Allergic reactions
Anaphylaxis
Fever
Nausea and vomiting

Dosage: 30 units slow IV over 2–5 minutes

Route: IV (slow)

Pediatric Dosage: Not recommended

Aspirin

Class: Platelet inhibitor/Anti-inflammatory

Action: Blocks platelet aggregation

Indications: New chest pain suggestive of acute MI
Signs and symptoms suggestive of recent stroke (CVA)

Contraindications: Patients with known hypersensitivity to the drug

Precautions: GI bleeding and upset

Side Effects: Heartburn
Nausea and vomiting
Wheezing

Dosage: 160 or 325 mg PO or chewed

Route: PO

Pediatric Dosage: Not recommended

Atropine

Class: Parasympatholytic (anticholinergic)

Actions: Blocks acetylcholine receptors
Increases heart rate
Decreases gastrointestinal secretions

Indications: Hemodynamically-significant bradycardia
Hypotension secondary to bradycardia
Asystole
Organophosphate poisoning

Contraindication: None when used in emergency situations

Precautions: Dose of 0.04 mg/kg should not be exceeded except in cases of organophosphate poisonings
Tachycardia
Hypertension

Side Effects: Palpitations and tachycardia
Headache, dizziness, and anxiety

Dry mouth, pupillary dilation, and blurred vision
Urinary retention (especially older males)

Dosage:
Bradycardia
0.5 mg every 3–5 minutes to maximum of 0.04 mg/kg
Asystole
1 mg
Organophosphate Poisoning
2–5 mg

Routes:
IV
Endotracheal (endotracheal dose 2 to 2.5 times IV dose)

Pediatric Dosage:
Bradycardia
0.02 mg/kg (minimum dose of 0.1 mg)
Maximum single dose (child 0.5 mg) (adolescent 1.0 mg)
Maximum total dose (child 1.0 mg) (adolescent 2.0 mg)

Bretylium (Bretylol)

Class:
Antiarrhythmic

Actions:
Increases ventricular fibrillation threshold
Blocks the release of norepinephrine from peripheral sympathetic nerves

Indications:
Ventricular fibrillation refractory to lidocaine
Ventricular tachycardia refractory to lidocaine
PVCs refractory to first-line medications

Contraindications:
None when used in the management of lifethreatening arrhythmias

Precautions:
Postural hypotension occurs in approximately 50 percent of patients receiving Bretylium
Patient must be kept supine
Decrease dosage in patients being treated with catecholamine sympathomimetics

Side Effects:
Hypotension, syncope, and bradycardia
Increased frequency of arrhythmias
Dizziness and vertigo

Dosage:
5 mg/kg. May be repeated at dose of 10 mg/kg up to a total dose of 30 mg/kg

Route:
Rapid IV bolus

Pediatric Dosage:
5 mg/kg

Bumetanide (Bumex)

Class:
Potent diuretic

Actions:
Inhibits reabsorption of sodium chloride
Promotes prompt diuresis
Slight vasodilation

Indications: Congestive heart failure
Pulmonary edema

Contraindications: Dehydration
Pregnancy

Precautions: Should be protected from light
Dehydration

Side Effects: Few in emergency usage

Dosage: 0.5–1.0 mg

Routes: IV
IM

Pediatric Dosage: Safety in children has not been established

Butorphanol (Stadol)

Class: Synthetic analgesic

Actions: Central nervous system depressant
Decreases sensitivity to pain
2 mg Stadol equivalent to 10 mg morphine

Indication: Moderate to severe pain

Contraindications: Patients with a history of hypersensitivity to the drug
Head injury
Use with caution in patients with impaired respiratory function

Precautions: Respiratory depression (naloxone should be available)
Patients dependent on narcotics

Side Effects: May experience symptoms of withdrawal when administered to persons dependent on narcotics
Nausea
Altered levels of consciousness

Dosage: *IV*
1 mg
IM
2 mg

Routes: IV
IM

Pediatric Dosage: Rarely used

Calcium Chloride

Class: Electrolyte

Action: Increases cardiac contractility

Indications: Acute hyperkalemia (elevated potassium)
Acute hypocalcemia (decreased calcium)

Calcium channel blocker (nifedipine, verapamil, etc.) overdose
Abdominal muscle spasm associated with spider bite and Portuguese man-o-war stings
Antidote for magnesium sulfate

Contraindication: Patients receiving digitalis

Precautions: IV line should be flushed between calcium chloride and sodium bicarbonate administration
Extravasation may cause tissue necrosis

Side Effects: Arrhythmias (bradycardia and asystole)
Hypotension

Dosage: 2–4 mg/kg of a 10% solution; may be repeated at 10-minute intervals

Route: IV

Pediatric Dosage: 5–7 mg/kg of a 10% solution

Chlorpromazine (Thorazine)

Class: Major tranquilizer

Actions: Blocks dopamine receptors in brain associated with mood and behavior
Has antiemetic properties

Indications: Acute psychotic episodes
Mild alcohol withdrawal
Intractable hiccoughs
Nausea and vomiting

Contraindications: Comatose states
Should not be administered in the presence of sedatives
Should not be administered in the presence of hallucinogens or phencyclidine-like compounds

Precautions: Orthostatic hypotension
May cause extrapyramidal reactions (Parkinson-like), especially in children

Side Effects: Physical and mental impairment
Drowsiness

Dosage: 25–100 mg

Route: IM

Pediatric Dosage: 0.5 mg/kg

Dexamethasone (Decadron, Hexadrol)

Class: Steroid

Actions: Possibly decreases cerebral edema
Anti-inflammatory
Suppresses immune response (especially in allergic reactions)

Indications: Cerebral edema
Anaphylaxis (after epinephrine and diphenhydramine)
Asthma
COPD

Contraindications: None in the emergency setting

Precautions: Should be protected from heat
Onset of action may be 2–6 hours and thus should not be considered to be of use in the critical first hour following an anaphylactic reaction

Side Effects: Gastrointestinal bleeding
Prolonged wound healing

Dosage: 4–24 mg

Routes: IV
IM

Pediatric Dosage: 0.2–0.5 mg/kg

Dextrose (50%)

Class: Carbohydrate

Action: Elevates blood glucose level rapidly

Indication: Hypoglycemia

Contraindications: None in the emergency setting

Precaution: A blood sample should be drawn before administering 50% dextrose

Side Effect: Local venous irritation

Dosage: 25 grams (50 ml)

Route: IV

Pediatric Dosage: 0.5 g/kg slow IV; should be diluted 1:1 with sterile water to form a 25% solution

Diazepam (Valium)

Class: Tranquilizer

Actions: Anticonvulsant
Skeletal muscle relaxant
Sedative

Indications: Major motor seizures
Status epilepticus
Premedication before cardioversion
Skeletal muscle relaxant
Acute anxiety states

Contraindication: Patients with a history of hypersensitivity to the drug

Precautions: Can cause local venous irritation
Has short duration of effect

Do not mix with other drugs because of possible precipitation problems
Flumazenil (Romazicon) should be available

Side Effects: Drowsiness
Hypotension
Respiratory depression, apnea

Dosage: *Status Epilepticus*
5–10 mg IV
Acute Anxiety
2–5 mg IM or IV
Premedication before Cardioversion
5–15 mg IV

Routes: IV (care must be taken not to administer faster than 1 ml/min)
IM
Rectal

Pediatric Dosage: *Status Epilepticus*
0.1–0.2 mg/kg

Diazoxide (Hyperstat)

Class: Antihypertensive

Actions: Causes decrease in both systolic and diastolic pressures
Direct peripheral arterial dilation

Indication: Hypertensive emergency

Contraindications: None in the emergency setting

Precautions: Avoid overcorrection of blood pressure
Blood pressure must be constantly monitored
Patient should be supine

Side Effects: Hypotension
Syncope
Local venous irritation

Dosage: 1–3 mg/kg boluses by rapid injection (less than 30 seconds) repeated at 5–15-minute intervals up to 150 mg in a single injection

Route: IV only

Pediatric Dosage: 1–3 mg/kg

Digoxin (Lanoxin)

Class: Cardiac glycoside

Actions: Increases cardiac contractile force
Increases cardiac output
Reduces edema associated with congestive heart failure
Slows AV conduction

Indications: Congestive heart failure
Rapid atrial arrhythmias, especially atrial flutter and atrial fibrillation

Contraindications: Any patient with signs or symptoms of digitalis toxicity
Ventricular fibrillation

Precautions: Monitor for signs of digitalis toxicity
Patients who have recently suffered a myocardial infarction have greater sensitivity to the effects of digitalis
Calcium should not be administered to patients receiving digitalis

Side Effects: Nausea
Vomiting
Arrhythmias
Yellow vision

Dosage: 0.25–0.50 mg

Route: IV

Pediatric Dosage: 25–40 μ/kg

Diltiazem (Cardizem)

Class: Calcium channel blocker

Actions: Slows conduction through the AV mode
Causes vasodilation
Decreases rate of ventricular response
Decreases myocardial oxygen demand

Indications: To control rapid ventricular rates associated with atrial fibrillation and flutter
Angina pectoris

Contraindications: Hypotension
Wide-complex tachycardia
Conduction system disturbances

Precautions: Should not be used in patients receiving intravenous β-blockers
Hypotension
Diltiazem must be kept refrigerated

Side Effects: Nausea
Vomiting
Hypotension
Dizziness

Dosage: 0.25 mg/kg bolus (typically 20 mg) IV over two minutes. This should be followed by a maintenance infusion of 5–15 mg/hour.

Routes: IV
IV drip

Pediatric Dosage: Rarely used

Dimenhydrinate (Gravol, Dramamine)

Class: Antihistamine

Action: Antiemetic

Indications: Nausea and vomiting
Motion sickness
To potentiate the effects of analgesics

Contraindications: Comatose states
Patients who have received a large amount of depressants (including alcohol)

Precautions: Use with caution in patients with seizure disorders
Asthma

Side Effects: May impair mental and physical ability
Drowsiness

Dosage: 12.5–25.0 mg slow IV
50–100 mg IM or PO

Routes: IV
IM
PO

Pediatric Dosage: Pediatric data unavailable

Diphenhydramine (Benadryl)

Class: Antihistamine

Actions: Blocks histamine receptors
Has some sedative effects

Indications: Anaphylaxis
Allergic reactions
Dystonic reactions due to phenothiazines

Contraindications: Asthma
Nursing mothers

Precautions: Hypotension

Side Effects: Sedation
Dries bronchial secretions
Blurred vision
Headache
Palpitations

Dosage: 25–50 mg

Routes: Slow IV push
Deep IM

Pediatric Dosage: 2–5 mg/kg

Dobutamine (Dobutrex)

Class: Sympathomimetic

Actions: Increases cardiac contractility
Little chronotropic activity

Indication: Short-term management of congestive heart failure

Contraindication: Should only be used in patients with an adequate heart rate

Precautions: Ventricular irritability
Use with caution following myocardial infarction
Can be deactivated by alkaline solutions

Side Effects: Headache
Hypertension
Palpitations

Dosage: 2.5–20 μg/kg/minute
Method
250 mg should be placed in 500 ml of D_5W, which gives a concentration of 0.5 mg/ml

Route: IV drip

Pediatric Dosage: 2–20 μg/kg/min

Dopamine (Intropin)

Class: Sympathomimetic

Actions: Increases cardiac contractility
Causes peripheral vasoconstriction

Indications: Hemodynamically-significant hypotension (systolic blood pressure of 70–100 mmHg) not resulting from hypovolemia
Cardiogenic shock

Contraindications: Hypovolemic shock where complete fluid resuscitation has not occurred
Pheochromocytoma

Precautions: Should not be administered in the presence of severe tachyarrhythmias
Should not be administered in the presence of ventricular fibrillation
Ventricular irritability
Beneficial effects lost when dose exceeds 20 μg/kg/minute

Side Effects: Ventricular tachyarrhythmias
Hypertension
Palpitations

Dosage: 2–5 μ/kg/minute; increase as needed
Method
800 mg should be placed in 500 ml of D_5W giving a concentration of 1600 μg/ml

Route: IV drip only

Pediatric Dosage: 2–20 μg/kg/minute

Edrophonium (Tensilon)

Class: Anticholinesterase

Actions: Inhibits action of enzyme cholinesterase, thus potentiating acetylcholine
Increases parasympathetic tone

Indication:	PSVT refractory to vagal maneuvers; considered a second-line agent to verapamil or adenosine
Contraindication:	Patients with a history of hypersensitivity to the drug
Precautions:	Respirations must be constantly monitored Bradycardia Hypotension Avoid exposure to dextrose solutions
Side Effects:	Dizziness Syncope
Dosage:	5 mg
Route:	IV
Pediatric Dosage:	0.1–0.2 mg/kg

Epinephrine 1:1,000

Class:	Sympathomimetic
Action:	Bronchodilation
Indications:	Bronchial asthma Exacerbation of COPD Allergic reactions Pediatric cardiac arrest (after initial epinephrine dosage)
Contraindications:	Patients with underlying cardiovascular disease Hypertension Pregnancy Patients with tachyarrhythmias
Precautions:	Should be protected from light Blood pressure, pulse, and EKG must be constantly monitored
Side Effects:	Palpitations and tachycardia Anxiousness Headache Tremor
Dosage:	0.3–0.5 mg
Route:	Subcutaneous
Pediatric Dosage:	0.01 mg/kg up to 0.3 mg

Epinephrine 1:10,000

Class:	Sympathomimetic
Actions:	Increases heart rate and automaticity Increases cardiac contractile force Increases myocardial electrical activity Increases systemic vascular resistance Increases blood pressure Causes bronchodilation

Indications: Cardiac arrest
Anaphylactic shock
Severe reactive airway disease

Contraindications: Epinephrine 1:10,000 is for intravenous or endotracheal use; it should not be used in patients who do not require extensive resuscitative efforts

Precautions: Should be protected from light
Can be deactivated by alkaline solutions

Side Effects: Palpitations
Anxiety
Tremulousness
Nausea and vomiting

Dosage: *Cardiac Arrest*
0.5–1.0 mg repeated every 3–5 minutes; higher doses may be ordered by medical control
Severe Anaphylaxis
0.3–0.5 mg (3–5 ml); occasionally an epinephrine drip is required

Routes: IV
IV drip
Endotracheal (endotracheal dose 2 to 2.5 times IV dose)

Pediatric Dosage: 0.01 mg/kg initially. With subsequent doses, epinephrine 1:1,000 should be used at a dose of 0.1 mg/kg.

Esmolol (Brevibloc)

Class: Beta blocker (β_1 selective)

Actions: Decreases heart rate
Decreases AV conduction

Indications: Symptomatic supraventricular tachycardia (including atrial fibrillation and atrial flutter) as evidenced by chest pain, palpitations, or dizziness

Contraindications: Sinus bradycardia
Heart block greater than first degree
Cardiogenic shock
Overt congestive heart failure
Patients with bronchospastic disease (asthma)

Precautions: Hypotension is common, usually dose related
Patients with CHF may have worsening of their symptoms
May worsen bronchospastic disease

Side Effects: Dizziness, diaphoresis, and hypotension
Nausea

Dosage: *Preparation*
Place two 2.5-gram ampules in 500 ml D_5W yielding a concentration of 10 mg/ml
Loading Dose
500 μg/kg/min for 1 minute; then reduce to maintenance dose

Maintenance Dose

50 μg/kg/min; if ineffective after 4 minutes, repeat loading dose and increase maintenance dose to 100 μg/kg/min; may repeat as needed until a total maintenance dose of 200 μg/kg/minute has been achieved

Route: IV infusion only

Pediatric Dosage: Safety in children has not been established

Fentanyl Citrate (Sublimaze)

Class: Narcotic

Actions:
Central nervous system depressant
Decreases sensitivity to pain

Indications:
Severe pain
Adjunct to rapid sequence intubation
Maintenance of analgesia

Contraindications:
Shock
Severe hemorrhage
Undiagnosed abdominal pain
Patients with history of hypersensitivity to the drug

Precautions:
Respiratory depression (naloxone should be available)
Hypotension
Nausea

Side Effects:
Dizziness
Altered level of consciousness
Bradycardia

Dosage: 25–100 μg

Route: IV

Pediatric Dosage:
2–12 years
1.7–3.3 μg/kg

Flumazenil (Romazicon)

Class: Benzodiazepine antagonist

Action: Reverses the effects of benzodiazepines

Indication: To reverse CNS respiratory depression associated with benzodiazepines

Contraindications:
Flumazenil should not be used as a diagnostic agent for benzodiazepine overdose in the same manner naloxone is used for narcotic overdose
Known hypersensitivity to the drug

Precautions: Administer with caution to patients dependent on benzodiazepines as it may induce life-threatening benzodiazepine withdrawal

Side Effects: Fatigue, headache, nervousness, dizziness

Dosage: 0.2 mg IV over 30 seconds; repeated as needed to a maximum dose of 1.0 mg

Route: IV

Pediatric Dosage: Pediatric data unavailable

Furosemide (Lasix)

Class: Potent diuretic

Actions: Inhibits reabsorption of sodium chloride
Promotes prompt diuresis
Vasodilation

Indications: Congestive heart failure
Pulmonary edema

Contraindications: Pregnancy
Dehydration

Precautions: Should be protected from light
Dehydration

Side Effects: Few in emergency usage

Dosage: 40–80 mg

Route: IV

Pediatric Dosage: 1 mg/kg

Glucagon

Class: Hormone (antihypoglycemic agent)

Actions: Causes breakdown of glycogen to glucose
Inhibits glycogen synthesis
Elevates blood glucose level
Increases cardiac contractile force
Increases heart rate

Indication: Hypoglycemia

Contraindication: Hypersensitivity to the drug

Precautions: Only effective if there are sufficient stores of glycogen within the liver
Use with caution in patients with cardiovascular or renal disease
Draw blood glucose before administration

Side Effects: Few in emergency situations

Dosage: 0.25–0.5 unit IV
1.0 mg IM

Routes: IV
IM

Pediatric Dosage: 0.03 mg/kg

Haloperidol (Haldol)

Class: Major tranquilizer

Actions: Blocks dopamine receptors in brain responsible for mood and behavior
Has antiemetic properties

Indication: Acute psychotic episodes

Contraindications: Should not be administered in the presence of other sedatives
Should not be used in the management of dysphoria caused by Talwin

Precaution: Orthostatic hypotension

Side Effects: Physical and mental impairment
Parkinson-like reactions have been known to occur, especially in children

Dosage: 2–5 mg

Route: IM

Pediatric Dosage: Rarely used

Hydralazine (Apresoline)

Class: Antihypertensive (potent vasodilator)

Actions: Relaxes vascular smooth muscle
Decreased arterial pressure (diastolic greater than systolic)
Increases cardiac output

Indications: Hypertensive emergency in which a prompt reduction in blood pressure is required
Hypertension accompanying pregnancy

Contraindications: Patients with a known history of coronary artery disease
Rheumatic heart disease involving the mitral valve
History of hypersensitivity to the drug

Precautions: May induce angina
May cause EKG changes and cardiac ischemia
Blood pressure, pulse rate, and EKG should be constantly monitored

Side Effects: Headache, nausea, vomiting, tachycardia, palpitations, and diarrhea

Dosage: 20–40 mg given by slow IV bolus
May be repeated, if required

Route: IV

Pediatric Dosage: Safety in children has not been established

Hydrocortisone (Solu-Cortef)

Class: Steroid

Actions: Anti-inflammatory
Suppresses immune response (especially in allergic/anaphylactic reactions)

Indications: Severe anaphylaxis
Asthma/COPD
Urticaria (hives)

Contraindications: None in the emergency setting

Precautions: Must be reconstituted and used promptly
Onset of action may be 2–6 hours and thus should not be expected to be of use in the critical first hour following an acute anaphylactic reaction

Side Effects: GI bleeding
Prolonged wound healing
Suppression of natural steroids

Dosage: 100–250 mg

Routes: IV
IM

Pediatric Dosage: 30 μg/kg

Hydroxyzine (Vistaril)

Class: Antihistamine

Actions: Antiemetic
Antihistamine
Antianxiety
Potentiates analgesic effects of narcotics and related agents

Indications: To potentiate the effects of narcotics and synthetic narcotics
Nausea and vomiting
Anxiety reactions

Contraindication: Patients with a history of hypersensitivity to the drug

Precautions: Orthostatic hypotension
Analgesic dosages should be reduced when used with hydroxyzine
Urinary retention

Side Effects: Drowsiness

Dosage: 50–100 mg

Route: Deep IM

Pediatric Dosage: 1 mg/kg

Insulin (Humulin, Novolin, Iletin)

Class: Hormone (hypoglycemic agent)

Actions: Causes uptake of glucose by the cells

	Decreases blood glucose level Promotes glucose storage
Indications:	Elevated blood glucose Diabetic ketoacidosis
Contraindications:	Avoid overcompensation of blood glucose level; if possible, administration should wait until the patient is in the emergency department
Precautions:	Administration of excessive dose may induce hypoglycemia Glucose should be available
Side Effects:	Few in emergency situations
Dosage:	10–25 units regular insulin IV followed by an infusion at 0.1 units/kg/hr
Routes:	IV SQ
Pediatric Dosage:	Dosage is based on blood glucose level

Ipecac

Class:	Emetic
Actions:	Irritates the enteric tract Acts on vomiting center in the brain
Indication:	Poisoning in conscious patient
Contraindications:	Vomiting should not be induced in any patient with impaired consciousness Poisonings involving strong acids, bases, or petroleum distillates Antiemetic poisonings, especially of the phenothiazine type
Precautions:	Monitor and assure a patent airway The risk of aspiration is increased when using ipecac
Side Effects:	Rare
Dosage:	30 ml (1 ounce) followed by 15 ml/kg of warm water
Route:	Oral
Pediatric Dosage:	*Less than 1 Year of Age* 10 ml *1–12 Years of Age* 15 ml *Greater Than 12 Years of Age* 30 ml

Ipratropium (Atrovent)

Class:	Anticholinergic
Actions:	Causes bronchodilation Dries respiratory tract secretions

Indications: Bronchial asthma
Reversible bronchospasm associated with chronic bronchitis and emphysema

Contraindications: Should not be used in patients with history of hypersensitivity to the drug
Should not be used as primary acute treatment of bronchospasm

Precautions: Monitor vital signs

Side Effects: Palpitations
Dizziness
Anxiety
Headache
Nervousness

Dosage: 500 μg placed in small-volume nebulizer (typically administered with a β agonist)

Route: Inhaled

Pediatric Dosage: Safety in children has not been established

Isoetharine (Bronkosol)

Class: Sympathomimetic (β_2 selective)

Actions: Bronchodilation
Increases heart rate

Indications: Asthma
Reversible bronchospasm associated with chronic bronchitis and emphysema

Contraindication: Patients with history of hypersensitivity to the drug

Precautions: Blood pressure, pulse, and EKG must be constantly monitored

Side Effects: Palpitations, tachycardia
Anxiety and tremors
Headache

Dosage: *Hand Nebulizer*
Four inhalations
Small-Volume Nebulizer
0.5 ml (1:3 with saline)

Route: Inhalation only

Pediatric Dosage: 0.25–0.5 ml diluted with 4 ml normal saline

Isoproterenol (Isuprel)

Class: Sympathomimetic

Actions: Increases heart rate
Increases cardiac contractile force
Causes bronchodilation

Indications: Bradycardias refractory to atropine (when transcutaneous pacing is unavailable)
Severe status asthmaticus

Contraindication: Should not be used to increase blood pressure in cardiogenic shock

Precautions: Can cause ventricular irritability
Can be deactivated by alkaline solutions
Should be used with caution for recent myocardial infarction
External pacing, if available, should be used instead of isoproterenol

Side Effects: Tachyarrhythmias and tremor
Palpitations and headache

Dosage: 1 mg should be placed in 500 ml of D_5W. This should then be slowly infused at 2–10 μg/min and titrated until the desired rate is obtained or until PVCs occur.

Route: IV drip only

Pediatric Dosage: 0.1 μg/kg/minute

Ketorolac (Toradol)

Class: Non-steroidal anti-inflammatory agent

Actions: Anti-inflammatory
Analgesic (peripherally acting)

Indication: Mild to moderate pain

Contraindications: Patients with a history of hypersensitivity to the drug
Patients allergic to aspirin

Precautions: GI irritation or hemorrhage can occur

Side Effects: Edema
Rash
Heartburn

Dosage: *IV*
15–30 mg
IM
30–60 mg

Routes: IV
IM

Pediatric Dosage: Rarely used

Labetalol (Trandate) (Normodyne)

Class: Sympathetic blocker

Actions: Selectively blocks α_1 receptors and nonselectively blocks β receptors

Indication: Hypertensive crisis

Contraindications: Bronchial asthma
Congestive heart failure
Heart block
Bradycardia
Cardiogenic shock

Precautions: Blood pressure, pulse, and EKG must be constantly monitored
Atropine should be available

Side Effects: Bradycardia
Heart block
Congestive heart failure
Bronchospasm
Postural hypotension

Dosage: 20 mg by slow IV infusion over 2 minutes; doses of 40 mg can be repeated in 10 minutes until desired supine blood pressure is obtained or until 300 mg of the drug has been given
200 mg placed in 500 ml D_5W to deliver 2 mg/minute

Route: IV infusion or slow IV bolus as described earlier

Pediatric Dosage: Safety in children has not been established

Lidocaine (Xylocaine)

Class: Antiarrhythmic

Actions: Suppresses ventricular ectopic activity
Increases ventricular fibrillation threshold
Reduces velocity of electrical impulse through conductive system

Indications: Malignant PVCs
Ventricular tachycardia
Ventricular fibrillation
Prophylaxis of arrhythmias associated with thrombolytic therapy

Contraindications: High-degree heart blocks
PVCs in conjunction with bradycardia

Precautions: Dosage should not exceed 300 mg/hr
Monitor for central nervous system toxicity
Dosage should be reduced by 50% in patients older than 70 years of age or who have liver disease
In cardiac arrest, use only bolus therapy

Side Effects: Anxiety, drowsiness, dizziness, and confusion
Nausea and vomiting
Convulsions
Widening of QRS

Dosage: *Bolus*
Initial bolus of 1.0–1.5 mg/kg; additional boluses of 0.5–0.75 mg/kg can be repeated at 3–5 minute intervals until the arrhythmia has been suppressed or until 3.0 mg/kg of the drug has been administered; reduce dosage by 50% in patients older than 70 years of age

Drip

After the arrhythmia has been suppressed, a 2–4 mg/minute infusion may be started to maintain adequate blood levels

Routes: IV bolus
IV infusion

Pediatric Dosage: 1 mg/kg

Lorazepam (Ativan)

Class: Tranquilizer

Actions: Anticonvulsant
Sedative

Indications: Major motor seizures
Status epilepticus
Premedication before cardioversion
Acute anxiety states

Contraindication: Patients with a history of hypersensitivity to the drug

Precautions: Has short duration of effect
Do not mix with other drugs because of possible precipitation problems
Flumazenil (Romazicon) should be available
Dilute with normal saline of D_5W prior to intravenous administration

Side Effects: Drowsiness
Hypotension
Respiratory depression, apnea

Dosage: 0.5–2.0 mg IV; may be increased to 1.0–4.0 mg IV

Routes: IV
IM
Rectal

Pediatric Dosage: 0.05–0.10 mg/kg (maximum dose 4 mg)

Magnesium Sulfate

Class: Anticonvulsant/Antiarrhythmic

Actions: Central nervous system depressant
Anticonvulsant
Antiarrhythmic

Indications: *Obstetrical*

Eclampsia (toxemia of pregnancy)

Cardiovascular

Severe refractory ventricular fibrillation/pulseless ventricular tachycardia
Post-myocardial infarction as prophylaxis for arrhythmias
Torsades de pointes (multi-axial ventricular tachycardia)

Contraindications: Shock
Heart block

Precautions: Caution should be used in patients receiving digitalis
Hypotension
Calcium chloride should be readily available as an antidote if respiratory depression ensues
Use with caution in patients with renal failure

Side Effects: Flushing
Respiratory depression
Drowsiness

Dosage: 1–4 g

Routes: IV
IM

Pediatric Dosage: Not indicated

Mannitol (Osmotrol)

Class: Osmotic diuretic

Actions: Decreases cellular edema
Increases urinary output

Indications: Acute cerebral edema
Blood transfusion reactions

Contraindications: Pulmonary edema
Patients who are dehydrated
Hypersensitivity to the drug

Precautions: Rapid administration can cause circulatory overload
Crystallization of the drug can occur at lower temperatures
An in-line filter should be used

Side Effects: Pulmonary congestion
Sodium depletion
Transient volume overload

Dosage: 1.5–2.0 g/kg

Route: IV (slow bolus or infusion)

Pediatric Dosage: 0.25–0.5 g/kg IV over 60 minutes

Meperidine (Demerol)

Class: Narcotic

Actions: Central nervous system depressant
Decreases sensitivity to pain

Indication: Moderate to severe pain

Contraindications: Patients receiving monoamine oxidase inhibitors
Undiagnosed abdominal pain
Patients with history of hypersensitivity to the drug

Precautions: Respiratory depression (Naloxone should be available)
Hypotension
Nausea

Side Effects: Dizziness
Altered level of consciousness

Dosage: *IV*
25–50 mg
IM
50–100 mg

Routes: IV
IM

Pediatric Dosage: 1 mg/kg

Metaproterenol (Alupent)

Class: Sympathomimetic (β_2 selective)

Actions: Bronchodilation
Increases heart rate

Indications: Bronchial asthma
Reversible bronchospasm associated with chronic bronchitis and emphysema

Contraindications: Patients with cardiac dysrhythmias or significant tachycardia

Precautions: Blood pressure, pulse, and EKG must be constantly monitored; occasional nausea and vomiting reported

Side Effects: Palpitations, anxiety, headache, nausea, vomiting, dizziness, and tremor

Dosage: *Metered-Dose Inhaler*
2–3 inhalations; can be repeated in 3–4 hours if required
Small-Volume Nebulizer
0.2–0.3 ml diluted in 2–3 ml normal saline administered over 5–15 minutes

Route: Inhalation only

Pediatric Dosage: 0.05–0.3 ml in 4 ml normal saline

Metaraminol (Aramine)

Class: Sympathomimetic (indirect acting)

Actions: Causes release of endogenous stores of norepinephrine
Increases cardiac contractile force
Increases cardiac rate
Causes peripheral vasoconstriction

Indication: Hemodynamically significant hypotension not due to hypovolemia

Contraindication: Hypotensive states due to hypovolemia

Precautions: Constant monitoring of blood pressure is essential
Not effective in catecholamine-depleted patients

Side Effects: Palpitations, tachycardia, and PVCs
Hypertension, tremor, and dizziness

Dosage: 200 mg should be placed in 500 ml of D_5W; this gives a concentration of 0.4 mg/ml, which should be slowly infused and titrated to blood pressure response
5–10 mg can be administered IM when an IV cannot be placed

Routes: IV drip
IM

Pediatric Dosage: Safety in children has not been established

Methylprednisolone (Solu-Medrol)

Class: Steroid

Actions: Anti-inflammatory
Suppresses immune response (especially in allergic reactions)

Indications: Severe anaphylaxis
Asthma/COPD
Possibly effective as an adjunctive agent in the management of spinal cord injury

Contraindications: None in the emergency setting

Precautions: Must be reconstituted and used promptly
Onset of action may be 2–6 hours and thus should not be expected to be of use in the critical first hour following an anaphylactic reaction

Side Effects: GI bleeding
Prolonged wound healing
Suppression of natural steroids

Dosage: *General Usage*
125–250 mg
Spinal Cord Injury
Initial bolus of 30 mg/kg administered over 15-minute period; this is followed by a maintenance infusion of 5.4 mg/kg/hour

Routes: IV
IM

Pediatric Dosage: 30 μg/kg

Metoclopramide (Reglan)

Class: Phenothiazine antiemetic

Actions: Antiemetic
Reduces gastroesophageal reflux

Indications: Nausea and vomiting
Gastroesophageal reflux

Contraindications: GI hemorrhage
Bowel obstruction or perforation
Patients with a history of hypersensitivity to the drug

Precaution: EPS (dystonic) symptoms have been reported

Side Effects: May impair mental and physical ability
Drowsiness

Dosage: 10–20 mg IM
10 mg by slow IV push over 1–2 minutes

Routes: IV
IM

Pediatric Dosage: Rarely indicated

Metoprolol (Lopressor)

Class: Sympathetic blocker (β2 selective)

Action: Selectively blocks β2-adrenergic receptors (cardioprotective)

Indications: Suspected or definite acute myocardial infarction in patients who are hemodynamically stable

Contraindications: Heart rate less than 45 beats per minute
Systolic blood pressure < 100 mmHg
Heart block
Shock
History of asthma

Precautions: Blood pressure, pulse, and EKG must be constantly monitored
Atropine and transcutaneous pacing should be available

Side Effects: Bradycardia
Heart block
Congestive heart failure
Depression
Bronchospasm

Dosage: Initial bolus of 5 mg slow IV injection
May repeat 5 mg bolus in 5 minutes if vital signs are stable
May repeat 5 mg bolus in 10 minutes if vital signs are stable

Route: Slow IV bolus

Pediatric Dosage: Safety in children has not been established

Midazolam (Versed)

Class: Tranquilizer

Actions: Hypnotic
Sedative

Indications: Premedication before cardioversion
Acute anxiety states

Contraindications: Patients with a history of hypersensitivity to the drug
Narrow-angle glaucoma
Shock

Precautions: Emergency resuscitative equipment must be available
Flumazenil (Romazicon) should be available
Dilute with normal saline of D_5W prior to intravenous administration
Respiratory depression more common with midazolam than with other benzodiazepines

Side Effects: Drowsiness
Hypotension
Amnesia
Respiratory depression, apnea

Dosage: 1.0–2.5 mg IV

Routes: IV
PO
Intranasal

Pediatric Dosage: 0.03 mg/kg

Morphine

Class: Narcotic

Actions: Central nervous system depressant
Causes peripheral vasodilation
Decreases sensitivity to pain

Indications: Severe pain
Pulmonary edema

Contraindications: Head injury
Volume depletion
Undiagnosed abdominal pain
Patients with history of hypersensitivity to the drug

Precautions: Respiratory depression (Naloxone should be available)
Hypotension
Nausea

Side Effects: Dizziness
Altered level of consciousness

Dosage: *IV*
2–5 mg followed by 2 mg every few minutes until the pain is relieved or until respiratory depression ensues
IM
5–15 mg based on patient's weight

Routes: IV
IM

Pediatric Dosage: 0.1–0.2 mg/kg IV

Nalbuphine (Nubain)

Class: Synthetic analgesic

Actions: Central nervous system depressant
Decreases sensitivity to pain

Indication: Moderate to severe pain

Contraindication: Patients with a history of hypersensitivity to the drug

Precautions: Use with caution in patients with impaired respiratory function
Respiratory depression (Naloxone should be available)
Patients dependent on narcotics may experience symptoms of withdrawal
Nausea

Side Effects: Dizziness
Altered mental status

Dosage: 5–10 mg

Routes: IV
IM

Pediatric Dosage: Rarely used

Naloxone (Narcan)

Class: Narcotic antagonist

Action: Reverses effects of narcotics

Indications: Narcotic overdoses including the following:

morphine	Dilaudid	fentanyl
Demerol	Paregoric	methadone
heroin	Percodan	Tylox

Synthetic analgesic overdoses including the following:

Nubain	Stadol	Talwin
Darvon	Alcoholic coma	

To rule out narcotics in coma of unknown origin

Contraindication: Patients with a history of hypersensitivity to the drug

Precautions: Should be administered with caution to patients dependent on narcotics as it may cause withdrawal effects
Short-acting, should be augmented every 5 minutes

Side Effects: Rare

Dosage: 1–2 mg

Routes: IV
IM
Endotracheal (endotracheal dose 2 to 2.5 times IV dose)

Pediatric Dosage:

< 5 years old	*> 5 years old*
0.1 mg/kg	2.0 mg

Nifedipine (Procardia)

Class: Calcium channel blocker

Actions: Relaxes smooth muscle causing arteriolar vasodilation
Decreases peripheral vascular resistance

Indications: Severe hypertension
Angina pectoris

Contraindications: Known hypersensitivity to the drug
Hypotension

Precautions: Blood pressure should be constantly monitored
May worsen congestive heart failure
Nifedipine should not be administered to patients receiving intravenous beta blockers

Side Effects: Dizziness, flushing, nausea, headache, and weakness

Dosage: 10 mg sublingually; puncture the capsule several times with a needle and place it under the patient's tongue and have them withdraw the liquid medication

Routes: Oral
Sublingual

Pediatric Dosage: 0.25–0.5 mg/kg

Nitroglycerin (Nitrostat)

Class: Antianginal

Actions: Smooth-muscle relaxant
Reduces cardiac work
Dilates coronary arteries
Dilates systemic arteries

Indications: Angina pectoris
Chest pain associated with myocardial infarction

Contraindications: Children younger than 12 years of age
Hypotension

Precautions: Constantly monitor blood pressure
Syncope
Drug must be protected from light
Expires quickly once bottle is opened

Side Effects: Headache
Dizziness
Hypotension

Dosage: 1 tablet repeated at 3–5 minute intervals up to 3 times

Route: Sublingual

Pediatric Dosage: Not indicated

Nitroglycerin Spray (Nitrolingual Spray)

Class: Antianginal

Actions: Smooth-muscle relaxant
Decreases cardiac work
Dilates coronary arteries
Dilates systemic arteries

Indications: Angina pectoris
Chest pain associated with myocardial infarction

Contraindication: Hypotension

Precautions: Constantly monitor vital signs
Syncope can occur

Side Effects: Dizziness
Hypotension
Headache

Dosage: One spray administered under the tongue; may be repeated in 3–5 minutes; no more than three sprays in 15-minute period; spray should not be inhaled

Route: Sprayed under tongue on mucous membrane

Pediatric Dosage: Not indicated

Nitroglycerin Paste (Nitro-Bid)

Class: Antianginal

Actions: Smooth-muscle relaxant
Decreases cardiac work
Dilates coronary arteries
Dilates systemic arteries

Indications: Angina pectoris
Chest pain associated with myocardial infarction

Contraindications: Children younger than 12 years of age
Hypotension

Precautions: Constantly monitor blood pressure
Syncope
Drug must be protected from light
Expires quickly once bottle is opened

Side Effects: Dizziness
Hypotension

Dosage: 1/2 to 1 inch

Route: Topical

Pediatric Dosage: Not indicated

Nitrous Oxide (Nitronox)

Class: Gas

Action: Central nervous system depressant

Indications: Pain of musculoskeletal origin, particularly fractures
Burns
Suspected ischemic chest pain
States of severe anxiety including hyperventilation

Contraindications: Patients who cannot comprehend verbal instructions
Patients intoxicated with alcohol or drugs
Head-injury patients who exhibit an altered mental status
COPD (increased oxygen concentration may cause respiratory depression)
Thoracic injury suspicious for pneumothorax

Abdominal pain and distension suggestive of bowel obstruction

Precautions: Use only in well-ventilated area
Gas-scavenging system is recommended
May not operate properly at low temperatures

Side Effects: Headache, dizziness, giddiness, nausea, and vomiting

Dosage: Self-administered only using fixed 50% nitrous oxide/50% oxygen blender

Route: Inhalation only

Pediatric Dosage: Self-administered only

Norepinephrine (Levophed)

Class: Sympathomimetic

Action: Causes peripheral vasoconstriction

Indications: Hypotension (systolic blood pressure < 70 mm Hg refractory to other sympathomimetics)
Neurogenic shock

Contraindications: Hypotensive states due to hypovolemia

Precautions: Can be deactivated by alkaline solutions
Constant monitoring of blood pressure is essential
Extravasation can cause tissue necrosis

Side Effects: Anxiety
Palpitations
Headache
Hypertension

Dosage: 0.5 to 30 µg/minute
Method
8 mg should be placed in 500 ml of D_5W, giving a concentration of 16 µg/ml

Route: IV drip only

Pediatric Dosage: 0.01–0.5 µg/kg/minute (rarely used)

Oxygen

Class: Gas

Action: Necessary for cellular metabolism

Indication: Hypoxia

Contraindications: None

Precautions: Use cautiously in patients with COPD
Humidify when providing high-flow rates

Side Effect: Drying of mucous membranes

Dosage: *Cardiac Arrest*
100%
Other Critical Patients
100%

	COPD
	35% (increase as needed)
Route:	Inhalation
Pediatric Dosage:	24–100% as required

Oxytocin (Pitocin)

Class:	Hormone (oxytocic)
Actions:	Causes uterine contraction Causes lactation Slows postpartum vaginal bleeding
Indication:	Postpartum vaginal bleeding
Contraindications:	Any condition other than postpartum bleeding Cesarean section
Precautions:	Essential to assure that the placenta has delivered and that there is not another fetus before administering oxytocin Overdosage can cause uterine rupture Hypertension
Side Effects:	Anaphylaxis Cardiac arrhythmias
Dosage:	*IV* 10–20 units in 500 ml of D_5W administered according to uterine response *IM* 3–10 units
Routes:	IV drip IM
Pediatric Dosage:	Not indicated

Pancuronium Bromide (Pavulon)

Class:	Neuromuscular blocking agent (non-depolarizing)
Actions:	Skeletal muscle relaxant Paralyzes skeletal muscles including respiratory muscles
Indication:	To achieve paralysis to facilitate endotracheal intubation
Contraindication:	Patients with known hypersensitivity to the drug
Precautions:	Should not be administered unless persons skilled in endotracheal intubation are present Endotracheal intubation equipment must be available Oxygen equipment and emergency resuscitative drugs must be available Paralysis occurs within 3–5 minutes and lasts for approximately 60 minutes
Side Effects:	Prolonged paralysis Hypotension Bradycardia

Dosage: 0.04–0.1 mg/kg. Repeat doses of 0.01–0.02 mg/kg intravenously as required every 20–40 minutes

Route: IV

Pediatric Dosage: 0.1 mg/kg

Phenobarbital (Luminal)

Class: Barbiturate

Actions: Suppresses spread of seizure activity through the motor cortex
Central nervous system depressant

Indications: Major motor seizures
Status epilepticus
Acute anxiety states

Contraindication: History of hypersensitivity to the drug

Precautions: Respiratory depression
Hypotension
Can cause hyperactivity in children
Extravasation may cause tissue necrosis

Side Effects: Drowsiness
Children may become hyperactive

Dosage: 100–250 mg

Routes: IV (slowly)
IM

Pediatric Dosage: 10 mg/kg

Phenytoin (Dilantin)

Class: Anticonvulsant/Antiarrhythmic

Actions: Inhibits spread of seizure activity through motor cortex
Antiarrhythmic

Indications: Major motor seizures
Status epilepticus
Arrhythmias due to digitalis toxicity

Contraindications: Any arrhythmia except those due to digitalis toxicity
High-grade heart blocks
Patients with history of hypersensitivity to the drug

Precautions: Should not be administered with glucose solutions
Hypotension
EKG monitoring during administration is essential

Side Effects: Local venous irritation
Itching
Central nervous system depression

Dosage: *Status Epilepticus*
150–250 mg (10–15 mg/kg) not to exceed 50 mg/minute

Digitalis Toxicity
100 mg over 5 minutes until the arrhythmia is suppressed or until a maximum dose of 1,000 mg has been administered or symptoms or central nervous system depression occur

Route: IV (dilute with saline)

Pediatric Dosage:
Status Epilepticus
8–10 mg/kg IV
Digitalis Toxicity
3–5 mg/kg IV over 100 minutes

Physostigmine (Antilirium)

Class: Cholinesterase inhibitor

Actions:
Inhibits cholinesterase
Potentiates acetylcholine

Indications:
Tricyclic overdoses including the following:
Tofranil Norpramin Sinequan
Elavil Adapin Triavil
Atropine/Belladonna overdoses

Contraindications:
Asthma and COPD
Gangrene
Diabetics
Cardiovascular disease

Precautions:
Monitor for bronchospasm and laryngospasm
Seizures

Side Effects:
Excessive salivation
Bradycardia
Emesis

Dosage: 0.5–2.0 mg

Route: IV

Pediatric Dosage: 0.5–1.0 mg over 5 minutes

Pralidoxime (2-PAM) (Protopam)

Class: Cholinesterase reactivator

Actions:
Reactivates cholinesterase in cases of organophosphate poisoning
Deactivates certain organophosphates by direct chemical reaction

Indications:
Severe organophosphate poisoning as characterized by muscle twitching, respiratory depression, and paralysis

Contraindications:
Poisonings due to inorganic phosphates
Poisonings other than organophosphates

Precautions:
Always assure safety and protection of rescue personnel

Laryngospasm, tachycardia, and muscle rigidity have occurred following rapid administration
Should only follow atropinization

Side Effects: Excitement
Manic behavior

Dosage: 1–2 grams in 250–500 ml of normal saline infused over 30 minutes

Route: IV drip

Pediatric Dosage: 20–40 mg/kg by the same method

Procainamide (Pronestyl)

Class: Antiarrhythmic

Actions: Slows conduction through myocardium
Elevates ventricular fibrillation threshold
Suppresses ventricular ectopic activity

Indications: Persistent cardiac arrest due to ventricular fibrillation and refractory to lidocaine
PVCs refractory to lidocaine
Ventricular tachycardia refractory to lidocaine

Contraindications: High-degree heart blocks
PVCs in conjunction with bradycardia

Precautions: Dosage should not exceed 17 mg/kg
Monitor for central nervous system toxicity

Side Effects: Anxiety
Nausea
Convulsions
Widening of QRS

Dosage: *Initial*
20 mg/minute until:
- Arrhythmia abolished
- Hypotension ensues
- QRS widened by 50% of original width
- Total of 17 mg/kg has been given

Maintenance
- 1–4 mg/minute

Routes: Slow IV bolus
IV drip

Pediatric Dosage: Rarely used

Prochlorperazine (Compazine)

Class: Phenothiazine antiemetic

Action: Antiemetic

Indications: Nausea and vomiting
Acute psychosis

Contraindications: Comatose states
Patients who have received a large amount of depressants (including alcohol)
Patients with a history of hypersensitivity to the drug

Precaution: EPS (dystonic) symptoms have been reported

Side Effects: May impair mental and physical ability
Drowsiness

Dosage: 5–10 mg slow IV or IM

Routes: IV
IM

Pediatric Dosage: Not recommended

Promethazine (Phenergan)

Class: Antihistamine (H_1 antagonist)

Actions: Mild anticholinergic activity
Antiemetic
Potentiates actions of analgesics

Indications: Nausea and vomiting
Motion sickness
To potentiate the effects of analgesics
Sedation

Contraindications: Comatose states
Patients who have received a large amount of depressants (including alcohol)

Precaution: Avoid accidental intra-arterial injection

Side Effects: May impair mental and physical ability
Drowsiness

Dosage: 12.5–25.0 mg

Routes: IV
IM

Pediatric Dosage: 0.5 mg/kg

Propranolol (Inderal)

Class: Sympathetic blocker

Action: Nonselectively blocks β-adrenergic receptors

Indications: Ventricular tachyarrhythmias refractory to lidocaine and bretylium
Recurrent ventricular fibrillation refractory to lidocaine and bretylium
Tachyarrhythmias due to digitalis toxicity

Contraindications: Asthma/COPD
Patients dependent on sympathetic agonists
CHF

Precautions: Should not be given concurrently with verapamil
Atropine and transcutaneous pacing should be readily available

Side Effects: Bradycardia
Heart blocks
Congestive heart failure
Bronchospasm

Dosage: 1–3 mg diluted in 10–30 ml of D_5W given slowly IV

Route: Slow IV bolus

Pediatric Dosage: 0.01 mg/kg

Racemic Epinephrine (MicroNEFRIN)

Class: Sympathomimetic

Actions: Bronchodilation
Increases heart rate
Increases cardiac contractile force

Indication: Croup (laryngotracheobronchitis)

Contraindications: Epiglottitis
Hypersensitivity to the drug

Precautions: Vital signs should be constantly monitored
Should be used only once in the prehospital setting

Side Effects: Palpitations
Anxiety
Headache

Dosage: 0.25–0.75 ml of a 2.25% solution in 2.0 ml normal saline

Route: Inhalation only (small-volume nebulizer)

Pediatric Dosage: 0.25–0.75 ml of a 2.25% solution in 2.0 ml normal saline

Sodium Bicarbonate

Class: Alkalinizing agent

Actions: Combines with excessive acids to form a weak volatile acid
Increases pH

Indications: Late in the management of cardiac arrest, if at all
Tricyclic antidepressant overdose
Severe acidosis refractory to hyperventilation

Contraindication: Alkalotic states

Precautions: Correct dosage is essential to avoid overcompensation of pH
Can deactivate catecholamines
Can precipitate with calcium
Delivers large sodium load

Side Effect: Alkalosis

Dosage: 1 mEq/kg initially followed by 0.5 mEq/kg every 10 minutes as indicated by blood gas studies

Route: IV

Pediatric Dosage: 1 mEq/kg initially followed by 0.5 mEq/kg every 10 minutes

Sodium Nitroprusside (Nipride, Nitropress)

Class: Potent vasodilator

Actions:
Peripheral arterial and venous vasodilator
Decreases blood pressure
Increases cardiac output in CHF

Indication: Hypertensive emergency

Contraindications: None when used in the management of life-threatening emergency

Precautions:
Bottle must be wrapped in foil to protect from light
Should not be administered to children or pregnant women in the prehospital setting
Reduce the dosage in elderly patients
Blood pressure, pulse, and EKG must be diligently monitored

Side Effects: Nausea, retching, vomiting, palpitations, diaphoresis, tachycardia, and dizziness; side effects often diminish as dosage is reduced

Dosage: 0.5 μg/kg/minute

Route: IV infusion only

Pediatric Dosage: Not indicated in prehospital setting

Streptokinase (Strepase)

Class: Thrombolytic

Action: Dissolves blood clots

Indication: Acute MI

Contraindications:
Persons with internal bleeding
Suspected aortic dissection
Traumatic CPR
Severe persistent hypertension
Recent head trauma or known intracranial tumor
History of stroke in the last 6 months
Pregnancy

Precautions:
May be ineffective if administered within 12 months of prior streptokinase of anistreplase therapy
Antiarrhythmic and resuscitative drugs should be available

Side Effects:
Bleeding
Allergic reactions
Anaphylaxis

	Fever Nausea and vomiting
Dosage:	1.5 million units over 1 hour
Route:	IV drip
Pediatric Dosage:	Not recommended

Succinylcholine (Anectine)

Class:	Neuromuscular blocking agent (depolarizing)
Actions:	Skeletal muscle relaxant Paralyzes skeletal muscles including respiratory muscles
Indication:	To achieve paralysis to facilitate endotracheal intubation
Contraindication:	Patients with known hypersensitivity to the drug
Precautions:	Should not be administered unless persons skilled in endotracheal intubation are present Endotracheal intubation equipment must be available Oxygen equipment and emergency resuscitative drugs must be available Paralysis occurs within 1 minutes and lasts for approximately 8 minutes
Side Effects:	Prolonged paralysis Hypotension Bradycardia
Dosage:	1–1.5 mg/kg (40–100 mg in an adult)
Route:	IV
Pediatric Dosage:	1 mg/kg

Terbutaline (Brethine)

Class:	Sympathomimetic
Actions:	Bronchodilator Increases heart rate
Indications:	Bronchial asthma Reversible bronchospasm associated with COPD Preterm labor
Contraindication:	Patients with known hypersensitivity to the drug
Precautions:	Blood pressure, pulse, and EKG must be constantly monitored
Side Effects:	Palpitations, tachycardia, and PVCs Anxiety, tremor, and headache
Dosage:	*Metered-Dose Inhaler* Two inhalations, 1 minute apart *Subcutaneous Injection* 0.25 mg; may be repeated in 15–30 minutes

Routes: Inhalation
Subcutaneous injection
IV drip (in pre-term labor)

Pediatric Dosage: 0.01 mg/kg subcutaneously

Thiamine (Vitamin B_1)

Class: Vitamin

Action: Allows normal breakdown of glucose

Indications: Coma of unknown origin
Alcoholism
Delirium tremens

Contraindications: None in the emergency setting

Precaution: Rare anaphylactic reactions have been reported

Side Effects: Rare, if any

Dosage: 100 mg

Routes: IV
IM

Pediatric Dosage: Rarely indicated

Tissue Plasminogen Activator (tPA) (Activase)

Class: Thrombolytic

Action: Dissolves blood clots

Indication: Acute MI

Contraindications: Persons with internal bleeding
Suspected aortic dissection
Traumatic CPR
Severe persistent hypertension
Recent head trauma or known intracranial tumor
History of stroke in the last 6 months
Pregnancy

Precautions: Antiarrhythmic and resuscitative drugs should be available

Side Effects: Bleeding
Allergic reactions
Anaphylaxis
Fever
Nausea and vomiting

Dosage: *Front-Loaded Regimen*
15 mg IV bolus over 1–2 minutes; followed by infusion of 50 mg over the first hour and 35 mg over the second hour (total dose = 100 mg)
Standard Regimen
10 mg IV bolus over 1–2 minutes; followed by 50 mg over the first hour, 20 mg over the second hour, and 20 mg over the third hour

Route: IV (slow) and IV infusion

Pediatric Dosage: Not recommended

Trimethobenzamide (Tigan)

Class: Antiemetic

Action: Antiemetic with fewer sedative effects than other common antiemetic drugs

Indication: Nausea and vomiting

Contraindications: Children (injectable form only)
Patients with a history of hypersensitivity to the drug

Precaution: EPS (dystonic) symptoms have been reported

Side Effects: May impair mental and physical ability
Drowsiness

Dosage: 200 mg IM

Route: IM

Pediatric Dosage: Parenteral administration not recommended

Vecuronium (Norcuron)

Class: Neuromuscular blocking agent (non-depolarizing)

Action: Skeletal muscle relaxant
Paralyzes skeletal muscles including respiratory muscles

Indication: To achieve paralysis to facilitate endotracheal intubation

Contraindication: Patients with known hypersensitivity to the drug

Precautions: Should not be administered unless persons skilled in endotracheal intubation are present
Endotracheal intubation equipment must be available
Oxygen equipment and emergency resuscitative drugs must be available
Paralysis occurs within 1 minute and lasts for approximately 30 minutes

Side Effects: Prolonged paralysis
Hypotension
Bradycardia

Dosage: 0.08–0.1 mg/kg

Route: IV

Pediatric Dosage: 0.1 mg/kg

Verapamil (Isoptin) (Calan)

Class: Calcium channel blocker

Actions: Slows conduction through the AV node

Inhibits reentry during PSVT
Decreases rate of ventricular response
Decreases myocardial oxygen demand

Indication: PSVT

Contraindications: Heart block
Conduction system disturbances

Precautions: Should not be used in patients receiving intravenous β-blockers
Hypotension

Side Effects: Nausea, vomiting, hypotension, and dizziness

Dosage: 2.5–5 mg. A repeat dose of 5–10 mg can be administered after 15–30 minutes if PSVT does not convert. Maximum dose is 30 mg in 30 minutes

Route: Intravenous

Pediatric Dosage: *0–1 Year*
0.1–0.2 mg/kg (maximum of 2.0 mg) administered slowly
1–15 Years
0.1–0.3 mg/kg (maximum of 5.0 mg) administered slowly

appendix D

Home Medication Reference Guide

TABLE D-1

Home Medication Classes

Class	*Actions*
Analgesics	Raise pain threshold Alleviate anxiety and fear Alter physiological response to pain
Anorexiants	Control appetite
Antacids	Reduce stomach and duodenal activity Raise stomach pH
Antianginals	Dilate peripheral and coronary arterioles Decrease cardiac work
Antiarrhythmics	Suppress ectopic activity Control rhythm of heart
Antiarthritics	Control joint inflammation and pain associated with arthritis
Antibiotics	Combat microorganisms
Anticoagulants	Prolong blood-clotting time
Anticholinergics	Block actions of acetylcholine, thus potentiating sympathetic nervous system
Anticonvulsants	Suppress seizure activity in the brain Suppress spread of seizure activity in motor cortex
Antidepressants	Tricyclic compounds potentiate sympathetic effects by preventing the uptake of norepinephrine in the central nervous system Monoamine oxidase inhibitors prevent impulse transmission at the neurons and inhibit catecholamine breakdown
Antidiarrheals	Reduce bowel motility
Antiemetics	Relieve or prevent nausea and vomiting Stimulate H_2 histamine receptors

TABLE D-1

Home Medication Classes (continued)

Class	*Actions*
Antihistamines	Block release of histamine
Antihypertensives	Lower blood pressure Cause peripheral vasodilation
Antipsychotics	Phenothiazines are thought to block dopamine receptors in the brain associated with mood and behavior
Antispasmodics	Relieve pain Block acetylcholine in parts of the parasympathetic nervous system
Antituberculosis	Deactivates the tubercle bacillus
Bronchodilators	Relax smooth muscle of bronchioles
Cardiac Glycosides	Increase cardiac output Slow SA and AV conduction Positive inotrope Control certain rhythm disorders
Diuretics	Stimulate release of water and sodium chloride from kidneys Inhibit reabsorption of sodium in nephron
Hypnotics and Sedatives	Induce sleep Depress central nervous system
Hypoglycemics	Provide insulin to promote uptake of glucose by the cells
Laxatives and Stool Softeners	Stimulate peristalsis Alter fecal consistency
Steroids	Control inflammatory response
Sulfamides	Antibiotics for urinary tract infections
Tranquilizers	Induce calmness without depression of level of consciousness Depress central nervous system

TABLE D-2

Common Home Medications

Medication	*Use*
A/T/S	Topical antibiotic
Accupril	Antihypertensive
Accutane	Acne agent
acebutalol	β blocker
acetaminophen	Analgesic
acetazolamide	Diuretic
Achromycin	Antibiotic
Actibine	Impotence agent
Actifed	Antihistamine and decongestant
Actigall	Gallstone dissolution agent
Acyclovir	Antiviral
Adalat	Calcium channel blocker
Adipex	Appetite suppressant
Aerobid	Steroid inhaler
Agyestin	Progesterone
Akineton	Anti-Parkinson agent
albuterol	Bronchodilator
Aldactazide	Diuretic
Aldactone	Diuretic
Aldoclor	Antihypertensive and diuretic
Aldomet	Antihypertensive
Aldoril	Antihypertensive and diuretic
allopurinol	Antigout
alprazolam	Benzodiazepine
Alupent	Bronchodilator

TABLE D-2

Common Home Medications (continued)

Medication	*Use*
amantadine	Anti-Parkinson agent and antiviral
Ambenyl	Narcotic cough suppressant
Ambien	Sedative/Hypnotic
Amen	Progesterone
amiloride	Diuretic
Aminophyllin	Theophylline
amiodarone	Antiarrhythmic
amitriptyline	Tricyclic antidepressant
amlodipine	Calcium channel blocker
amoxapine	Antidepressant
amoxicillin	Antibiotic
Amoxil	Antibiotic
Anaprox	Analgesic and antiarthritic
Anexia	Analgesic
Ansaid	Antiarthritic
Anspor	Antibiotic
Antabuse	Antialcoholism agent
Antivert	Antidizziness agent
Anturane	Antigout
Apresazide	Antihypertensive and diuretic
Apresoline	Antihypertensive
Aristocort	Steroid
Artane	Anti-Parkinson
Asendin	Antidepressant
aspirin	Analgesic
astemizole	Antihistamine
Astramorph	Narcotic
Atarax	Antihistamine
atenolol	β Blocker
Ativan	Benzodiazepine
Atrohist	Antihistamine
Atromid	Lipid-lowering agent
Atrovent	Bronchodilator
Augmentin	Antibiotic
Axid	Antiulcer
Axotal	Analgesic
azathioprine	Immunosuppressant
Azdone	Narcotic analgesic
azithromycin	Antibiotic
Bactrim	Antibiotic
Bactroban	Antibiotic
Bancap HC	Narcotic analgesic
beclomethasone	Steroid
Beclovent	Steroid inhaler
Beconase	Steroid
Benadryl	Antihistamine
benazapril	Antihypertensive
Benemid	Antigout
Bentyl	Gastrointestinal antispasmodic
benzonatate	Cough suppressant
benzotropine	Anti-Parkinson
bepridil	Antihypertensive
Betaoptic	Antiglaucoma and β blocker
betaxolol	Antiglaucoma and β blocker
Biaxin	Antibiotic
Bicillin	Antibiotic
bisoprolol	β blocker
Blocadren	β Blocker

TABLE D-2

Common Home Medications (continued)

Medication	*Use*
Bontril	Appetite suppressant
Breathaire	Bronchodilator
Brethine	Bronchodilator
Brevicon	Birth control
Bricanyl	Bronchodilator
bromocriptine	Anti-Parkinson
brompheniramine	Antihistamine
Bronkodyl	Theophylline
Brontex	Narcotic cough suppressant
bumetanide	Diuretic
Bumex	Diuretic
Buprenex	Narcotic analgesic
bupropion	Antidepressant
Buspar	Anxiolytic
buspirone	Anxiolytic
butalbital	Analgesic
Butazolidin	Antiarthritic
Butisol	Hypnotic
Cafergot	Migraine headache agent
Calan	Calcium channel blocker
Cantil	Antiulcer
Capital	Analgesic
Capoten	Antihypertensive
Capozide	Antihypertensive and diuretic
captopril	Antihypertensive
Carafate	Antiulcer
carbamazepine	Anticonvulsant
carbidopa	Anti-Parkinson
Cardene	Calcium channel blocker
Cardilate	Antianginal
Cardizem	Calcium channel blocker
carisoprodol	Muscle relaxant
carteolol	β Blocker
Cartrol	β Blocker
Cataflam	Antiarthritic
Catapres	Antihypertensive
Ceclor	Antibiotic
Cedilanid	Digitalis
cefaclor	Antibiotic
cefadroxil	Antibiotic
cefixime	Antibiotic
cefpodoxime	Antibiotic
cefprozil	Antibiotic
Ceftin	Antibiotic
cefuroxime	Antibiotic
Cefzil	Antibiotic
Centrax	Benzodiazepine
Cesamet	Antiemetic
chlordiazepoxide	Benzodiazepine
Chloromycetin	Antibiotic
chlorpromazine	Antiulcer
chlorpropamide	Oral hypoglycemic agent
chlorthalidone	Diuretic
Choledyl	Theophylline
cholestyramine	Lipid lowering agent
Choloxin	Thyroid preparation
Chronulac	Laxative
Cibalith	Lithium (anti-mania)

TABLE D-2

Common Home Medications (continued)

Medication	*Use*
cimetadine	Antiulcer
Cinobac	Antibiotic
Cipro	Antibiotic
ciprofloxacin	Antibiotic
cisapride	Antiulcer
cladribine	Lipid lowering agent
Claritin	Antihistamine
Cleocin	Antibiotic
clindamycin	Antibiotic
Clinoril	Antiarthritic
clofazimine	Antileprosy
clofibrate	Lipid lowering agent
clonazepam	Antiseizure and benzodiazepine
clonidine	Antihypertensive
clorazepate	Benzodiazepine
Codiclear	Narcotic cough suppressant
Codimal	Decongestant
Cogentin	Anti-Parkinson
CoIBENEMID	Antigout
Colace	Stool softener
Combipress	Antihypertensive and diuretic
Comhist	Antihistamine and decongestant
Comtrex	Decongestant
Constant-T	Theophylline
Cordarone	Antiarrhythmic
Corgard	β Blocker
Corzide	β Blocker/diuretic
Coumadin	Anticoagulant
cromolyn sodium	Allergy suppressant
Crystodigin	Digitalis
Cyclert	Central nervous system stimulant
cyclizine	Antiemetic
cycloserine	Antituberculosis
cyclosporine	Immunosuppressant
cycobenzaprine	Muscle relaxant
Cycrin	Progesterone
cyproheptadine	Antihistamine
Cystospaz	Urinary antispasmodic
Cytadren	Adrenal suppressant
Cytomel	Thyroid
Cytotec	Antiulcer
Dalmane	Benzodiazepine
Damason	Analgesic
Dantrium	Antispasmodic
Dapsone	Antileprosy
Daraprim	Antiparasitic
Darbid	Antiulcer
Darvon	Narcotic-type analgesic
Datril	Antiarthritic
Decadron	Steroid
Declomycin	Antibiotic
Deconamine	Decongestant
Deconsal	Decongestant
Delsym	Cough suppressant
Deltasone	Steroid
democycline	Antibiotic
Demulen	Birth control
Depakene	Anticonvulsant

TABLE D-2

Common Home Medications (continued)

Medication	*Use*
Depakote	Anticonvulsant
Deponit	Nitroglycerin antianginal
deserpidine	Antihypertensive
desipramine	Tricyclic antidepressant
Desoxyn	Amphetamine
Desyrel	Antidepressant
dexamethasone	Steroid
Dexedrine	Amphetamine
Diabeta	Oral hypoglycemic
Diabinase	Oral hypoglycemic agent
Diamox	Diuretic
diazepam	Benzodiazepine
diclofenac	Antiarthritic
Dicumarol	Anticoagulant
dicyclomine	Gastrointestinal antispasmodic
Didrex	Appetite suppressant
diethylproprion	Appetite suppressant
diethylstilbestrol	Estrogen
Diflucan	Antifungal
diflunisal	Antiarthritic
digoxin	Digitalis
Dilacor XR	Calcium channel blocker
Dilantin	Anticonvulsant
Dilatrate	Antianginal
Dilaudid	Narcotic analgesic
Dilor	Theophylline
diltiazem	Calcium channel blocker
Dimetame	Decongestant
diphenhydramine	Antihistamine
dipyridamone	Anticoagulant
Disalcid	Antiarthritic
disopyramide	Antiarrhythmic
disulfirim	Antialcoholism agent
Ditropan	Bladder antispasmodic
Diulo	Diuretic
Diupres	Antihypertensive and diuretic
Diurel	Diuretic
Diutensin	Antihypertensive
divalproex sodium	Anticonvulsant
docusate	Laxative
Dolobid	Antiarthritic
Dolophine	Narcotic
Donnatal	Gastrointestinal antispasmodic
Doral	Benzodiazepine
Doriden	Hypnotic
Dorx	Antibiotic
doxepin	Antidepressant
doxycycline	Antibiotic
Dramamine	Antihistamine
Dulcolax	Laxative
Duocet	Analgesic
Dura-Vent	Decongestant
Duratuss	Decongestant
Duratuss HD	Narcotic cough suppressant
Duricef	Antibiotic
Dyazide	Diuretic
Dynacirc	Calcium channel blocker
Dyrenium	Diuretic

TABLE D-2

Common Home Medications (continued)

Medication	*Use*
E.E.S.	Antibiotic
Easprin	Aspirin
Ecotrin	Aspirin
Edecrin	Diuretic
Effexor	Antidepressant
Elavil	Tricyclic antidepressant
Eldepryl	Anti-Parkinson agent
Elixophyllin	Theophylline
Emetrol	Antiemetic
Empirin	Analgesic
enalapril	Antihypertensive
encainaide	Antiarrhythmic
Endal HD	Narcotic cough suppressant
Endep	Tricyclic antidepressant
Enduron	Diuretic
Enduronyl	Antihypertensive and diuretic
Enkaid	Antiarrhythmic
Enovid	Birth control
Entex	Decongestant
Entolase	Digestive enzyme supplement
Equagesic	Analgesic
Ergostat	Migraine headache agent
ERYC	Antibiotic
Eryderm	Topical antibiotic
erythrityl	Antianginal
Erythrocin	Antibiotic
erythromycin	Antibiotic
Ery-Tab	Antibiotic
Esgic	Analgesic
Esidrix	Diuretic
Eskalith	Antimania agent
Esmil	Antihypertensive and diuretic
estazolam	Benzodiazepine
Estinyl	Estrogen
Estrace	Estrogen
Estraderm	Estrogen
estradiol	Estrogen
Estratab	Estrogen
estropipate	Estrogen
Estrovis	Estrogen
ethacrynic acid	Diuretic
Ethatab	Vasodilator
ethaverine	Vasodilator
ethchlorvynol	Hypnotic
ethinamate	Hypnotic
Ethmozine	Antiarrhythmic
ethosuximide	Antiseizure
ethotoin	Anticonvulsant
etodolac	Antiarthritic
Etrafon	Antianxiety and tricyclic antidepressant
Euthroid	Thyroid
E-mycin	Antibiotic
famotidine	Antiulcer
Fastin	Appetite suppressant
felbamate	Anticonvulsant
Felbatol	Anticonvulsant
Feldene	Antiarthritic
felodipine	Calcium channel blocker

TABLE D-2

Common Home Medications (continued)

Medication	*Use*
fenfluramine	Appetite suppressant
Feosol	Iron
Fergon	Iron
Fero-Folic	Iron tablets
Fero-Grad	Iron tablets
Fero-Gradumer	Iron tablets
finasteride	Antihypertensive
Fioricet	Analgesic
Fiorinal	Analgesic
Flagyl	Antibiotic
flecanine	Antiarrhythmic
Flexeril	Muscle relaxant
Floxin	Antibiotic
fluconazole	Antifungal
fluoxetine	Antidepressant
fluphenazine	Antipsychotic
flurazepam	Benzodiazepine
flurbiprofen	Antiarthritic
fosinopril	Anthypertensive
Fulvicin	Antifungal
furazolidone	Antibiotic
furosemide	Diuretic
Furoxone	Antibiotic
Gantrisin	Antibiotic
gemfibrozil	Lipid-lowering agent
Genora	Birth control
Geocillin	Antibiotic
glipizide	Oral hypoglycemic agent
Glucotrol	Oral hypoglycemic agent
glyburide	Oral hypoglycemic agent
glycopyrrolate	Antiulcer
Glynase	Oral hypoglycemic agent
Grisactin	Antifungal
guanethidine	Antihypertensive
guanfacine	Antihypertensive
Halcion	Benzodiazepine
Haldol	Antipsychotic
haloperidol	Antipsychotic
Harmonyl	Antihypertensive
Hexadrol	Steroid
Hismanal	Antihistamine
Histaspan	Antihistamine
Humibid	Decongestant
Humulin N	Insulin
Humulin R	Insulin
Hycodan	Narcotic cough suppressant
hycomine	Narcotic cough suppressant
Hycotuss	Narcotic cough suppressant
hydralazine	Antihypertensive
Hydrocet	Narcotic analgesic
hydrochlorthiazide	Diuretic
hydrocodone	Analgesic
Hydrocortone	Steroid
HydroDIURIL	Diuretic
hydroflumethazide	Diuretic
hydromorphone	Narcotic analgesic
Hydromox	Diuretic

TABLE D-2

Common Home Medications (continued)

Medication	*Use*
Hydromox	Antihypertensive and diuretic
Hydropres	Antihypertensive and diuretic
hydroxyzine	Antihistamine
Hygroton	Diuretic
Hytrin	Antihypertensive/Prostate agent
Iberet-Folic-500	Iron tablets
ibuprofen	Antiarthritic
Ilosone	Antibiotic
Ilotycin	Antibiotic
Imetrex	antimigraine agent
imipramine	Tricyclic antidepressant
Imodium	Antidiarrheal
Imodium A-D	Antidiarrheal
Imuran	Immunosuppressant
indapamide	Antihypertensive
Inderal	β Blocker
Inderide	β Blocker and diuretic
Indocin	Antiarthritic
indomethacin	Antiarthritic
INH	Antituberculosis
Insulatard	Insulin
Intal	Allergy suppressant
Inversine	Antihypertensive
ipratropium	Bronchodilator
Ismelin	Antihypertensive
isocarboxazid	Antidepressant (monoamine oxidase-inhibitor)
isoproterenol	Bronchodilator
Isoptin	Calcium channel blocker
isorbide	Antianginal
Isordil	Antianginal
isotretinoin	Acne agent
isradipine	Calcium channel blocker
Janimine	Tricyclic antidepressant
Kaochlor	Potassium supplement
Kaon	Potassium supplement
Kaopectate	Antidiarrheal
Kato	Potassium supplement
Keflit	Antibiotic
Keftab	Antibiotic
Kemadrin	Anti-Parkinson agent
Kerlone	β blocker
ketoconazole	Antifungal
ketoprofen	Antiarthritic
Kinesed	Antiulcer
Klonapin	Antiseizure/Benzodiazepine
Klorvess	Potassium supplement
Klor-Con	Potassium supplement
Klotrix	Potassium supplement
K-DUR	Potassium supplement
K-Lor	Potassium supplement
K-Lyte	Potassium supplement
K-Phos	Urinary acidifier
K-Tab	Potassium supplement
labetalol	β Blocker
Lamprene	Antileprosy

TABLE D-2

Common Home Medications (continued)

Medication	*Use*
Lanoxicaps	Digitalis
Lanoxin	Digitalis
Larodopa	Anti-Parkinson
Lasix	Diuretic
Lente	Insulin
Leustatin	Lipid-lowering agent
Levatol	β Blocker
levodopa	Anti-Parkinson
Levothroid	Thyroid
Levoxine	Thyroid
Librax	Gastrointestinal antispasmodic/Benzodiazepine
Librium	Benzodiazepine
lidocaine	Local anesthetic
Lincocin	Antibiotic
lincomycin	Antibiotic
Lioresal	Muscle relaxant
lisinopril	Antihypertensive
Lithane	Antimania agent
Lithobid	Lithium (antimania)
Lo/Ovral	Birth control
Lodine	Antiarthritic
Loestrin	Birth control
Lomotil	Antidiarrheal
Loniten	Antihypertensive
loperamide	Antidiarrheal
Lopid	Lipid-lowering agent
Lopressor	β Blocker
lorazepam	Benzodiazepine
Lorcet	Narcotic analgesic
Lorelco	Cholesterol-lowering agent
Lortab	Narcotic analgesic
Lotensin	Antihypertensive
lovastatin	Cholesterol-lowering agent
loxapine	Antipsychotic
Loxitane	Antipsychotic
Lozol	Antihypertensive
Ludiomil	Antidepressant
Lufyllin	Theophylline
Macrodantin	Antibiotic
Magan	Antiarthritic
magnesium salicylate	Antiarthritic
maprotiline	Antidepressant
Marax	Bronchodilator
Marezine	Antiemetic
Marinol	Antiemetic
Marplan	Antidepressant (monoamine oxidase inhibitor)
Materna	Vitamins
Maxair	Inhaled bronchodilator
Maxzide	Diuretic
Mebaral	Barbiturate hypnotic
mebendazole	Antiparasitic
mecamylamine	Antihypertensive
meclazine	Antidizziness agent
meclofenamate	Antiarthritic
Meclomen	Antiarthritic
Medrol	Steroid
mefenmic	Analgesic
Mellaril	Antipsychotic

TABLE D-2

Common Home Medications (continued)

Medication	*Use*
mepenzolate	Antiulcer
meprobamate	Anxiolytic
Mesantoin	Anticonvulsant
mesoridazine	Antipsychotic
Mestinon	Myasthenia gravis agent
Metandren	Testosterone
Metaprel	Bronchodilator
metaproterenol	Bronchodilator
methadone	Narcotic
methamphetamine	Amphetamine
methocarbamol	Muscle relaxant
Methotrexate	Antiarthritic
methyclothiazide	Diuretic
methyldopa	Antihypertensive
methylphenidate	Central nervous system stimulant
metoclopramide	Gastric stimulant
metolazone	Antihypertensive
metoprolol	β Blocker
metronidazole	Antibiotic
Mevacor	Cholesterol-lowering agent
mexiletine	Antiarrhythmic
Mexitil	Antiarrhythmic
Micro K	Potassium supplement
Micronase	Oral antihypoglycemic agent
Micronor	Birth control
Midamor	Diuretic
Midrin	Analgesic
Milontin	Antiseizure
Miltown	Anxiolytic
Minipress	Antihypertensive
Minitran	Nitroglycerin antianginal
Minizide	Antihypertensive and diuretic
Minocin	Antibiotic
minocycline	Antibiotic
minoxidil	Antihypertensive
misprostol	Antiulcer
Mixtard	Insulin
Moban	Antipsychotic
Modane	Laxative
Moderil	Antihypertensive
Modicon	Birth control
Moduretic	Diuretic
molindone	Antipsychotic
Monopril	Anthypertensive
Mongesic	Antiarthritic
moricizine	Antiarrhythmic
Motofen	Antidiarrheal
Motrin	Antiarthritic
MS Contin	Narcotic analgesic
MSIR	Narcotic analgesic
Myambutol	Antituberculosis
Mycostatin	Antifungal
Mykrox	Antihypertensive
Mysoline	Antiseizure
nabilone	Antiemetic
nadolol	β Blocker
Naldecon	Decongestant
Nalfon	Antiarthritic

TABLE D-2

Common Home Medications (continued)

Medication	*Use*
Naphcon	Ophthalmic antihistamine and decongestant
Naprosyn	Antiarthritic
Nardil	Antidepressant (monoamine oxidase-inhibitor)
Nasalcrom	Allergy suppressant
Nasalide	Steroid
Natalins	Vitamins
Naturetin	Diuretic
Navane	Antipsychotic
Nembutal	Barbiturate
Neosporin	Topical antibiotic
nicardipine	Calcium channel blocker
Niclocide	Antiparasitic
Nicorette	Nicotine gum
nifedipine	Calcium channel blocker
nimodipine	Calcium channel blocker
Nimotop	Calcium channel blocker
Nitrgard	Nitroglycerin antianginal
Nitrodisc	Nitroglycerin antianginal
nitrofurantoin	Antibiotic
nitroglycerin	Antianginal
Nitrol	Nitroglycerin antianginal
Nitrolingual	Nitroglycerin antianginal
Nitrospan	Nitroglycerin antianginal
Nitrostat	Nitroglycerin antianginal
Nitro-Bid	Nitroglycerin antianginal
Nitro-Dur	Nitroglycerin antianginal
Nix	Antiparasitic (lice)
nizatidine	Antiulcer
Nizoral	Antifungal
Nolamine	Decongestant
Nolex	Decongestant
Noluldar	Hypnotic
Norcept	Birth control
Nordette-21	Birth control
Norethin	Birth control
Norflex	Muscle relaxant
norfloxacin	Antibiotic
Norgesic	Analgesic
Norinyl	Birth control
Norisodrine	Bronchodilator
Norlestrin	Birth control
Norlutate	Progesterone
Norlutin	Progesterone
Normodyne	β blocker
Normozide	β blocker and diuretic
Noroxin	Antibiotic
Norpace	Antiarrhythmic
Norpramin	Tricyclic antidepressant
nortriptyline	Tricyclic antidepressant
Norvasc	Calcium channel blocker
Norzine	Antiemetic
Novafed	Decongestant
Novahistine	Decongestant and antihistamine
Novolin	Insulin
Nucofed	Narcotic cough suppressant
Octamide	Gastric stimulant
Ogen	Estrogen
Omnipen	Antibiotic

TABLE D-2

Common Home Medications (continued)

Medication	*Use*
omperazole	Antiulcer
Orap	Antipsychotic
Oretic	Diuretic
Oreticyl	Antihypertensive and diuretic
Organidin	Decongestant
Orinase	Oral hypoglycemic agent
Ornade	Decongestant and antihistamine
orphrnadrine	Muscle relaxant
Ortho-Novum	Birth control
Orudis	Antiarthritic
Ovcon	Birth control
Ovral	Estrogen
Ovral-28	Birth control
oxazepam	Benzodiazepine
oxybutynin	Bladder antispasmodic
oxycodone	Narcotic analgesic
oxytetracycline	Antibiotic
Pamelor	Tricyclic antidepressant
Pancrease	Digestive enzyme supplement
pancrelipase	Digestive enzyme supplement
Panwarfin	Anticoagulant
Paradione	Antiseizure
Parafon Forte	Muscle relaxant
paramethadione	Antiseizure
Parlodel	Anti-Parkinson
Parnate	Antidepressant (monoamine oxidase-inhibitor)
Pavabid	Peripheral vascular antispasmodic
PBZ	Antihistamine
PCE	Antibiotic
Pediacare	Decongestant and antihistamine
Pediapred	Steroid
Pediazole	Antibiotic
Peganone	Anticonvulsant
pemoline	Central nervous system stimulant
penicillin	Antibiotic
Penntuss	Narcotic cough suppressant
pentazocine	Narcotic-like analgesic
Pentids	Antibiotic
pentobarbital	Barbiturate
pentoxifylline	Decreases blood viscosity
Pepcid	Antiulcer
Percocet	Narcotic analgesic
Percodan	Narcotic analgesic
Periactin	Antihistamine
Peritrate	Antianginal
Peri-Colace	Stool softener and laxative
Permax	Anti-Parkinson
Permitil	Antipsychotic
Persantine	Anticoagulant
Pertofrane	Antidepressant
Pfizerpen	Antibiotic
phenacemide	Anticonvulsant
Phenaphen	Analgesic
phenazopyridine	Urinary tract analgesic
phenelzine	Antidepressant (monoamine oxidase-inhibitor)
Phenergan	Antiemetic
phenmetrazine	Appetite suppressant
phenolphthalein	Laxative

TABLE D-2

Common Home Medications (continued)

Medication	*Use*
phensuximide	Antiseizure
phentermine	Appetite suppressant
Phenurone	Anticonvulsant
phenylbutazone	Antiarthritic
phenyltoloxoamine	Antihistamine
phenytoin	Anticonvulsant
pimozide	Antipsychotic
pindolol	β Blocker
piroxicam	Antiarthritic
Placidyl	Hypnotic
Plendil	Calcium channel blocker
Plegine	Appetite suppressant
PMB	Estrogen
Polaramine	Antihistamine
Polysporin	Topical antibiotic
Pondimin	Appetite suppressant
Ponstel	Analgesic
potassium chloride	Potassium supplement
prazepam	Benzodiazepine
prazosin	Antihypertensive
prednisolone	Steroid
prednisone	Steroid
Preluden	Appetite suppressant
Premarin	Estrogen
Prilosec	Antiulcer
Primatene	Inhaled bronchodilator
primidone	Antiseizure
Principen	Antibiotic
Prinivil	Antihypertensive
Prinzide	Antihypertensive and diuretic
probenecid	Antigout
probucol	Cholesterol-lowering agent
procainamide	Antiarrhythmic
Procan SR	Antiarrhythmic
Procardia	Antihypertensive and antianginal
procyclidine	Anti-Parkinson agent
Prolixin	Antipsychotic
Proloid	Thyroid
promethazine	Antiemetic
Pronestyl	Antiarrhythmic
propafenone	Antiarrhythmic
Propagest	Decongestant
propoxyphene	Narcotic-type analgesic
propranolol	β Blocker
Propulsid	Antiulcer
Proscar	Antihypertensive
Protostat	Antibiotic
protriptyline	Antidepressant
Proventil	Bronchodilator
Provera	Progesterone
Prozac	Antidepressant
Pro-Banthine	Antiulcer
pseudoephedrine	Decongestant
PV Tussin	Narcotic cough suppressant
Pyridium	Urinary tract analgesic
pyridostigmine	Myasthenia gravis agent
Quadrinal	Combination bronchodilator
Quarzan	Antiulcer

TABLE D-2

Common Home Medications (continued)

Medication	*Use*
quazepam	Benzodiazepine
Questran	Lipid-lowering agent
Quibron	Theophylline
Quinamm	Muscle cramp analgesic
quinapril	Antihypertensive
quinethazone	Diuretic
Quinidex	Antiarrhythmic
quinidine	Antiarrhythmic
Quiniglute	Antiarrhythmic
Quinora	Antiarrhythmic
ranitidine	Antiulcer
Raudixin	Antihypertensive
Rauzide	Antihypertensive and diuretic
Regitine	Antihypertensive
Reglan	Stomach stimulant
Regroton	Antihypertensive
Renese	Antihypertensive and diuretic
reserpine	Antihypertensive
Respid	Theophylline
Restoril	Benzodiazepine
Retrovir	Antiviral agent (AIDS)
Ridaura	Antiarthritic (gold)
Rifadin	Antituberculosis
Rifamate	Antituberculosis
Rimactane	Antibiotic
Ritalin	Central nervous system stimulant
ritodrine	Tocolytic (suppresses labor)
Robaxin	Muscle relaxant
Robinul	Antiulcer
Rogaine	Baldness treatment
Rondec	Decongestant
Roxanol	Narcotic analgesic
Rufen	Antiarthritic
Ru-Tuss	Cough and decongestant
Rynatuss	Cough suppressant and decongestant
Rythmol	Antiarrhythmic
Salflex	Antiarthritic
salmeterol	Bronchodilator inhaler
salsalate	Antiarthritic
Saluron	Diuretic
Salutensin	Antihypertensive and diuretic
Sanorex	Appetite suppressant
Sectral	β blocker
Seldane	Antihistamine
Semilente	Insulin
Septra	Antibiotic
Serax	Benzodiazepine
Serentil	Antipsychotic
Serevent	Bronchodilator inhaler
Seromycin	Antituberculosis
Serpasil	Antihypertensive
SER-AP-ES	Antihypertensive
sertraline	Antidepressant
Sinemet	Anti-Parkinson
Sinequan	Antidepressant
Sinulin	Decongestant
Skelaxin	Muscle relaxant

TABLE D-2

Common Home Medications (continued)

Medication	*Use*
Slo-Bid	Theophylline
Slo-Phyllin	Theophylline
Soma	Muscle relaxant
Spectrobid	Antibiotic
spironolactone	Diuretic
Stelazine	Antipsychotic
sucralfate	Antiulcer
Sudafed	Decongestant
sulfamethoxazole	Antibiotic
sulfinpyrazone	Antigout
sulfisoxazole	Antibiotic
sulindac	Antiarthritic
sumatriptin	Antimigraine agent
Sumycin	Antibiotic
Suprax	Antibiotic
Surbex	Vitamin
Surmontil	Tricyclic antidepressant
Symmetrel	Anti-Parkinson and antiviral
Synalgos-DC	Narcotic analgesic
Synthroid	Thyroid preparation
Tagamet	Antiulcer
Talwin	Narcotic-like analgesic
Tambocor	Antiarrhythmic
TAO	Antibiotic
Tavist	Antihistamine
Tegretol	Anticonvulsant
temazepam	Benzodiazepine
Tenex	Antihypertensive
Tenoretic	β Blocker and diuretic
Tenormin	β Blocker
Tenuate	Appetite suppressant
Ten-K	Potassium supplement
Tepanil	Appetite suppressant
terazosin	Antihypertensive/Prostate agent
terbutaline	Bronchodilator
tenadine	Antihistamine
Terramycin	Antibiotic
Tessalon	Cough suppressant
tetracycline	Antibiotic
Thalitone	Diuretic
Theobid	Theophylline bronchodilator
Theochron	Theophylline
Theoclear	Theophylline
Theolair	Theophylline
Theo-24	Theophylline
Theo-Dur	Theophylline
thiordazine	Antipsychotic
thiothixene	Antipsychotic
Thorazine	Antiulcer
Tigan	Antiemetic
Timolide	β Blocker and antihypertensive
timolol	β Blocker
tocainaide	Antiarrhythmic
Tofranil	Tricyclic antidepressant
tolazamide	Oral hypoglycemic agent
tolbutamide	Oral hypoglycemic agent
Tolectin	Antiarthritic
Tolinase	Oral hypoglycemic agent

TABLE D-2

Common Home Medications (continued)

Medication	*Use*
Toncard	Antiarrhythmic
Toradol	Analgesic
Torecan	Antiemetic
Tornalate	Inhaled bronchodilator
Trancopal	Anxiolytic
Trandate	β Blocker
Transderm-Nitro	Nitroglycerin antianginal
Transdern SCOP	Antiemetic
Tranxene	Benzodiazepine
tranylcypromine	Antidepressant (monoamine oxidase-inhibitor)
trazadone	Antidepressant
Trecator	Antituberculosis
Trental	Decreases blood viscosity
triamcinolone	Steroid
Triaminic	Decongestant
triamterene	Diuretic
Triavil	Tricyclic antidepressant
triazolam	Benzodiazepine
Tridil	Nitroglycerin antianginal
Tridione	Anticonvulsant
trifluoperazine	Antipsychotic
trihexyphenidyl	Anti-Parkinson
Trilafon	Antipsychotic
Trilisate	Antiarthritic
trimethadione	Anticonvulsant
trimethobenzamide	Antiemetic
trimethoprim	Antibiotic
trimipramine	Tricyclic antidepressant
Trimox	Antibiotic
Trimpex	Antibiotic
Trinalin	Antihistamine
Triphasil	Birth control
Tri-Levlen	Birth control
Tri-norinyl	Birth control
Tussigon	Narcotic cough suppressant
Tussionex	Narcotic cough suppressant
Tussi-Organidin	Cough suppressant
Tylenol	Analgesic
Tylenol with Codeine	Narcotic analgesic
Tylox	Narcotic analgesic
Tympagesic	Ear anesthetic
Ultracef	Antibiotic
Unipen	Antibiotic
Uniphyl	Theophylline
Urecholine	Bladder antispasmodic
Urised	Urinary antispasmodic
Urispas	Urinary antispasmodic
ursodiol	Gallstone dissolution agent
Valium	Benzodiazepine
Valmid	Hypnotic
Valpin	Antiulcer
valproic acid	Anticonvulsant
Valrelease	Benzodiazepine
Vancenase	Steroid
Vanceril	Steroid
vancomycin	Antibiotic
Vanocin	Antibiotic

TABLE D-2

Common Home Medications (continued)

Medication	*Use*
Vantin	Antibiotic
Vascor	Antihypertensive
Vasoretic	Antihypertensive and diuretic
Vasotec	Antihypertensive
Veetids	Antibiotic
Velosef	Antibiotic
Velosulin	Insulin
venlafaxine	Antidepressant
Ventolin	Bronchodilator
verapamil	Calcium channel blocker
Verelan	Calcium channel blocker
Vermox	Antiparasitic
Vibramycin	Antibiotic
Vicodin	Narcotic analgesic
Vicon	Vitamin
Visken	β Blocker
Vistaril	Antihistamine
Vivactil	Antidepressant
Voltaren	Antiarthritic
Vontrol	Antiemetic
warfarin	Anticoagulant
Wellbutrin	Antidepressant
Wigraine	Migraine headache agent
Wycillin	Antibiotic
Wygesic	Analgesic
Wymox	Antibiotic
Wymycin	Antibiotic
Wytensin	Antihypertensive
Xanax	Benzodiazepine
Xylocaine	Local anesthetic
yohimbine	Impotence agent
Yohimex	Impotence agent
Yutopar	Tocolytic (suppresses labor)
Zantac	Antiulcer
Zarontin	Antiseizure
Zebeta	β blocker
Zestoretic	Antihypertensive and diuretic
Zestril	Antihypertensive
Ziac	β blocker
zidovudine	Antiviral agent (AIDS)
Zithromax	Antibiotic
Zoloft	Antidepressant
zolpidem	Sedative/Hypnotic
ZORprin	Aspirin
Zovirax	Antiviral
Zydone	Narcotic analgesic
Zyloprim	Antigout
Zymase	Digestive enzyme supplement

Listing of the most commonly prescribed medications. If additional information is required concerning a drug, consult the *Physician's Desk Reference* or a similar source. Trade names are capitalized, and generic names are lowercased.

appendix E

Pediatric Drug Dosages

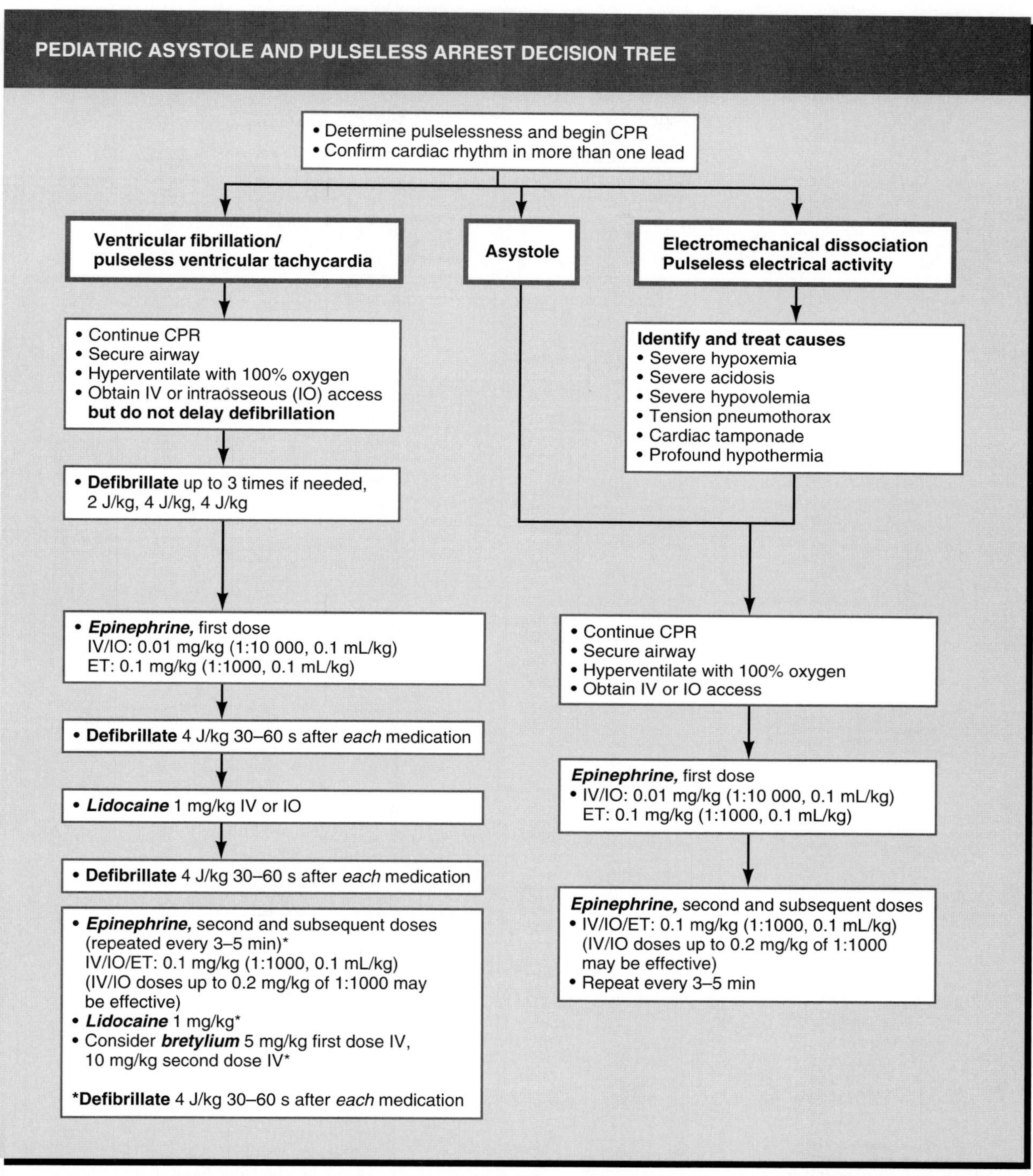

PEDIATRIC ASYSTOLE AND PULSELESS ARREST DECISION TREE
• Determine pulselessness and begin CPR
• Confirm cardiac rhythm in more than one lead
Ventricular fibrillation/ pulseless ventricular tachycardia
Asystole
Electromechanical dissociation Pulseless electrical activity
• Continue CPR
• Secure airway
• Hyperventilate with 100% oxygen
• Obtain IV or intraosseous (IO) access but do not delay defibrillation
Identify and treat causes
• Severe hypoxemia
• Severe acidosis
• Severe hypovolemia
• Tension pneumothorax
• Cardiac tamponade
• Profound hypothermia
• Defibrillate up to 3 times if needed, 2 J/kg, 4 J/kg, 4 J/kg
• Epinephrine, first dose IV/IO: 0.01 mg/kg (1:10 000, 0.1 mL/kg) ET: 0.1 mg/kg (1:1000, 0.1 mL/kg)
• Continue CPR
• Secure airway
• Hyperventilate with 100% oxygen
• Obtain IV or IO access
• Defibrillate 4 J/kg 30–60 s after each medication
Epinephrine, first dose
• IV/IO: 0.01 mg/kg (1:10 000, 0.1 mL/kg) ET: 0.1 mg/kg (1:1000, 0.1 mL/kg)
• Lidocaine 1 mg/kg IV or IO
• Defibrillate 4 J/kg 30–60 s after each medication
Epinephrine, second and subsequent doses
• IV/IO/ET: 0.1 mg/kg (1:1000, 0.1 mL/kg) (IV/IO doses up to 0.2 mg/kg of 1:1000 may be effective)
• Repeat every 3–5 min
• Epinephrine, second and subsequent doses (repeated every 3–5 min)* IV/IO/ET: 0.1 mg/kg (1:1000, 0.1 mL/kg) (IV/IO doses up to 0.2 mg/kg of 1:1000 may be effective)
• Lidocaine 1 mg/kg*
• Consider bretylium 5 mg/kg first dose IV, 10 mg/kg second dose IV*
*Defibrillate 4 J/kg 30–60 s after each medication

Figure E-1 *Journal of the American Medical Association (JAMA),* October 28, 1992. Volume 268, Number 16 (pages 2171–2302). Copyright 1992, American Medical Association. Reproduced with permission.

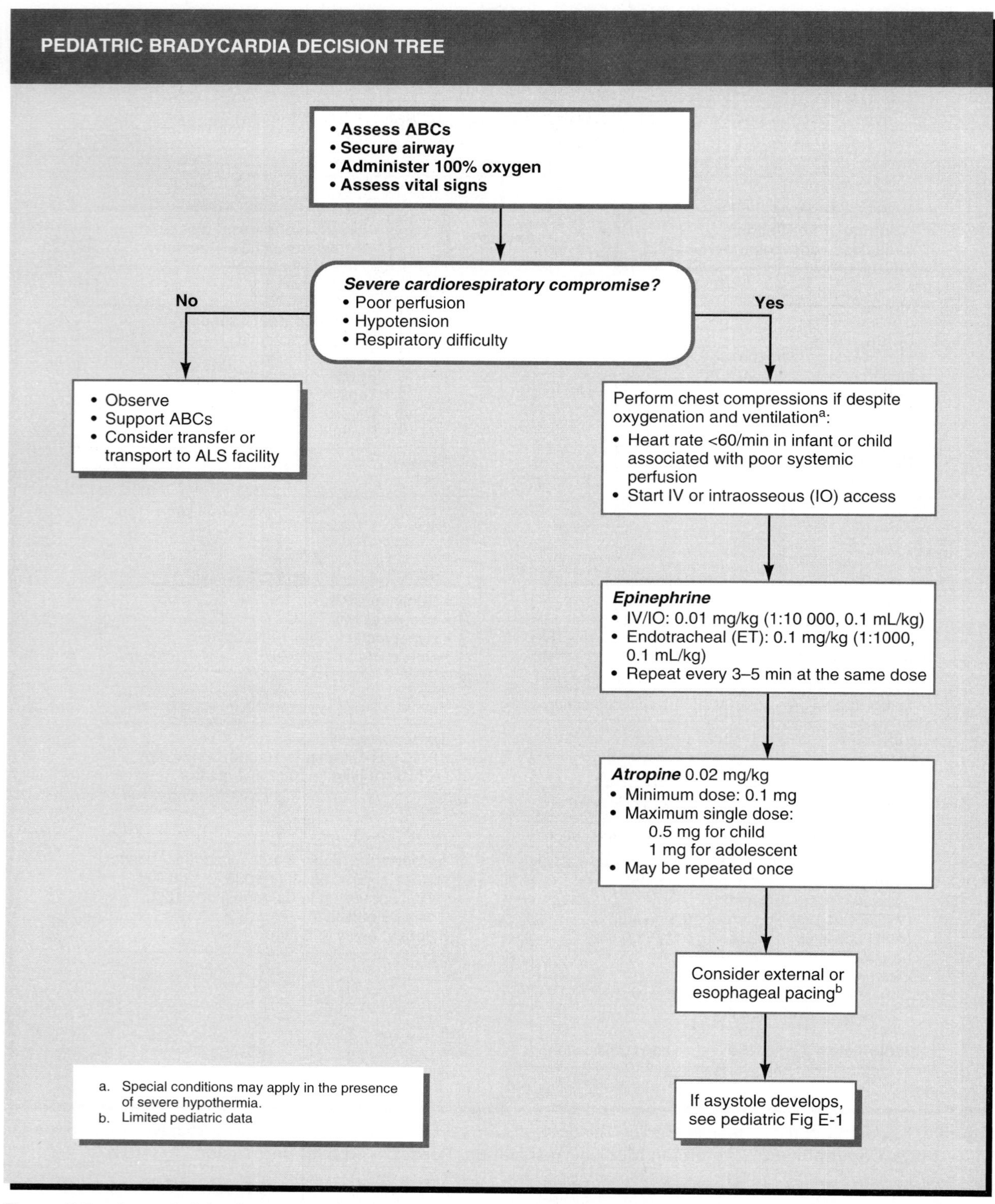

Figure E-2 *Journal of the American Medical Association (JAMA),* October 28, 1992. Volume 268, Number 16 (pages 2171–2302). Copyright 1992, American Medical Association. Reproduced with permission.

Figure E-3

Drugs Used in Pediatric Advanced Life Support

Drugs	*Dosage (Pediatric)*	*Remarks*
Adenosine	0.1–0.2 mg/kg Maximum single dose: 12 mg	Rapid IV bolus
Atropine sulfate*	0.02 mg/kg	Minimum dose: 0.1 mg Maximum single dose: 0.5 mg in child, 1.0 mg in adolescent
Bretylium	5 mg/kg; may be increased to 10 mg/kg	Rapid IV
Calcium chloride 10%	20 mg/kg	Give slowly.
Dopamine hydrochloride	2–20 μg/kg per min	α-Adrenergic action dominates at ≥15–20 μg/kg per min.
Dobutamine hydrochloride	2–20 μg/kg per min	Titrate to desired effect.
Epinephrine for bradycardia*	IV/IO: 0.01 mg/kg (1:10 000, 0.1 mL/kg) ET: 0.1 mg/kg (1:1000, 0.1 mL/kg)	Be aware of total dose of preservative administered (if preservatives are present in epinephrine preparation) when high doses are used.
Epinephrine for asystolic or pulseless arrest*	*First dose:* IV/IO: 0.01 mg/kg (1:10 000, 0.1 mL/kg) ET: 0.1 mg/kg (1:1000, 0.1 mL/kg) IV/IO doses as high as 0.2 mg/kg of 1:1000 may be effective. *Subsequent doses:* IV/IO/ET: 0.1 mg/kg (1:1000, 0.1 mL/kg) • Repeat every 3–5 min. IV/IO doses as high as 0.2 mg/kg of 1:1000 may be effective.	Be aware of total dose of preservative administered (if preservatives are present in epinephrine preparation) when high doses are used.
Epinephrine infusion	Initial at 0.1 mg/kg per min Higher infusion dose used if asystole present	Titrate to desired effect (0.1–1.0 mg/kg per min).
Lidocaine*	1 mg/kg	
Lidocaine infusion	20–50 μg/kg per min	
Naloxone*	If ≤ 5 years old or ≤ 20 kg: 0.1 mg/kg If > 5 years old or > 20 kg: 2.0 mg	Titrate to desired effect.
Sodium bicarbonate	1 mEq/kg per dose or 0.3 × kg × base deficit	Infuse slowly and only if ventilation is adequate.

*For ET administration dilute medication with normal saline to a volume of 3 to 5 mL and follow with several positive-pressure ventilations.

From *Pediatric Advanced Life Support*. American Heart Association, Dallas, TX. 1994 (Reproduced with Permission).

Figure E-4

Preparation of Catecholamine Infusions in Infants and Children*

Medication	*Dilution*	*Delivery Rate*
Isoproterenol Epinephrine	0.6 × body weight (kg) is the mg dose added to sufficient diluent to create a total volume of 100 mL†	1 mL/h delivers 0.1 µg/kg/min
Dopamine Dobutamine	6 × body weight (kg) is the mg dose added to sufficient diluent to create a total volume of 100 mL†	1 mL/h delivers 1 µg/kg/min

*This provides an initial concentration only. Drug concentration can be adjusted based on the patient's fluid requirements or limitations.

†In large patients the amount of drug used to create 100 mL of the drug infusion may deplete the available supply of the drug. To reduce the volume of drug needed to prepare the infusion, decrease the drug concentration by a factor of 10 and increase the hourly infusion rate by a factor of 10. For example, according to the formula above, a 20-kg child would require 12 mg (20 × 0.6) or 60 mL (0.2 mg/mL) of isoproterenol per 100 mL. Instead, dilute 1.2 mg (6mL) in a solution totaling 100 mL and infuse the final solution at 10 mL/h (instead of 1 mL/h).

If high doses of the drug are required (eg, greater than or equal to 10 µg/kg per minute), the resulting amount of fluid delivered may be excessive for small infants or children. Under these conditions the concentration of the drug may be *increased* by a factor of 3, 5, or 10 and the rate of infusion *decreased* by the same factor.

From *Pediatric Advanced Life Support.* American Heart Association, Dallas, TX. 1994 (Reproduced with Permission).

appendix F

Additional Practice Problems

DRUG CALCULATION WORKSHEET

Convert the following:

1.	1 milligram	=	_______	micrograms
2.	5 micrograms	=	_______	milligrams
3.	10 grams	=	_______	micrograms
4.	250 milliliters	=	_______	liters
5.	2 grams	=	_______	micrograms
6.	0.005 grams	=	_______	milligrams
7.	0.15 liters	=	_______	milliliters
8.	20 milligrams	=	_______	grams
9.	0.5 milligrams	=	_______	micrograms
10.	0.0005 grams	=	_______	micrograms
11.	154 pounds	=	_______	kilograms
12.	165 pounds	=	_______	kilograms
13.	121 pounds	=	_______	kilograms
14.	100 kilograms	=	_______	pounds
15.	60 kilograms	=	_______	pounds

16. If a solution has a concentration of 1 mg/ml, how many ml must be given to achieve a dose of 0.3 mg?

17. If a solution has a concentration of 20 mg/ml, how many ml must be given to achieve a dose of 50 mg?
18. If 25 ml of a drug contains 1 gram of medication, what is the solution concentration in mg/ml?
19. How many ml of a drug, which is supplied in a concentration of 20 mg/ml, must be given to achieve a dose of 1 mg/kg for a 176 lb patient?
20. If 1 mg of medication is added to a 250 ml IV bag, what is the solution concentration in mg/ml?
21. If you want to give 90 mg of a drug that is supplied in a 2% solution, how many ml must you give?
22. If you want to give 100 mg of a drug that is supplied in a concentration of 80 mg/ml, how many ml must you give?
23. If you add 4 mg of a drug to 500 ml of IV solution, what is the drip rate necessary to achieve a 6 mcg/min infusion?
24. If you add 500 mg of a drug to 250 ml of IV solution, what is the drip rate necessary to achieve a 800 mcg/min infusion?
25. If you add 80 mg of a drug to 500 ml of IV solution, what is the drip rate necessary to achieve a 90 mcg/min infusion?
26. How many ml of a 4% solution must be added to 500 ml of IV solution to achieve a solution concentration of 4 mg/ml?
27. You find a patient with dopamine running at 45 gtts per minute. You know that 400 mg of dopamine was added to 500 ml of IV solution and the patient is receiving 5 mcg/kg/min. How much does the patient weigh in pounds?
28. You have added 1 mg of a drug to 250 ml of IV solution. What is the drip rate necessary to achieve an infusion of 7 mcg/min?
29. You have added 100 mg of a drug to 250 ml of IV solution. What is the drip rate necessary for the patient to receive 50 mg over the next 5 hours?
30. You are asked to give 25 mg of a drug that is supplied in a 2% 50 ml vial. How many ml must you draw up?
31. You are asked to give 0.01 mg/kg epinephrine to a 65 kg child. The epinephrine is supplied in a 1:1000 in a 1 ml ampule. How many ml do you need?
32. You are asked to administer 5 mcg/min of Isuprel. You add 1 mg of the drug to 250 ml of D_5W. What is the drip rate (minidrip set)? The effects of the drug are such that you have to slow the rate to 2 mcg/min. What is the drip rate?
33. How many mg of NaCl are in a 1,000 cc bag of 0.9% solution?
34. You have to give 4 mg/min Lidocaine drip. You have a 250 ml bag of D_5W to which you add 250 mg Lidocaine. What is the drip rate (minidrip)? What is the drip rate if you switch to a 15 gtts/ml administration set? To a 10 gtts/ml set?
35. You have to deliver 4 mcg/kg/min of dopamine to a 165 lb patient. You add 400 mg of the drug to 250 ml of D_5W. What is the drip rate?
36. You are asked to administer 15 mg of a drug that is supplied 50 mg in a 10 ml vial. How many ml must you draw up?
37. How many ml of a drug supplied as 2% in a 25 ml vial would you need to administer 75 mg?
38. If you add 1mg of isoproterenol to a 250 ml bag of D_5W, what is the drip rate for an infusion of 5 mcg/min?

39. If a drug is supplied as 5:1000, how many ml are needed to supply a dose of 1.5 mg?
40. If a 250 ml solution contains 2000 mg of medication, what is the solution concentration in percent (%)?
41. You have to deliver 5 mcg/kg/min of dopamine to a 165 pound patient. You add 400mg dopamine to a 250 ml bag of D_5W. What is the drip rate?
42. How many mg of lidocaine are in a 2% solution in a 250 ml bag?
43. You are ordered to give 50 mg Lasix supplied 15 mg/ml. How many ml do you draw up and administer?
44. Give 1 mg/kg of 2% lidocaine to a 187 lb patient. How many ml do you administer?
45. If 500 ml of solution contains 2000mg, what is its concentration (mg/ml)?
46. Give 35 mg of a 2% drug. How many ml do you administer?
47. Give 1 mg/kg of a 2% drug to a 99 lb patient. How many ml do you administer?
48. If you put 1 g lidocaine in 250 cc D_5W, what is the drip rate necessary for 1 mg/min? for 2 mg/min? for 3 mg/min? for 4 mg/min?
49. Give 0.01 mg/kg atropine to a 55 lb patient. How many ml do you administer if supplied 0.5mg/5ml?
50. If drug Y is supplied in a concentration of 1600 mcg, how many gtts/min are required to administer 6 mcg/kg/min to a 176 lb patient?

Worksheet provided courtesy of Eric L. Golpe, NREMT-P, Knoxville, TN (adenocard @aol.com)

DRUG CALCULATION WORKSHEET ANSWERS

Note: All minidrips are 60 gtts/min; otherwise assume 10 gtts/min.

1. 1000 mcg
2. 0.005 mg
3. 10,000,000 mcg
4. 0.25 L
5. 2,000,000 mcg
6. 5 mg
7. 150 ml
8. 0.02 G
9. 500 mcg
10. 500 mcg
11. 70 kg
12. 75 kg
13. 55 kg
14. 220 lbs
15. 132 lbs
16. 0.3 ml
17. 2.5 ml
18. 40 mg/ml

19. 4 ml
20. 0.004 mg/ml
21. 4.5 ml
22. 1.25 ml
23. 45 gtts/min
24. 150 gtts/min
25. 135 gtts/min
26. 50 ml
27. 264 lbs
28. 105 gtts/min
29. 25 gtts/min
30. 1.25 ml
31. 0.3 ml
32. 75 gtts/min; 30 gtts/min
33. 9,000 mg
34. 240 gtts/min; 60 gtts/min; 40 gtts/min
35. 10.8 gtts/min (if you work it out with 4 places instead of 2, you get 11.25 gtts/min)
36. 3 ml
37. 3.75 ml
38. 75 gtts/min
39. 0.3 ml
40. 0.8%
41. 14 gtts/min
42. 5,000 mg
43. 2.6 ml
44. 4.25 ml
45. 4 mg/ml
46. 1.75 ml
47. 2.25 ml
48. 15 gtts/min; 30 gtts/min; 45 gtts/min; 60 gtts/min
49. 2.5 ml
50. 18 gtts/min

Glossary

absorb—to take into the body.

acidosis—state in which the pH is lower than normal because of an increased hydrogen ion concentration.

acute myocardial infarction—death and subsequent necrosis of the heart muscle caused by inadequate blood supply.

addiction—physical or psychological dependence on a substance.

adrenergic—see *sympathomimetic.*

afterload—pressure or resistance against which the heart must pump.

agonist—drug or other substance that causes a physiological response.

air embolism—presence of an air bubble in the circulatory system.

albumin—protein found in all animal tissues that constitutes one of the major proteins in human blood.

alkalosis—state in which the pH is higher than normal because of a decreased hydrogen ion concentration.

allergic reaction—hypersensitivity to a given antigen; a reaction more pronounced than would occur in the general population.

amphetamine—substance that acts on the central nervous system as a stimulant.

anaphylaxis—acute, generalized, and violent antigen-antibody reaction that may be rapidly fatal.

antagonism—opposition of effect between two or more medications.

antagonist—drug or other substance that blocks a physiological response or that blocks the action of another drug or substance.

antiadrenergic—see *sympatholytic.*

antibiotics—medications effective in inhibiting the growth or killing of bacteria. They have no impact on viruses.

anticholinergic—see *parasympatholytic.*

antidote—substance that neutralizes a poison or the effects of a poison.

antigen—any substance capable of inducing an immune response.

apothecary's system—an antiquated system of weights and measures used widely in early medicine.

arrhythmia—absence of cardiac electrical activity, often used interchangeably with dysrhythmia.

autonomic nervous system—part of the nervous system controlling involuntary bodily functions; separated into the sympathetic and the parasympathetic divisions.

barbiturates—organic compounds derived from barbituric acid that depress the central nervous system, respirations, and heart rate, and decrease blood pressure.

benzodiazepines—general term to describe a group of tranquilizing drugs with similar chemical structures.

biotransformation—process of changing a drug into a different form, either active or inactive, by the body.

blood brain barrier—protective mechanism that selectively allows the entry of only a few compounds into the brain.

bolus—single, oftentimes large, dose of a medication.

bradycardia—heart rate less than 60 beats per minute.

buffer—substance that neutralizes or weakens a strong acid or base.

cardiac contractile force—force generated by the heart during each contraction.

cardiac output—amount of blood pumped by the heart in 1 minute.

cardiogenic shock—inability of the heart to meet the metabolic needs of the body, resulting in inadequate tissue perfusion.

cardioversion—passage of a current through the heart during a specific part of the cardiac cycle to terminate certain dysrhythmias.

catecholamines—class of hormones that act on the autonomic nervous system including epinephrine, norepinephrine, and similar compounds.

cholinergic—see *parasympathomimetic.*

chronotrope—drug or other substance that affects the heart rate.

chronotropy—pertaining to heart rate.

colloid osmotic pressure—pressure generated by the presence of colloids in the vascular system or in the interstitial spaces.

contraindications—medical or physiological conditions present in a patient that would make it harmful to administer a medication of otherwise known therapeutic value.

COPD—Chronic obstructive pulmonary disease characterized by a decreased ability of the lungs to perform the function of ventilation.

croup—laryngotracheobronchitis, a common viral infection of young children resulting in edema of the subglottic tissues; characterized by barking cough and inspiratory stridor.

defibrillation—the passage of a DC electrical current through a fibrillating heart to depolarize a "critical mass" of myocardial cells allowing them to depolarize uniformly, resulting in an organized rhythm.

dehydration—abnormal decrease in total body water.

delirium tremens (DT's)—disorder found in habitual and excessive users of alcoholic beverages after cessation of drinking for 48 to 72 hours; patients experience visual, tactile, and auditory hallucinations.

depressant—medication that decreases or lessens a body function.

diffusion—movement of solutes (substances dissolved in a solution) from an area of greater concentration to an area of lesser concentration.

drug—chemical agent used in diagnosis, treatment, and prevention of disease.

dysrhythmia—any deviation from the normal electrical rhythm of the heart.

electrolytes—chemical substances that dissociate into charged particles when placed in water.

endocrine gland—gland that secretes hormones directly into the blood.

epiglottitis—bacterial infection of the epiglottis, usually occurring in children older than age 4; a serious medical emergency.

FiO_2—concentration of oxygen in inspired air.

habituation—physical or psychological dependence on a drug.

half-life—time required for level of a drug in the blood to be reduced by 50 percent of its beginning level.

hematocrit—percentage of the blood consisting of the red blood cells, or erythrocytes (usually 35 to 45 percent).

histamine—chemical released by mast cells and basophils on stimulation; one of the most powerful vasodilators known and a major mediator of anaphylaxis.

homeostasis—body's natural tendency to keep the internal environment constant.

hormone—chemical substance released by a gland that controls or affects other glands or body systems.

hypersensitivity—reaction that is more profound than seen in the normal population.

hypertension—common disorder characterized by elevation of the blood pressure persistently exceeding 140/90 millimeters of mercury.

hypertensive emergency—acute elevation of blood pressure that requires the blood pressure to be lowered within 1 hour, characterized by end-organ changes such as hypertensive encephalopathy, renal failure, or blindness.

hypertensive encephalopathy—cerebral disorder of hypertension indicated by severe headache, nausea, vomiting, and altered mental status; neurological symptoms may include blindness, muscle twitches, inability to speak, weakness, and paralysis.

hypertensive urgency—an acute elevation of blood pressure that requires the blood pressure to be lowered in 24 hours, usually unaccompanied by end-organ changes.

hypertonic—state in which a solution has a higher solute concentration on one side of a semipermeable membrane compared with the other side.

hypoglycemia—complication of diabetes characterized by low levels of blood glucose; often occurs from too high a dose of insulin or from inadequate food intake following a normal insulin dose; sometimes called insulin shock, hypoglycemia is a true medical emergency.

hypotonic—state in which a solution has a lower solute concentration on one side of a semipermeable membrane compared with the other side.

hypoxemia—reduction in the oxygen content in the arterial blood or in the PaO_2.

hypoxia—state in which insufficient oxygen is available to meet the oxygen requirements of the cells.

idiosyncrasy—reaction to a drug that is unusually different from that seen in the rest of the population.

indication—medical condition(s) in which a drug has proved to be of therapeutic value.

ingestion—entrance of a substance into the body through the gastrointestinal tract.

inhalation—entrance of a substance into the body through the respiratory tract.

injection—entrance of a substance into the body through a break in the skin.

inotrope—drug or other substance that affects the contractile force of the heart.

inotropy—pertaining to cardiac contractile force.

intractable—resistant to cure, relief, or control.

intraosseous injection—to administer into the bone marrow, an alternative to venous access in children under the age of 6 years.

isotonic—state in which solutions on opposite sides of a semipermeable membrane are in equal concentration.

ketoacidosis—complication of diabetes owing to decreased insulin secretion or intake, which is characterized by high levels of glucose in the blood, metabolic acidosis, and, in advanced stages, coma; ketoacidosis is often called diabetic coma.

Korsakoff's syndrome—psychosis characterized by disorientation, muttering delirium, insomnia, delusions, and hallucinations; symptoms include painful extremities, bilateral wrist drop (rarely), bilateral foot drop (frequently), and pain or pressure over the long nerves.

logarithm—mathematical concept that eases calculation of large numbers; the log of a number is the exponent of the power to which a given base must be raised to equal that number—for example, the log of 100 is 2 ($100 = 10^2$), and the log of 1000 is 3 ($1000 = 10^3$).

metric system—system of weights and measures widely used in science and medicine, and based on a base unit of 10.

milliequivalent—number of grams of a solute contained in 1 milliliter of a normal solution.

neurotransmitter—substance that is released from the axon terminal of a presynaptic neuron on excitation that travels across the synaptic cleft to either excite or inhibit the target cell; examples include acetylcholine, norepinephrine, and dopamine.

osmosis—movement of a solvent (water) across a semipermeable membrane from an area of lesser (solute) concentration to an area of greater (solute) concentration; osmosis is a form of diffusion.

overdose—dose of a drug in excess of that usually prescribed, which can potentially adversely affect the patient's health.

overhydration—excess of total body water.

parasympathetic nervous system—division of the autonomic nervous system that is responsible for controlling vegetative functions.

parasympatholytic—drug or other substance that blocks or inhibits the actions of the parasympathetic nervous system (also called anticholinergic).

parasympathomimetic—drug or other substance that causes effects like those of the parasympathetic nervous system (also called cholinergic).

parenteral drugs—drugs administered into the body without going through the digestive tract.

peripheral vascular resistance—resistance to blood flow owing to the peripheral blood vessels; this pressure must be overcome for the heart to pump blood effectively.

pH—scientific method of expressing the acidity or alkalinity of a solution, which is the logarithm of the hydrogen ion concentration divided by 1; the higher the pH the more alkaline the solution, and the lower the pH the more acidic the solution.

pharmacodynamics—study of a drug's action on the body.

pharmacokinetics—study of how drugs enter the body, reach their site of action, and are eventually eliminated.

pharmacology—study of drugs and how they affect the body.

physiology—study of body function.

plasma—fluid portion of the blood consisting of serum and protein substances in solution.

Poiseuille's law—law of physiology that states that blood flow through a vessel is directly proportional to the diameter of the vessel to the fourth power.

poison control center—information center staffed by trained personnel that provides up-to-date toxicological information.

poisoning—taking any substance into the body that interferes with normal physiological functions.

postpartum—period after delivery of the fetus.

preload—pressure within the ventricles at the end of diastole, commonly called the end-diastolic volume.

psychosis—any major mental disorder of organic or emotional origin that is usually evidenced by derangement of the personality or loss of contact with reality.

refractory—disorder or condition that resists treatment.

seizure—disorder of the nervous system owing to a sudden, excessive, disorderly discharge of brain neurons.

semipermeable membrane—specialized biological membrane, such as that which encloses the body's cells, that allows the passage of certain substances and restricts the passage of others.

shock—state of inadequate tissue perfusion.

side effects—unavoidable, undesirable effects frequently seen even in therapeutic drug dosages.

status epilepticus—act of having two or more seizures in succession without intervening periods of consciousness.

stimulant—drug that enhances a bodily function.

surface absorption—entrance of a substance into the body directly through the skin.

sympathetic nervous system—division of the autonomic nervous system that prepares the body for stressful situations.

sympatholytic—drug or other substance that blocks the actions of the sympathetic nervous system (also called antiadrenergic).

sympathomimetic—drug or other substance that causes effects like those of the sympathetic nervous system (also called adrenergic).

syncope—transient loss of consciousness caused by inadequate blood flow to the brain.

synergism—combined action of two drugs that is much stronger than the effects of either drug administered separately.

tachycardia—heart rate greater than 100 beats per minute.

therapeutic action—desired, intended action of a drug given in the appropriate medical condition.

therapeutic index—index of a drug's safety profile, which is determined by calculating the difference between the drug's therapeutic threshold and toxic level. It is typically determined in the laboratory.

therapeutic threshold—minimum amount of drug needed in the bloodstream to cause the desired therapeutic effect.

titration—estimation of the appropriate dosage by slowly changing the rate of administration.

tonicity—number of particles present per unit volume.

universal precautions—set of procedures and precautions published by the Centers for Disease Control to assist health care personnel in protecting themselves from infectious disease.

Valsalva's maneuver—forced exhalation against a closed glottis that increases the intra-abdominal and intrathoracic pressure, causing slowing of the pulse.

Wernicke's syndrome—condition characterized by loss of memory and disorientation, associated with chronic alcohol intake and a diet deficient in thiamine.

Wolff-Parkinson-White syndrome—disorder of the heart characterized by early contraction of part of the heart muscle.

References

AMERICAN HEART ASSOCIATION, *Textbook of Advanced Cardiac Life Support*, 3rd ed. Dallas, TX: American Heart Association, 1994.

AMERICAN HEART ASSOCIATION AND AMERICAN ACADEMY OF PEDIATRICS, *Textbook of Neonatal Resuscitation.* Dallas, TX: American Heart Association, 1987.

AMERICAN HEART ASSOCIATION AND AMERICAN ACADEMY OF PEDIATRICS, *Textbook of Pediatric Advanced Life Support.* Dallas, TX: American Heart Association, 1994.

BLEDSOE, BRYAN E., CHERRY, RICHARD A., AND PORTER, ROBERT S., *Intermediate Emergency Care.* Englewood Cliffs, NJ: Prentice-Hall, 1995.

BLEDSOE, BRYAN E., PORTER, ROBERT S., AND SHADE, BRUCE, *Paramedic Emergency Care, 2nd ed.* Englewood Cliffs, NJ: Prentice Hall, 1993.

GONSOULIN, SHERYL M. AND RAYNOVICH, WILLIAM, *Prehospital Drug Therapy.* Saint Louis, MO: Mosby Lifeline, 1994.

MEDICAL ECONOMICS COMPANY, *Physician's Desk Reference, 49th ed.* Oradell, NJ: Medical Economics Company, 1995.

Microsoft Encarta. Redmond, WA: Microsoft Corporation and Funk and Wagnall's Corporation, 1993.

SHADE, BRUCE, ET AL, *Advanced Cardiac Life Support: Certification, Preparation, and Review.* Englewood Cliffs, NJ: Brady Communications, 1988.

TINTINALLI, JUDITH E., KROME, RONALD L., AND RUIZ, ERNEST, *Emergency Medicine: A Comprehensive Study Guide, 3rd ed.* New York: McGraw-Hill, 1992.

UNITED STATES DEPARTMENT OF TRANSPORTATION, NATIONAL HIGHWAY TRAFFIC SAFETY ADMINISTRATION, *Emergency Medical Technician-Paramedic: National Standard Curriculum.* Washington, DC: U.S. Government Printing Office, 1985.

Index